SEXUALIZED VIOLENCE
against Women and Children

SEXUALIZED VIOLENCE
against Women and Children

A PSYCHOLOGY AND LAW PERSPECTIVE

Edited by B. J. CLING

THE GUILFORD PRESS
New York   London

© 2004 The Guilford Press
A Division of Guilford Publications, Inc.
72 Spring Street, New York, NY 10012
www.guilford.com

Chapter 7 © 2004 Erna Olafson

Printed in the United States of America

This book is printed on acid-free paper.

Last digit is print number: 9 8 7 6 5 4 3 2 1

Library of Congress Cataloging-in-Publication Data
Sexualized violence against women and children : a psychology and law
perspective / edited by B. J. Cling.
    p. cm.
  Includes bibliographical references and index.
  ISBN 1-59385-061-1 (hardcover : alk. paper)
  1. Women—Crimes against—United States.   2. Abused women—Legal
status, laws, etc.—United States.   3. Children—Crimes against—United
States.   4. Child abuse—United States.   5. Abused children—Legal
status, laws, etc.—United States.   6. Sex crimes—United States.
  HV6250.4.W65S49 2004
  362.883'0973—dc22
                                                        2004012745

*To the memory of my lawyer father, Irving Rosenbaum,
who, although he died many years before this book,
always had confidence that I could produce it*

*And to my husband, Phillip Shinnick,
and my son, Kent,
for being the bedrock of my life*

About the Editor

B. J. Cling, PhD, JD, is a clinical psychologist and a lawyer in private practice in New York City. She is also an associate adjunct professor at John Jay College of Criminal Justice and St. John's University, where she teaches forensic psychology in the MA and PhD programs, respectively. Dr. Cling received two postdoctoral certificates, one in psychiatry and law from the University of Southern California and one in psychoanalysis from New York University. A member of the New York State Psychological Association's Committee on Ethical Practice, she publishes in the area of psychology and law. She is currently helping to develop a postgraduate program in forensic psychology and science at St. John's University.

Contributors

Julie Blackman, PhD, social psychologist, private practice, New York, New York

Laura S. Brown, PhD, Department of Psychology, Argosy University Seattle, Seattle, Washington

B. J. Cling, PhD, JD, John Jay College of Criminal Justice and St. John's University, New York, New York

Carrie L. Hempel, JD, University of Southern California Law School, Los Angeles, California

Nancy Kaser-Boyd, PhD, Department of Psychiatry and Behavioral Science, University of California–Los Angeles School of Medicine, Los Angeles, California

William D. Murphy, PhD, Department of Psychiatry, University of Tennessee Health Science Center, Memphis, Tennessee

Maureen O'Connor, PhD, JD, Department of Psychology, John Jay College of Criminal Justice, New York, New York

Erna Olafson, PhD, PsyD, The Childhood Trust, Cincinnati Children's Hospital, and University of Cincinnati College of Medicine, Cincinnati, Ohio

Barry Rosenfeld, PhD, Department of Psychology, Fordham University, Bronx, New York

Karen Terry, PhD, Department of Criminal Justice, City University of New York Graduate Center, New York, New York

Brigitte Vallabhajosula, MA, doctoral candidate, Department of Psychology, John Jay College of Criminal Justice, New York, New York

Acknowledgments

As we all know, a book is never authored by one person alone. I want to thank not only my wonderful contributing authors and coauthors, but also my students over the years at John Jay College of Criminal Justice and, more recently, at St. John's University for helping me develop the ideas embodied in the book. The materials for my class in Psychology and Law, and the students' responses to those materials, are the backbone of my ideas on this subject. In particular, I had the much-needed help of two extraordinary John Jay graduate students—Kim Reeves and Kelly Egan. In different ways, they each put in long, hard hours helping me with the research and writing of my chapters and were generally helpful in putting the whole volume together. Hopefully, they are on their way to bigger and better things: Kim to a PhD program and Kelly to law school. I also want to acknowledge my former graduate student Angela Solimo, who helped with the early phase of my work.

I would like to thank James Wulach, Director of the MA program in Forensic Psychology at John Jay College of Criminal Justice, for hiring me and giving me great teaching assignments, and also Jack Zlotnick and Maureen O'Connor, the former and current chairs of the Psychology Department, which has supported me through this process. And a thank you to Raphael Javier, the Director of the Center for Psychological Services and Clinical Studies at St. John's University, who has enthusiastically supported my work and has given me the opportunity to help develop a postgraduate training program in forensic psychology.

I also appreciate The Guilford Press for publishing my book and want to offer special thanks to Jim Nageotte, who is the most pleasant and supportive editor I can imagine having.

Lastly, on a personal note, I would like to thank my husband, Phillip Shinnick, for his unstinting and selfless support of me and my work for all the many years it has taken to get this book to the finish line, and my son, Kent, whose life has certainly taken many hours away from this book, and yet whose birth has been a rebirth for me.

Contents

1 Introduction

B. J. CLING

This book is about wrongs—often sexual wrongs—perpetrated against women and children. Although all of these have been written about separately at length, this is the first time they have been gathered into one volume that examines them as new psychological syndromes, and as legal causes of action that protect women and children against sexualized violence. The recent "discovery" or identification of these psychological harms and these recently enacted (or actively prosecuted) laws are directly linked to the recent wave of feminism. Because it has become possible for women in significant numbers to train as doctors and lawyers—in part by making it illegal to refuse to admit them to professional schools and then illegal to deny them professional jobs—women have moved into the professions in droves. The new recognition of age-old psychological problems that result from various traumas, in particular sexual traumas, and the new outrage against perpetrators of these traumas, are directly related to the presence of women in roles that aid victims of these traumas. As professional women have noticed and objected to these wrongs, professional men have focused more interest and energy on these problems as well. Social change has been brought about by focusing on such evils as rape, spousal abuse, and child sexual abuse and by heightening awareness of their presence and their devastating effects. Part of that social change is embodied in the emergence of these new psychological syndromes and laws. And, in turn, their recognition has continued the process of social change.

1

However, underlying the investigation of this new "outbreak" of psychological syndromes and protective laws is the assumption that the fields of psychology and law intersect and interact. This chapter now examines that assumption.

In my own case, I entered the field of law after training first as a clinical psychologist, then as a forensic psychologist. One of my first challenges as a forensic psychology trainee (or postdoctoral fellow, as I was then) was to look at the two fields and try to understand their differences, particularly the mindset of lawyers and the legal profession (judges included), so that I could speak their language and make my points more effectively in their venue. I quickly came to see that my training in psychology was radically different from legal thinking, and I could see why many psychologists and psychiatrists had difficulty giving credible testimony in court.

Psychology, and all the social sciences, are fundamentally empirical. Obviously, experimental psychology, for example, is more empirically based than clinical work. But even clinical work is based on observation of patients, and on a view that the practitioner looks to see what is out there in the world to know what to do. This contrasts sharply with the field of law. In law, what follows logically is king. Thus, although the law may make some empirical assumptions (e.g., that people reasonably expect not to be searched in their homes), it rarely if ever looks at the empirical data that might back this up (or refute it). The law is also indifferent to probabilistic notions (e.g., that something is *likely* to have happened as opposed to definitely having happened), and looks for possibility, not probability.[1] In addition to its assumption that people are logical in their thinking (which is empirically questionable), the law assumes that people are emotionally neutral and have no biases. Thus, except for the *voir dire* examination of a jury (where possible bias is explored and obviously biased jurors eliminated) attitudinal bias is rarely addressed. Yet empirical research clearly shows general prejudice in the population on many issues. These prejudices are probably shared by the lawmakers who make the laws as well. However, if psychological realities were acknowledged instead of ignored, laws could be devised that counteract prejudice, instead of wrongly assuming it does not exist.

Another interesting difference between psychology and law is that there is a high degree of (perhaps healthy) skepticism among lawyers that is not characteristic of mental health professionals. Clinical psychologists, for example, are used to believing their patients, who have no obvious motive to lie to their therapists. However, in most arenas of law, there is a win–lose situation (i.e., if one side wins, the other loses). Law is fundamentally adversarial. In fact, our justice system is founded on the premise that, by having two opposing sides argue against each other, the truth will out. Thus, one side always has a motivation to shade things to its advantage. This is also true in most areas of forensic psychology, where people being evaluated have a lot to gain or lose by the outcome of the forensic evaluation. Thus, a *forensic* psychologist must also be skeptical and be prepared to deal with the issue of malingering.

Interestingly, the mode of presentation in psychology and in law are different as well. Generally, in science, you present the history of the area you are investigating, describe what you did, and then present the results and conclusions. In law, you present the conclusion first, then you go back and prove how you came to it, and then you repeat it at the end. Judges and lawyers are not used to having general considerations presented first and then narrowed down until finally a conclusion is reached. In fact, they tend to have the impression that the reasoning is fuzzy and unclear if the conclusion is not immediately in sight. Thus, mental health testimony may be discounted if it is presented in the wrong format.

Another problem created by the overlap, and yet also the differences, between psychology and law is that when laws are made or used in the courtroom, they often do not take into consideration the psychological realities of the areas with which they are dealing. For example, empirical research shows us that child victims of sexual abuse have difficulty reporting their abuse. As a result, appropriate questioning has to take place in a context that helps the victim tell the truth. Only recently have such new legal adaptations as closed-circuit TV questioning of child victims in court taken place, so that a young child does not have to be in the same room as the terrifying defendant who abused him or her (and thereby be frightened into silence).

Another example is the considerable difficulty faced by those trying to help battered women who have struck back and killed their abusers. First, the notion of self-defense, as it has usually been used in law, assumes two people fighting each other, often people who are not very involved with each other and who have little history together. In the case of spousal abuse, for example, a long history of a man physically punching and kicking his wife provides a different context for hearing threats such as "When I come home I'm going to kill you." Thus, although from the battered woman's point of view it is self-defense when she shoots the battering spouse when he comes home, from a traditional prosecutor's point of view it is not, as the spouse did not threaten her just minutes before she shot him. Thus, the wife is the aggressor. And such women are regularly charged with murder, even though their husbands had repeatedly put them in the hospital with extreme violence. The psychological context within which the threat occurs provides an explanation for this normal reaction to an atmosphere of violence. In an effort to bring psychological knowledge into the legal arena, feminist lawyers have attempted to introduce expert testimony on battered woman syndrome and the effects of battering to help a jury understand why, from the battered woman's perspective, her actions were self-defense.

Another good example of an area in which the fields of psychology and law should successfully meet, but do not completely, is sexual harassment. Sexual harassment in the workplace is now illegal, in large measure due to the efforts of Catherine MacKinnon in her seminal book *Sexual Harassment of Working Women*, in which she outlines the harm to women of being harassed at work. However, it is now a near requirement that credible cases of sexual harassment be filed quickly by a woman who has been harassed. A delay in filing against an employer is usually seen as a sign that the woman was not really harmed, or that the harassment never took place.[2] Yet, if lawmakers and judges looked at the psychological research on typical victim reaction, they would find that it is typical, when sexually assaulted or harassed, to feel traumatized. Victims of trauma (or posttraumatic stress disorder) try to minimize their emotional reactions in an effort to contain the flood of out-of-control feelings they feel. As a result they often are not psychologically able to report these wrongs right away. They need to detach emotionally from the stress of the event(s). Then they are ready to take legal action. In such a case, the normal psychological reaction to a true event (and one which is illegal) is to wait a bit. The law should understand this and take it into consideration when thinking about how to maximize the reporting and prosecuting of these crimes.

It is the view of this book that it is important to have knowledge of both psychology and law in order to be effective in the area of forensic psychology. As a psychologist, it is essential to understand what the law is, how it operates, and how those practicing it think in order to influence proceedings in a court of law. And, as a lawyer, it is helpful to understand the psychological context in which crimes and various mental states occur, in order to know how to use expert testimony effectively and how to craft laws that address pertinent issues. Too often, laws are narrowly drawn, ignoring the true nature of an offense and not looking to empirical evidence that tells you what is really occurring in the mind of a perpetrator or the damage in terms of the psychological effect on a victim. It is only by having a good understanding of both disciplines that their overlap can be productive in protecting our society from harm. This book attempts to foster that understanding.

NOTES

1. Thus a court might find it reasonable to exclude as prejudicial expert testimony that a woman had PTSD as a result of sex with an accused rapist. The court's reasoning might

be that although the victim's response of PTSD made it very likely (i.e., *probable*) that she was raped, it was *possible* that she had PTSD for some other reason, and thus the jury should not hear this testimony at all. (For a full discussion of this type of reasoning, see Chapter 2 on rape and rape trauma syndrome.)

2. This view is also true for cases of rape, where an early report of rape is viewed as more likely to be true than one filed after a delay.

PART I

Sexualized Violence against Women

In general, it is hard to know which sexual and/or violent behaviors toward women and children are older—rape, spousal abuse, or sexual abuse of children. These types of what we now feel are "wrongs" seem to be part of the fabric of human society and to date as far back as there are records of human behavior. It appears that none of them were viewed as crimes against women or children until relatively recently. Thus, sex with a woman without her permission, and physical harm to a wife or a child, were apparently viewed as part of a man's allowable relationships.

Early attempts to identify rape as a "crime" defined it as a violation against a man—the man to whom the female victim of the rape belonged, as either a daughter or a wife.[1] Thus the "crime" of rape was really a property crime against the controlling man, whose property was defiled by the rape. A virgin daughter would lose her value as a potential wife, or a wife would lose her value as the sole sexual property of her husband. These views are reflected in the early punishments for rape, which included, in some cases, marriage to the rapist (for example, if he paid the proper bride-price for the raped virgin), or death to both the rapist and the raped wife (who was considered an adulteress). In the latter case, in some societies, the husband could choose to save the wife if he wanted to. As odd as some of these laws may now seem, a disregard or distrust of the female victim continued well into recent times, as reflected by the slowly evolving laws of rape. For example, in modern history, even after rape came to be seen as a criminal act against the female victim, it required proof that the sex in question took place while the victim "resisted to the utmost." Thus, for a legal judgment of rape, coerced sex with a stranger in an alley would require, in addition to the woman's charge that it was rape, proof that she showed utmost resistance. There are few witnesses to rape, and proof of utmost resistance would be in the form of serious physical injury to the woman sustained while she was "resisting." It is hard to see how women, who generally perceive themselves as significantly weaker than men and are not trained to fight, might resist in the right kind of way to produce enough marks to satisfy the legal requirement. In some cases, proof was required that the woman resisted the entire time. Thus, if she could not show that she *continually* resisted, her resistance would not meet the legal standard and, although she certainly had not consented, legally she would not have been raped.

Underlying the resistance standard for rape is the unstated assumption that every man has permission from every woman to have sex with her. Logically and legally, it is after the man tries and the woman affirmatively resists that the man knows he does not have permission to have sex with her.[2] Today, the standard for rape in most jurisdictions is consent. The consent standard is an improvement for women because it shifts the initial presumption, so that men must get permission (consent) for sex beforehand. Even so, it is still difficult to prove rape. In fact, the reality is the opposite of the common belief that it is easy for women to "cry rape." It is so difficult to prove rape that most women do not report it when it happens. The police, the prosecuting attorneys,[3] and the defense are so harsh that many rape victims do not press charges. They do not want to be abused further by the legal system in their effort to punish the perpetrator.

Recent reforms have been instituted (such as specially trained police sex crimes units and rape shield laws) to increase the likelihood that rape victims will report these crimes against them. However, many still do not. In addition, society in general, as reflected by juries, is quite unsympathetic to rape victims, somehow holding them responsible for their rapists' behavior. (For example, many believe that going to a singles bar or wearing sexy clothing is "asking" for rape.)

This book looks at a relatively recent psychological syndrome, rape trauma syndrome, which is now considered a subset of posttraumatic stress disorder (PTSD), from which many rape victims suffer. Where allowed into court, evidence of the presence of this syndrome has been very helpful in showing the unlikelihood that the victim consented to sex when she suffered PTSD as a result. However, perhaps predictably, it has proven difficult for this very reliable testimony to be accepted into court. The book's section on rape and rape trauma syndrome also explores what the legal problems have been, and some societal reasons for them.

Spousal abuse, like rape, has been with us a long time.[4] The concept that a man cannot legally beat his wife is so new that court cases exist at least through the mid-1800s of men being acquitted after horsewhipping their spouses.[5] Sadly, even after spousal abuse became a crime, it was rarely prosecuted or even taken seriously by the police when reported. An example is the relatively recent case of O.J. Simpson, the well-known football star, whose undisputed physical abuse of his wife, Nicole, and the lack of seriousness with which the police and the court dealt with it, became public as a result of the unsuccessful case against him for her murder. The prevalence of spousal abuse, the relatively recent understanding of it as a problem, and the even more recent characterization of it as a crime are all important. Yet this book focuses, as well, on the psychological effect on a woman of being repeatedly beaten by the man she lives with, may have children with, and often will continue to live with. The psychological syndrome originally identified as battered woman syndrome, now often seen as a type of PTSD, has only recently been explored as a common phenomenon suffered by women who have experienced this maltreatment. The psychological ramifications of this type of repeated trauma are feelings of powerlessness, terror, and helplessness, in addition to problems making long-range plans and focusing on anything but surviving one day at a time. For these reasons, women in physically abusive relationships often do not leave their batterers; the ones who try are often stalked by the batterers, not supported by external systems, and ultimately threatened and beaten back into submission. While it is overwhelmingly more likely that a battered woman will ultimately be killed by her batterer than the reverse, there are some rare exceptions. Those cases, which often receive publicity and have interested feminist scholars in their efforts to help these women, involve battered women who strike back and kill their abusers.

Battered women who kill their abusers are often charged with murder.[6] Sometimes these women are able to kill their abusers during an assault. But more often (and understandably, since they are not of equal strength with their batterers), the women strike back during a quiet moment, before the batterer attempts to strike again. For example, a battered woman might shoot her batterer when he returns home after credibly threatening to kill her when he comes back. Historically, the police and district attorneys have not viewed these situations as ones justifying a plea of self-defense by the woman. Feminists have attempted to assist battered women who kill their abusers by helping them mount a special case for self-defense. Usually, self-defense law requires that the perpetrator reasonably believe she is in either imminent or immediate danger (depending on the legal jurisdiction). Feminists have tried to extend this legal definition to include the circumstances (i.e., actual violence) under which the woman has lived to help judges and juries understand why the threats and behavior of the batterer would reasonably be perceived as dangerous. To this end, some have advocated introducing expert testimony to show that the woman had been battered and, as such, suffered from battered woman syndrome. There is some controversy as to how successful this approach has been and some desire on the part of feminist scholars to bypass a characterization of the woman as having a psychological syndrome. Instead they advocate simply presenting expert testimony on battering and its effects. In any case, all those working to help these women feel that an introduction in court of the real situation in which the women live, and the psychological ramifications of this situation, will help judges and jurors understand how these women reasonably believe they are defending themselves as best they can.

There are two new areas of harm that have only recently (the past 15–20 years) been considered illegal. They are stalking,[7] and sexual harassment.[8] Prior to the 1990s, men were free to stalk women and, unless they physically assaulted them, could threaten the women in that way with impunity. Likewise, prior to the social and legal aftermath of Catherine MacKinnon's 1979 book *Sexual Harassment of Working Women*, male bosses and even coworkers could intimidate female employees at work with lewd behavior, and even demand sexual favors, with no repercussions. Likely as a result of the new wave of feminism, these behaviors were ultimately viewed as not acceptable. As more women joined the workforce, more were in positions to experience sexual harassment. And as more women became professionals, they were better able to identify these problems and advocate for change. Interestingly, it took a spate of high-profile celebrity stalker killings in California to create the first anti-stalking law, after which other states followed suit. Although it is helpful to have anti-stalking statutes currently on the books, it is unclear even now whether women are well protected from the harms that come from stalking, including violence. In the case of sexual harassment, working women are certainly better protected now. At a minimum, there is a heightened awareness in the workplace that sexually harassing behaviors should be stopped. This is particularly true for employers, who, since the passage of the Civil Rights Act of 1991 which allows victims of sexual harassment to collect damages, do not want to suffer the negative financial consequences of lawsuits. Even though there is controversy over whether the courts protect women sufficiently, or rather make it difficult for women to bring successful lawsuits, it is still a positive move for women to have anti-discrimination laws in place that now apply to sexual harassment as well.

The issues of rape, spousal abuse, stalking, and sexual harassment are addressed in the following chapters, which constitute Part I of this volume.

NOTES

1. For details on rape, rape trauma syndrome, and related references, see Chapter 2, this volume.
2. The opposite is true for most other crimes, for example, robbery. There is no assumption that a man has permission to take a woman's wallet or that she must affirmatively prove that she resisted when he took it.
3. Often the District Attorney's office, which would press charges against a rapist, will only proceed if the prosecutors believe they are likely to win. Thus, often in the past they have not been responsive to rape victims without airtight cases.
4. For details on spousal abuse, battered woman syndrome, and related references, see Chapter 3, this volume.
5. For example, the case of *Joyner v. Joyner,* 59 N.C. (1862).
6. For details on the use of expert testimony on battered woman syndrome in homicide trials, along with related references, see, Chapter 4, this volume.
7. For details on stalking, and related references, see Chapter 5, this volume.
8. For details on sexual harassment, see Chapter 6, this volume.

2 Rape and Rape Trauma Syndrome

B. J. CLING

This chapter is an in-depth examination of the issues surrounding rape trauma syndrome and its use in court to validate the truthfulness of a rape victim when prosecuting a rapist. However, in order to do that effectively, it is important first to have an understanding of the crime of rape, and particularly its long and somewhat strange history.

RAPE LAW

Early History of Rape

The most striking feature of very early rape law is the absence of regard for women as victims who suffered. As this chapter elaborates, virtually all of the known laws deal with rape of a woman as defilement of a man's property. In addition, some of the punishments reflect an utter disregard of the effect on the woman victim—for example, in the case of a raped virgin, forced marriage to her rapist, or, in the case of a married rape victim, characterization of rape as adultery and equal punishment of death along with her rapist.

The first known written rape law was contained in the ancient Babylonian Code of Hammurabi, circa 2250 B.C. (Harper, 1994). Women had social status only in relation to men. Thus a woman might be a virgin living with her father, or a married woman living with her husband. In this code, rape of a virgin was punished by death, and the virgin was held blameless. Rape of a married woman was considered adultery, and the woman was held equally responsible. Deaths of the rapist and victim were by drowning. The victim's husband had the option of rescuing his wife by pulling her out of the river. The king could excuse the rapist.

Other early rape laws were equally draconian. The ancient Assyrians followed the principle of an eye for an eye very strictly. Thus, the father of a raped virgin could rape the rapist's wife as punishment (Brownmiller, 1975). The Hebrews punished rape by stoning. If a virgin was raped within the city walls, where she could have cried for help, she was stoned along with the rapist. If outside the city, she had to marry her rapist, and he was forced to pay the bride-price to her father. On the other hand, if the raped virgin was already betrothed, the rapist was stoned, and the girl was sold into marriage for a low price. Any married woman who was raped was stoned with her rapist for adultery, and the husband was not permitted to rescue her (Brownmiller, 1975). The ancient Greeks considered rape of males as well as females, and punished the crime more humanely, mostly with fines (Brundage, 1987).

Early pre-British law in England follows a similar pattern. The earliest known law is Celtic law (approximately 1000–55 B.C.) (Ellis, 1995), and it is an interesting exception to the lack of regard for female victims of rape. Not only was rape recognized as a crime against the woman, punishable by fines, but two kinds of rape were defined: forcible rape (against the woman's will) and rape where the woman was incapable of consent (due to intoxication or mental illness). There were certain exceptions—the woman had to cry for help if possible, and had to report the rape immediately. Also, promiscuous and adulterous women were not protected.

Roman law initially viewed rape as a violent property crime ("raptus") that involved the abduction of a female who was under the protection of a man but did not necessarily include sex (Burgess-Jackson, 1999). During the fourth century A.D., Constantine made *raptus* punishable by death (Brundage, 1982). This punishment included the woman, if she consented to the abduction. Later, raptus was defined as forceful abduction or forced sex. In the sixth century, Justinian revised the law of raptus by making it a sexual crime against a woman. Thus, in addition to the crime of *raptus* of a married woman, which was effectively a crime against her husband, was added *raptus* of an unmarried woman, a widow, or a nun, which was a crime against the woman herself. However, prostitutes were not included (Burgess-Jackson, 1999).

Interestingly, a man could be prosecuted for raping his wife (there was no marital rape exemption) (Brundage, 1982).

During the Anglo-Saxon period, there were some changes to the law of rape (Bracton, 1968). In the 10th century, different levels of sexual assault were established, with different punishments. The most severe punishment, for forced intercourse, was death plus castration, and castration to the rapist's male animals as well (i.e., his horse, dog, etc.). The rapist's possessions were then given to the victim. Prostitutes were not exempted. Realistically, though, this level of punishment was rare, and applied in cases of high-born victims protected by powerful men (Brownmiller, 1975). Following this, William the Conqueror reduced the most extreme punishment to castration and blinding (Brownmiller, 1975).

In the 11th and 12th centuries, canon law began to view rape less as a property crime and more as a violent, sexual crime against an individual (Brundage, 1982). Four elements of rape were identified: violence, abduction, intercourse, and lack of consent. The victim was required to cry out, but did not have to evidence strong resistance. There was a marital rape exemption (i.e., no rape if the man was married to the woman), and prostitutes were excluded. Rapists could not marry their victims, to prevent them from benefiting from their crime. Although rape was treated as a serious crime that was technically against the woman, it was still treated practically as a crime against her father.

Starting in the 12th century, female rape victims were allowed to file a civil suit, which could result in a trial by jury (Bracton, 1968). However, bringing this suit was an extremely onerous burden for the victim, including showing everyone the physical results of the rape immediately after. In addition, if the rapist denied the rape, four women had to examine the victim to see if she were no longer a virgin. Some of the defenses the rapist could raise were to argue that the victim had slept with him before, or that she consented (Bracton, 1968).

The Statutes of Westminster at the end of the 13th century significantly changed the law of rape (Brownmiller, 1975). They provided that the crime of rape applied to all women, virgin or married, including concubines and prostitutes. Further, if the suit against the rapist was not pressed by the victim's family, the crown could prosecute. Fundamentally, this defined rape as a crime against the state, and not just against a family (as a property crime) (Brownmiller, 1975). However, rape victims were viewed with suspicion: Their reputations were examined; they had to have third-party support to their claim; they had to report the rape right away; they had to have cried out for help, and so on (Blackstone, 1983).

At the end of the 16th century, rape became carnal knowledge of a woman 10 years or older, forcibly and against her will (Blackstone, 1983). This is known as the common-law definition of rape, and was picked up by the American colonies. Early statutes in Massachusetts reflect the common-law definition of rape, which also provided a marital rape exemption, but it did not require corroboration of the victim's testimony (which later statutes did). Oddly, this is still the law in Georgia.[1]

Although the common-law definition of rape was an improvement for female rape victims, they were still viewed with suspicion. This is reflected in a well-known statement made by Sir Matthew Hale, Lord Chief Justice of the King's Bench (published in the United States in 1847), and not only repeated often but included in many jury instructions in the United States, that rape "is an accusation easy to be made, hard to be proved, and harder to be defended by the party accused though ever so innocent" (as cited in Soshnick, 1987, p. 650).

Early American rape statutes incorporated the common-law definition of rape, and were known as carnal knowledge statutes (Shapo, 1975). These statutes defined forcible rape as intercourse by force and against the woman's will. This focused on the response of the victim, and led to the interpretation that sex was only rape if the woman resisted to the utmost ("utmost resistance") and resisted in this manner during the entire rape (Anderson, 1998).

Modern Rape Law

Changing the standard of what constituted rape was a centerpiece of rape reform (Shapo, 1975).[2] "Utmost resistance" gave way to "earnest resistance," finally followed by "reasonable resistance under the circumstances" (Fried, 1996). This too has changed in most jurisdictions to date, and the "consent" standard is largely the rule today.[3] This represents a change in focus. Instead of focusing on the victim's response to the sex in question (i.e., how much she resisted it), consent requires that the man get the consent of the woman beforehand.

Modern rape reform began in the 1950s, with the introduction of an early draft of the Model Penal Code (MPC) (1962), which, in addition to other reforms, looked at rape in terms of the perpetrator's behavior, not the victim's response (Shapo, 1975). This model, written by the American Law Institute, served as a model for the laws of the states and the federal government. Other influential legal models that have affected modern rape law include the New York Penal Law,[4] adopted in 1961, and Michigan's revised laws of 1975 (Shapo, 1975).[5] New York defined rape in terms of a woman's lack of consent, although until the 1970s also required corroboration of various aspects of the rape, including lack of consent. Michigan's revisions were more progressive. They eliminated the resistance requirement, labeled the crime as "criminal sexual conduct," made it gender-neutral, and introduced a rape shield law that makes evidence of the victim's past sexual history with third parties inadmissible.

At the present time, many states have reformed their rape laws, and most now use the consent standard. However, in many ways a rape victim's credibility is still at the center of every rape trial, and while Lord Hale's warnings about lying rape victims is no longer included in jury instructions, there is a suspicion of victims of rape that does not apply to other crime victims, such as those who are robbed. Thus, while strict corroboration (such as an eyewitness to the rape) is not required, it is helpful to have medical corroboration to bolster the rape victim's credibility. In the absence of bruises and cuts, verifiable psychological damage, if present, is helpful in proving the likelihood of nonconsent.

RAPE TRAUMA SYNDROME

Gradually, rape became a more prosecuted crime as the standard of rape changed from resistance to consent. Thus the prosecution of not just stranger rape, but also acquaintance and date rape, was facilitated. The same societal and political forces pressing for a lower standard of recognition as a crime also pressed for more vigorous prosecution of rapists. While more rapes were now being prosecuted, some of the old problems of trying to get convictions persisted, or were even more acute. Usually, there are no witnesses to a rape. In fact, the acquaintance and date rape variety often take place in a car or home, where the victim thinks she is safe from such assault. When the issue in a rape prosecution is whether or not the victim consented, and not whether or not the particular defendant was the "guy who did it" (i.e., not a case of mistaken identity), it is the victim's word against the defendant's that the sex that occurred was rape. The credibility of the parties is crucial to a guilty versus not guilty verdict—and juries are historically and presently prejudiced against rape victims. Old, frankly misogynistic stereotypes abound, even today. Juries often feel that women who go on dates with relative strangers (e.g., someone they just met in a singles bar), dress in sexy clothing, or get into a young man's car are "asking for it." In spite of the fact that the law requires that the woman consent to intercourse, not just dinner, juries are harsh in their condemnation of women who find themselves in rapable situations, and are quick to blame the victim. As a result, the discovery/development of the psychological syndrome of rape trauma syndrome (RTS) was a tremendous benefit to rape victims, and also to prosecutors.

Because of the neutral, third-party nature of expert testimony—that evidence of RTS is being offered by a mental health professional as a medical diagnosis which is the result of a traumatic event—juries are often swayed in the victim's favor, to believe that trauma has occurred because the woman was raped, not because she had willing sex.

At first, as is typical in the history of introducing new psychiatric diagnoses into court, it was difficult to get this evidence admitted. Slowly RTS gained momentum and acceptance in the mental health field. It was accepted into the *Diagnostic and Statistical Manual of Mental Disorders* (DSM) as posttraumatic stress disorder (PTSD) where the stressor is rape (discussed later in this chapter), and it was accepted in more courts. However, by the 1980s, a little more than half the courts in the United States rejected the use of RTS as expert testimony (Cling, 1988). The grounds for this were strong statements about its "unreliability" and its nonacceptance in the field, in spite of the fact that the relevant body of experts evaluating the diagnosis had accepted it. This circumstance raises the possibility that the courts were rejecting the use of RTS not because it was unreliable, but because it was so effective in swaying juries and prosecuting rapists.

In the 1990s, the legal standard for accepting expert medical evidence into court changed (see "Changing Legal Standards for Medical Expert Witness Testimony," below). Some analyze the change as making it more difficult, and some as making it easier, to get medical evidence in. However, little to date has changed in the courts' acceptance or rejection of RTS in spite of this change in the law. At the present time, only 20 states have accepted RTS as medical evidence to show that a woman did not consent to sex, and was raped.[6] Even as these figures have stayed the same, clinical and empirical research within the mental health field have even more strongly endorsed the fact that RTS is a reliable psychiatric phenomenon, and is a normal, traumatic response to nonconsensual sex (Frazier, 2002).

As a countervailing force to the endorsement of RTS as valid by the mental health experts who use it, some legal experts have raised objections to it as one of many psychological/psychiatric syndromes (known as "abuse excuse") that have developed in the past 30–40 years that tend to help women and children who have been the victims of abuse, sexual and otherwise, such as battered woman syndrome and child sexual abuse syndrome (Dershowitz, 1994; Morse, 1998).[7] Although these and other syndrome-like diagnoses are not as firmly established in the mental health field, they do help the same general class of victims. Interestingly, some of these less-accepted syndromes have had an easier time finding their way into the courts.

History of Rape Trauma Syndrome

RTS was first observed by Burgess and Holmstrom, a nurse and a sociologist, respectively, who worked in an emergency room in a Boston hospital (Burgess & Holmstrom, 1974). Through clinical observation they noted a group of psychological symptoms from which most rape victims seemed to suffer. Identifying a pattern of responses shared by most individuals who suffer this trauma alleviates the victim's sense of guilt and validates that she is not alone in what she is feeling. Further, it helps professionals, such as psychologists and other mental health workers, understand and identify the problems. It is also helpful to prosecutors in explaining to judges and juries in a court of law what the victim has experienced, and how those experiences statistically validate what the victim claims has happened, that is, that she was indeed raped.

Burgess and Holmstrom wrote about their discovery of RTS, and also testified early on in cases involving rape. Their early formulations of RTS focused on a two-stage process, an acute phase followed by a chronic phase, which is somewhat mirrored in the most recent formulation of RTS according to the DSM as a form of PTSD where the stressor is rape.[8] Following Burgess and Holmstrom's early work on RTS, various research groups tested the concept of RTS empirically, to see whether such symptomatology truly identified a separate group of people who had been raped, and also to see whether certain types of psychological reactions are likely as a result of rape (e.g., serious depression, intense anxiety, etc.) There is significant empirical research on RTS, which validates its existence, and the existence of various strong psychological reactions to rape (Frazier, 2002). Thus, there is no controversy in the field of psychology that RTS and other symptoms exist as a frequent reaction to rape. However, specific definitions of RTS used in different studies vary. Thus there has been some confusion as to what RTS is, and what symptoms are likely following a rape (see "Research on Rape Trauma Syndrome," below). This section outlines briefly the main characteristics of the various formulations of RTS and reports on the main research in the area. It should be noted that, while the various formulations discussed herein do differ somewhat, they are essentially similar in describing the usual reaction to rape.

Burgess and Holmstrom

RTS was first noticed as an organized set of psychological symptoms as a reaction to rape by Ann Burgess and Lynda Holmstrom, who published their original work on it in 1974 and 1976. Burgess, a professor of nursing, and Holmstrom, a professor of sociology, observed and treated rape victims in an emergency room in Boston. Their 1974 paper set out what had hitherto been ignored in writings on rape—the psychological reaction of the victim. In an attempt to document what they noted as uniform and predictable emotional reactions to rape, Burgess and Holmstrom described in detail the symptomotology they observed in the large number of rape victims they studied, and highlighted the similarity to symptoms experienced by people who have been traumatized. The second article focused on coping strategies in dealing with the trauma. A later article by Burgess (1983) discussed in detail how RTS can be viewed as a specific example of PTSD, with rape as the stressor. Burgess and Holmstrom were successful in illustrating with very good clinical studies that there was a common psychological reaction to rape, and that it was specific and typical. Their formulation was accepted and included in the DSM, published by the American Psychiatric Association. Ultimately, as indicated earlier, RTS was included as a form of PTSD where the stressor is rape. There has been discussion of the differences between the original formulation by Burgess and Holmstrom and PTSD (Frazier, 2002), but the differences are generally agreed to be small. The usual definition of RTS now used in the field, particularly in court, is that of PTSD with rape as the stressor.

Diagnostic and Statistical Manual of Mental Disorders

The DSM is recognized as the basic diagnostic manual for mental health professionals. It lists all the possible diagnoses of mental disorders, with detailed descriptions of the relevant symptomatology for each recognized disorder. It is used by psychiatrists, psychologists, and all other mental health professionals to communicate with each other about these disorders. Compiled by a professional committee with the help of many advisory committees who meet for a number of years, the final draft of each edition must be approved by the Board of Trustees of the American Psychiatric Association before it is published. It is also updated regularly.[9] Thus, for a problem to be addressed in the DSM, there must be agreement in the mental health community that the problem is a mental disorder, and what the nature of that disorder is.

PTSD has been listed in all the versions of the DSM, including the most updated version—the DSM-IV-TR.[10] Burgess and Holmstrom's original article identifying rape trauma syndrome as a disorder caused by rape which resembled PTSD was published in 1974. Following this article, and the subsequent clinical work and research involving RTS, the DSM-III (the third version of the DSM) was published in 1980. In this version, under "posttraumatic stress disorder, chronic or delayed,"[11] rape is given as an example of a trauma that could cause PTSD.[12] The next, revised version, the DSM-III-R (published in 1986), preserves unchanged the reference to rape as a trauma causing PTSD. In the DSM-IV (published in 1994), the section describing PTSD was expanded to include many specific references to rape and sexual assault as traumas or stressors that cause PTSD.[13] For example, under "Diagnostic features," it states, "*Traumatic events* that are experienced directly include, but are not limited to, military combat, *violent personal assault* (*sexual assault*, physical attack, robbery mugging)" (American Psychiatric Association, 1994, p. 424, emphasis added). The section continues, "The disorder [PTSD] may be especially severe or long lasting when the *stressor* is of human design (e.g., torture, *rape*)" (emphasis added). Further, explaining some of the typical symptomatology of PTSD, it states, "Intense psychological distress (criterion B4) or physiological reactivity (criterion B5) often occurs when the person is exposed to triggering events that resemble or symbolize an aspect of the *traumatic event* (e.g., . . . *entering an elevator for a woman who was raped in an elevator*)" (p. 424, emphasis added). This expansion was similarly included in the DSM-IV-TR, the text revision published in 2000.

It seems clear, in addition to the many articles on RTS dealing with clinical work and experimental research, that RTS, as PTSD where the trauma or stressor is rape, has been irrefutably accepted by the mental health community (Frazier, 2002). It is recognized as a verifiable disorder with specific symptomatology, which can be distinguished from other disorders and is included in the DSM as a subset of PTSD.[14]

Research on Rape Trauma Syndrome

Frazier (2002) conducted an exhaustive review of the relevant psychological literature on RTS and related symptomatology. There were methodological differences among studies measuring the prevalence of PTSD in rape victims. Some studies measured only short-term (within 1 year) effects, others measured long-term (lifetime) effects, and only some studies used matching comparison groups. However, the following data emerged.

For short-term effects, although no matched group studies were found, short-term symptoms were overwhelmingly reported by rape victims in non-comparison group studies. Statistical instances of symptomotology ranged from 94 to 47%, depending on the amount of time that had passed since the rape—the closer in time, the stronger and more likely the symptoms. Generally speaking, the majority of rape victims studied met the criteria for PTSD shortly after the rape, and approximately 50% continued to meet the criteria after 1 year. Longer, lifetime effects varied widely, ranging from 2 to 80%, based on the methodology of the various studies and, in particular, the preciseness of the definition of rape. Higher rates were associated with narrower definitions of rape, closer to the legal definition (as opposed to broader definitions such as unwanted sexual contact). In general, those studies measuring rape from a legal perspective found rates between 30 and 60%. Those studies using broad definitions, with large sample sizes, found a consistent long-term effect of approximately 10–20%. Even in many cases of lower prevalence rates of long-term symptomotology after rape, the amount and intensity of the PTSD symptoms tended to be stronger than that associated with PTSD caused by other stressors.

In addition to the research on PTSD specifically, Frazier also reviewed studies of rape victims involving other psychological symptomatology, such as depression, fear, anxiety, social adjustment, general health problems, and substance abuse. In general, although there were significant differences in the methodologies as well as the populations involved in the various studies, all of them supported a finding of increased psychological distress post rape. Differences across studies involved the duration of the negative effect. The closer in time to the rape, the more likely it was for studies to show a psychological problem on the part of the rape victim, although the time sequences varied.

In sum, a meta-analysis of the psychological research on RTS indicates that symptoms of PTSD do appear in a large number of rape victims. The closer the definition of rape to the legal definition or the more recent the rape, the more likely the victim is to suffer from symptoms of PTSD. Rape victims suffering from PTSD tend to have more severe symptoms than individuals whose PTSD is due to other stressors.

Laws Affecting Rape Trauma Syndrome

Changing Legal Standards for Medical Expert Witness Testimony

The nexus between psychology and law usually occurs when a psychologist (or other mental health professional) appears in a court of law either to testify about the psychological state of someone involved in the case at hand or to give the trier of fact (the judge or the jury) general information about the field that they would not otherwise have. This is *expert* testimony, and is governed by special rules in court. Much of the controversy over whether RTS evidence can be introduced in court revolves around the standard that the court uses to admit such evidence, and the way that the standard is applied.

The relevant standards currently being used follow either one of two leading cases,[15] or the Federal Rules of Evidence. In all instances, expert testimony must be relevant and helpful. The original case that governed the admissibility of expert testimony is an old circuit court case,[16] *Frye v. United States*, 293 F. 1013 (D.C. Cir. 1923). Under this case, expert testimony was admissible in a case if the nature of the expert evidence was *generally accepted in the field*. Thus, in the case of psychological evidence, if the majority of psychologists thought that evidence of this kind was acceptable, and indeed used these terms and concepts professionally, then presumably that type of evidence would be admissible in court.

Until 1993, states and the federal courts tended to adopt the *Frye* standard, even though technically it is a D.C. Circuit Court decision and is required to apply only to those courts under its jurisdiction Then the Supreme Court decided the case of *Daubert v. Merrell Dow Pharmaceuticals, Inc.*, 509 U.S. 579, 113 S. Ct. 2786, 125 L. Ed. 2d 469 (1993), which changed the standard somewhat, at least for federal criminal cases. Following *Daubert*, the Federal Rules of Evidence were revised in 2000 to accommodate that decision.[17] Although these rules only apply to federal cases, they often serve as a model for states to adopt. The Federal Rules are particularly interesting because the Court in *Daubert* did not follow the *Frye* standard primarily because the Federal Rules did not incorporate *Frye*. The revised Federal Rules 701, 702, and 703 follow *Daubert* explicitly, and incorporate its principles into the language of the Rules. At this point, the states and federal courts are quite divided about which standard they are applying, although the practical effect may in fact be quite minimal.[18]

Under *Daubert*, expert testimony must *rest on a reliable foundation*, that is, be based on valid science. It is up to the court to determine directly whether the testimony is valid (as opposed to determining whether experts in the field accept it as valid, as required under *Frye*). This is often referred to as the new "gatekeeping" function of the court. *Daubert* also offers some nonexclusive guidelines on how to evaluate whether the science that particular testimony is based on is valid. The court can examine whether it is (1) testable (i.e., falsifiable), (2) what the error rate is, (3) whether it has been subjected to peer review and publication, and (4) whether is is generally accepted in the field (the old *Frye* standard). A further question as to how to apply *Daubert* arose when testimony was thought to be not really "scientific," but more "technical"—a distinction made in the Federal Rules of Evidence.[19] This uncertainty was decided by a later Supreme Court case, *Kumho Tire, Ltd. v. Carmichael*, 526 U.S. 137, 119 S. Ct. 1167, 143 L. Ed. 2d 238 (1999). Under *Kumho* the Court held that the same examination should be given to both scientific as well as technical evidence. This was particularly rele-

vant for the mental health profession, which largely considered itself
more "technical" than "scientific." There is voluminous writing on the
true meaning of *Daubert*, and what the courts should be doing as a result (Faigman, Kaye, Saks, & Sanders, 2002a).[20] However, to date, the
courts do not seem to have changed their behavior in admitting expert
testimony, regardless of what standard they presumably are following.

Use of Rape Trauma Syndrome in Court

Traditionally, it has been difficult to prosecute rapists because there is a
fair amount of bias against rape victims by juries (as well as prosecutors
and the police). Even if the police do investigate and arrest a suspect and
the prosecutor decides to try the case, it is often a matter of the victim's
word against the defendant's. Rarely are there witnesses to the crime,
and even independent evidence of assault does not necessarily prove
rape. (Consider the "preppie murder" of some years ago in New York,
where the defendant argued that he strangled the woman accidentally
because she wanted rough sex.) Thus it is very advantageous to have
medical evidence that indicates the likelihood of rape. RTS evidence can
serve that function and for that reason is supported by prosecutors, who
would like to show that the victim is so traumatized by the sex in question that she has PTSD as a result.[21] Even to a somewhat biased jury, the
likelihood would seem low that the victim consented to such sex. Although this is powerful evidence favorable to the victim, many courts
have been reluctant to let it in. At the current writing, only 20 states in
the United States allow medical evidence of RTS when the issue is
whether the victim consented to the sex in question.[22] The arguments
given by the various courts are discussed in the next section, and I would
argue that their conclusions about this evidence also indicate a bias
against rape victims.

Court Arguments against the Use of Rape Trauma Syndrome Evidence [23]

Even in jurisdictions that do not allow RTS evidence to prove nonconsent (and thus rape), courts generally allow it in for other purposes.
For example, it is allowed in as rebuttal evidence. Thus, when the defense argues that the victim did not show typical rape victim-like behavior, the prosecution can introduce evidence to show that this is the way a
person suffering from RTS will act. Also, if the case is a civil one (e.g.,
the victim is suing a parking lot for monetary damages because it did not
properly guard her safety), RTS can be introduced as evidence to show
how the victim has been harmed. Thus, the legally contentious area for

the introduction of RTS as evidence is in criminal cases to prove nonconsent.

There are three arguments that courts have raised to keep testimony on RTS out of court. The first is that it is not *scientifically reliable*, or does not meet the criteria for allowing scientific or technical information into court to help the jury understand a relevant issue. The second is that it is possible that, even if the victim is suffering from RTS, and even if such testimony is scientifically reliable, RTS could have been caused by another, *extraneous stressor*—such as an automobile accident—and thus should not be admitted. The last argument is that RTS was *developed as a clinical tool*, to help rape victims, and not as an evidentiary tool for conviction. Thus it should not be used in the latter capacity. Each argument is examined in the following sections. In addition, there is the possibility (not necessarily raised by the courts) that a victim could be malingering (faking RTS), or that she really believed that she was raped but was mistaken (somehow consented without realizing it). These arguments will also be considered.

Scientific Reliability [24]

As discussed in the section "Changing Legal Standards for Medical Expert Testimony," any changes in the legal standard for admissibility of RTS as evidence have had little if any practical effect to date. Jurisdictions that kept RTS evidence out under *Frye* continue to do so under the *Daubert* standard, and those that allowed it in continue to do so as well. Thus, the original (and still relevant) arguments against admitting RTS as scientific or technical data will be considered here.[25]

In many states, the charge that RTS is *scientifically unreliable* is the leading legal argument against admitting it as evidence of nonconsent.[26] Under *Frye*, courts argue that RTS is not generally accepted in its field (i.e., psychiatry, psychology, and mental health). Sadly, courts that assert this rarely, if ever, check with the field at issue. For example, the court in *State v. Saldana*, 324 N.W.2d 227, 320 (Minn. 1982), still a leading and oft-cited case for not admitting RTS as evidence, stated, "The scientific evaluation of rape trauma syndrome has not reached a level of reliability that surpasses the quality of common sense evaluation present in jury deliberations" (p. 320).[27] Similarly, in *State v. Taylor*, 663 S.W.2d 235 (Mo. 1984), the court held RTS evidence inadmissible because it was "not sufficiently based on a scientific technique, which is either parochially accepted or rationally sound" (p. 240).

However, for a long time, RTS has been completely accepted within the fields of psychiatry and psychology. It has been accepted into the DSM, which is used by practitioners and also health insurance companies as the basic text for diagnosing mental illness. In addition, there is now a large body of research on rape victims, which also documents that RTS is a reliable diagnostic category with specific, easily identifiable symptoms (see the earlier section "Research on Rape Trauma Syndrome"). There is no basis in fact for holding that RTS is not scientifically reliable, or generally accepted in the field, as required under *Frye*. And to the extent that psychological studies and psychiatric diagnoses, in general, "rest on a reliable foundation" as required under *Daubert* and the newly revised Federal Rules of Evidence, RTS evidence qualifies under that standard as well.

Extraneous Stressor

The second legal argument why RTS should not be admitted as evidence of nonconsent is that it may have been caused by some stressor other than rape. That is, the victim has PTSD as a result of some other trauma she may have experienced, and not as a result of sex with the alleged rapist.

There are two main arguments that counter this assertion. First, the diagnosis of PTSD itself has many requirements that investigate the nature of the traumatic event. Thus nightmares, flashbacks, and phobic reactions, for example, would be about the trauma itself, or related events (e.g., if the "rape" took place in an elevator, the victim might become claustrophobic in elevators). Thus, in the (unlikely) event that there were other stressors present in the recent history of the victim, such as a car accident, the specific content of the symptoms would help the mental health professional determine what the precipitating stressor was.

Second, and I believe most persuasively, even if there are other stressors that can be identified and shown, and the mental health professionals evaluating the victim cannot rule out the influence of these other stressors, this information can be brought to light by the defense. Thus, in an adversarial system, the other side can and will introduce into evidence the possibility of other stressors, the actual existence of these other stressors, and the mental health professional's inability to rule them out as precipitating factors in the victim's diagnosis of PTSD. In sum, it is best, and most in line with our notion of justice, to introduce RTS evidence and let the jury decide whether it indicates that the victim was raped or that the victim suffered other, more debilitating stressors.[28]

Development as a Clinical Tool

The third legal argument that courts raise to exclude RTS testimony is that it was not developed for evidence of rape in court, but for clinical

treatment of rape victims. However, this fact does not necessarily preclude using RTS testimony effectively and fairly in court. Indeed, few diagnoses or procedures are developed for the purpose of giving evidence
in court, and yet many medical and psychological procedures are testified to in court without this objection being raised. A good example of a
medical syndrome that was developed for clinical purposes yet is used
often and effectively in court for purposes of prosecution of wrongdoing
is battered child syndrome (Kempe, 1962). Radiologists looking at X-
rays of children were able to identify old healed broken bones in children presenting at clinics and hospitals with newly broken bones. The
X-rays revealed a pattern of child abuse that was otherwise hidden. Doctors were able to act on this information to help the child. Later, evidence of battered child syndrome (as it came to be called) was gradually
accepted in all jurisdictions as medical evidence in the prosecution of
child abusers, even though it was not developed for this purpose. The
singling out of RTS for this objection raises the issue that perhaps rape
victims are not being viewed neutrally by the courts and are being afforded less credibility than battered children.

Other Possible Legal Objections
to Rape Trauma Syndrome

Although not necessarily named as issues by leading courts in excluding
RTS as evidence, cogent arguments concerning *malingering* and *mistake*
can still be made against the introduction of RTS as medical evidence of
nonconsent.

Malingering

It can be argued that if a woman malingered, that is, faked the symptoms of RTS, she could fool a mental health professional, and for that
reason testimony about RTS should be barred.

Of course, successful malingering is always possible for many physical problems and most mental problems. Because there is no reliable
physical evidence of mental disturbance, psychiatrists and psychologists
must rely on interviews and testing of the person for diagnosis. Thus,
there is always the possibility that a person might be able to fool the professional in interviews and even on psychological tests. However, the
likelihood of successful malingering is generally quite low.

Because any mental problem could be faked, if RTS evidence is excluded on that basis, it follows logically that all psychological forensic
evidence should be kept out of court as well, since it is subject to the
same criticism. Yet evidence concerning competency to stand trial and
the plea of not guilty by reason of insanity are regularly admitted. Thus,

we have to ask what the precautions are that keep the likelihood of malingering low enough that our legal system generally admits psychiatric
and psychological evidence for juries to consider.

First, the expertise of the examiner is the first deterrent to malingering. Most of the people who do mental health evaluations for the court
are trained to reach appropriate diagnoses and conclusions given the
types of evidence usually considered to make these determinations. Psychiatrists and psychologists often interview the patient and examine test
results to determine what, if anything, he or she is suffering from.

Second, in order to malinger successfully, the patient has to be
aware of what to fake. Thus a successful malingerer would have to be familiar with the mental health standards used to evaluate whatever disorder they were faking—such as the DSM (see the earlier section "Diagnostic and Statistical Manual of Mental Disorders"). Also, he or she
would have to be familiar with various psychological tests and know
how to gauge answers to conform to the disorder being portrayed, a
more difficult task than the preceding one. It should be noted that several of the psychological tests often used to evaluate patients also have
scales designed to catch people who are trying to fake symptoms.

Third, the patient would have to be a very good actor to fake various symptoms convincingly for the trained examiner. Overacting would
probably be detected as malingering.

Thus, although it is always a logical possibility that one could fake
a disease such as RTS, it would be quite difficult to do it successfully. In
addition, in the case of RTS, a woman would have to be very motivated
to fake these symptoms simply to bring about a trial of a man she had
sex with. In contrast, in the case of competency to stand trial or not
guilty by reason of insanity, a defendant would have very strong motivation to fake various symptoms so as not to be tried and incarcerated.

Mistake

To my knowledge no court has ever considered the issue of a mistake,
but it is a logical possibility and thus should be addressed, even if ultimately dismissed. This is the possibility that a woman could have had
sex with a man under the circumstances where she believed that she did
not consent (i.e., said, "no"), but he reasonably believed she did (i.e.,
said, "yes").

One of the unusual circumstances of introducing RTS as evidence in
court is that it is evidence of the victim's state of mind. Most other forensic psychological determinations have to do with the defendant's state of
mind. Thus it is possible for the victim to have one state of mind, but the
state of mind of the defendant could still be innocent. If somehow a

woman who genuinely believed she did not consent to sex (and was traumatized by it) was mistaken, and a reasonable man would have believed that she did consent, she would have RTS but he would not have raped her under the law.

There are two reasons why RTS should still be admitted in court. First, the likelihood of a woman genuinely believing she is saying "no" and a man reasonably believing this is a "yes" is very low, so it does not make sense to bar all evidence of RTS in the event of this very unlikely scenario. Second, if the defense believes that this is the case, they may present supporting evidence in court. Our adversarial system was set up specifically to allow such controversy in front of a jury. I believe it is best to give the jury the expert information, and any counterinformation or arguments, and let them decide.

CONCLUSION

RTS, or PTSD where the stressor is rape, is a normal psychological reaction to the trauma of being raped. It was recognized by Burgess and Holmstrom in their groundbreaking work in the 1970s and was ultimately categorized in the DSM in the 1980s. There has been a significant amount of psychological research on it, and it has been validated as a verifiable phenomenon from which many rape victims suffer. Expert witness testimony on RTS has been used in rape trials, generally to inform the trier of fact (jury or judge) how a typical rape victim might react and specifically to inform the trier of fact that the particular victim in a rape trial suffers from this syndrome. The fact that a knowledgeable expert believes a victim suffers from RTS can be very persuasive to a jury in enhancing the credibility of the victim in rape trials where the issue is whether the victim was raped (i.e., did not consent) or consented to the sex at issue. Because there are rarely witnesses to a rape, and frequently little extrinsic evidence (bruises, etc.), many rape trials depend on the believability of the woman who says she was raped. For good reason, juries find it hard to believe that a woman who was traumatized by the sex in question actually consented to it. However, many courts have forbidden experts from testifying in these cases, even when they have firmly established that the woman has RTS. Those courts that do not allow this evidence to be heard argue that either it is not accepted in the field of mental health or it is generally unreliable, that other non-rape stressors could have caused this traumatic reaction, and that it was not developed for use in a court and thus should be barred.

This chapter gives the history of the development of RTS as a recognized phenomenon within the mental health field. It also briefly reviews the history and current law that determines whether expert witness testimony may be allowed into court. It evaluates the arguments courts have given for disallowing this testimony, and concludes that there is little basis for excluding such evidence, as follows:

1. RTS is clearly accepted in the field (the *Frye* standard).
2. RTS is as reliable as any other psychological phenomenon (the *Daubert* standard).
3. RTS is specific enough to allow in-court discussion on the likelihood that it could be due to another unrelated trauma.
4. RTS is no different from other clinical phenomena, such as battered child syndrome, that are regularly allowed into court and also were developed for clinical purposes.

This chapter further looks at the possibilities of malingering and mistake. It concludes that malingering is equally if not more likely in other forensic areas, such as competency to stand trial, that regularly allow psychological and psychiatric testimony. It also concludes that even in the rare circumstance that a victim is genuinely mistaken in her belief that she did not consent when a reasonable man might think she did, such evidence can always be introduced at trial, and is not a convincing reason to keep all RTS evidence out of every rape trial.

NOTES

1. Ga. Code Ann. § 16-6-1 (LexisNexis 2002).
2. In addition, some rape reforms focused on other important issues, such as the admissibility of the victim's sexual history (the "rape shield" laws), the corroboration requirement, the marital rape exemption, making rape a gender-neutral offense, the gradation of rape into degrees, and changing the name of "rape."
3. For states that use the consent standard, see Alaska Stat. § 11.41.470 (8)(a) (LexisNexis 2003); Ariz. Rev. Stat. § 13-1406 (LexisNexis 2003); Ark. Code Ann. § 5-14-103 (LexisNexis 2003); Cal. Penal Code § 261(a)(2) (LexisNexis 2003); Colo. Rev. Stat. § 18-3-402 (LexisNexis 2003); Conn. Gen. Stat. § 53a-70 (2003); D.C. Code § 22-3002 (2003); Fla. Stat. § 794.011(1)(a) (2002); Ga. Code Ann. § 16-6-1 (LexisNexis 2002); Hawaii Rev. Stat. § 707-730 (LexisNexis 2003); Ill. 720 ILCS 5/ 12-13 (2003); Ind. Code Ann. § 35-42-4-1 (LexisNexis 2003); Iowa Code § 709.5 (2003); Kan. Stat. Ann. § 21-3502 (LexisNexis 2002); Ky. Rev. Stat. § 510.010(2) (LexisNexis 2002); Me. Rev. Stat. tit. 17-A, § 251(E) (LexisNexis 2003); Md. Criminal Law Code Ann. § 3-303 (LexisNexis 2003); Mass. Gen. Laws Ann. ch. 265, § 22 (LexisNexis 2003); Mich. Comp. Laws § 750.520b (LexisNexis 2003); Minn. Stat. § 609.341, Subd. 4. (a)(2002); Miss. Code Ann. § 97-3-95 (2003); Mont. Code Ann, § 45-5-503 (2002); Nev. Rev. Stat. § 200.366 (LexisNexis 2003); N.H. Rev. Stat. Ann. § 632-A:2 (LexisNexis 2003); N.J. Stat. § 2C:14-2 (2003); N.M. Stat. Ann. § 30-9-10(A) (2003); N.Y. Penal Law § 130.35 (LexisNexis 2003); N.C. Gen. Stat. § 14-27.2

(2003); Ohio Rev. Code Ann. § 2907.02(C) (LexisNexis 2003); Okla. Stat. Ann. tit. 21, § 1111 (LexisNexis 2003); Or. Rev. Stat. § 163.305 and § 163.375 (LexisNexis 2001); R.I. Gen. Laws § 11-37-2 (2002); S.C. Code Ann. § 16-3-652 (2002); S.D. Codified Laws § 22-22-1 (2003); Tenn. Code Ann. § 39-13-503 (2003); Tex. Penal Code Ann. § 22.011 (LexisNexis 2003); Utah Code Ann. § 76-5-402 (2003); Vt. Stat. Ann. tit. 13, § 3252 (LexisNexis 2003); Va. Code Ann. § 18.2-61 (2003); Wis. Stat. § 940.225 (2002); and Wyo. Stat. § 6-2-302 (2003).

4. N.Y Penal Law §§ 130.00-.35 (McKinney, 1975).

5. Mich. Comp. Laws Ann. §§ 750.520(a)–(l) (Supp. 1975).

6. See Appendix 2.1 for states that do and do not allow experts to testify on RTS in criminal trials where the issue is whether or not the woman consented to sex.

7. For consideration of views opposing the "abuse excuse" position, see Taslitz (1999), supporting a feminist analysis of evidence, or Walker and Monahan (1987), endorsing the introduction of "social [science] framework" evidence.

8. See "Diagnostic and Statistical Manual of Mental Disorders" in this chapter, for a more detailed history of the gradual inclusion of RTS under PTSD.

9. The DSM was originally published in 1952. The DSM-II was published in 1968. It was followed by the DSM-III in 1980, and the DSM-III-R in 1986. The most recent version, the DSM-IV, was published in 1994, with a "text revision" (DSM-IV-TR) in 2000.

10. In the original DSM, and in the DSM-II, early versions of PTSD were represented ("gross stress reaction" in the DSM, and "transient situational disturbances" in the DSM-II). Starting with the publication of the DSM-III, PTSD in a form close to its current formulation has been included.

11. The DSM identifying number is 309.81.

12. The DSM-III states, "The *trauma* may be experienced alone (*rape* or assault) or in the company of groups of people (military combat) (American Psychiatric Association, 1980, p. 236, emphasis added).

13. Interestingly, in addition to the added inclusion of rape-specific references under PTSD, the introduction to the DSM-IV (and the DSM-IV-TR) specifically discusses the issue of the use of the DSM in forensic (i.e., legal) settings. Thus, there is an official awareness of the usefulness and inclusion of DSM categories in court when issues involving psychological functioning are involved.

14. It should be noted that a milder, more acute form of PTSD—acute stress disorder—could also be suffered as a result of rape. Acute stress disorder is similar in symptomatology to PTSD, but requires fewer symptoms for diagnosis, and lasts up to a month. If acute stress disorder persists, it is usually rediagnosed as PTSD.

15. There are two kinds of law that govern what the court must do—*black letter* law and *case* law. Black letter law refers to laws passed by legislatures and are most familiar to the lay public. For example, black letter law could be a statute defining what rape is, or it could be a Rule, determining what an expert may testify about. In addition, courts are also bound to follow case law—judges opinions in prior cases that interpret the black letter law and serve as precedent for the current courts. Lower courts must follow the interpretations of higher courts whose jurisdictions they are in, and the U.S. Supreme Court is the highest court of all, with the power to dictate how all courts must interpret the law.

16. The courts in the United States are hierarchically arranged. They are also separated into state and federal court systems. Generally speaking, federal courts are higher than state courts. In the federal court system, just below the U.S. Supreme Court are 13 "circuits" or areas, presided over by the various circuit courts.

17. Fed. R. Evid. 701–706.

18. See Appendix 2.2 for a list of which states are following which decision, if any.
19. "If *scientific, technical,* or other specialized knowledge will assist the trier of fact" (Fed. R. Evid. 702, emphasis added).
20. For a detailed look at *Frye, Daubert,* and their progeny, see Faigman, Kaye, Saks, and Sanders (2002a).
21. Interestingly, RTS has been used to some extent by the defense as well, to show that the alleged victim did *not* suffer from RTS, and thus presumably was *not* raped. The fact that a woman does not have a traumatic reaction to nonconsensual sex (which traumatizes most women) does not mean it did not occur. (PTSD requires not only a trauma but a traumatized *reaction* as well. See "Diagnostic criteria for 309.81 Post-traumatic Stress Disorder" A(2) in the DSM-IV-TR [American Psychiatric Association, 2000, p. 467]). For a discussion of this area, see Faigman et al. (2002b).
22. See Appendix 2.1 for a listing of states that do and do not allow this testimony.
23. The arguments in this chapter for admitting RTS testimony as evidence of nonconsent in a rape case are based on an earlier paper by this author on that subject (Cling, 1988). While at that time few papers addressed the issue, in the interim a number of articles have appeared viewing RTS testimony as evidence of nonconsent in what seems to be an increasingly favorable light. Readers interested in reviewing the history in this area may want to look at Frazier and Borgida (1988; 1992), Boeschen, Sales, and Koss (1998), and Faigman et al. (2002b).
24. For a more detailed legal discussion of this issue, see the earlier section "Changing Legal Standards for Medical Expert Witness Testimony."
25. Rape is usually a state crime and thus is tried in state court under state laws. Because the Unites States consists of 50 states, the laws on rape, and the admissibility of RTS as evidence, vary from state to state. See Appendix 2.2 for a listing of states and which standard each has adopted. In addition, of course, there is also federal court.
26. See Appendix 2.1 for a listing of which states allow and which states disallow such testimony.
27. Under *Daubert,* courts are now required to acquaint themselves with the relevant fields being evaluated, in order to determine what kind of evidence should and should not be admitted. However, courts, and the field of law generally, are averse to examining empirical data, and rarely check with the actual fields. Instead they seem to use their own logical sense of reliability, which is often inaccurate (see Faigman et al., 2002a). Some courts are hiring experts to help advise them as to what fields qualify for admissibility under *Daubert.*
28. The defense has begun to use RTS testimony more and more, to turn the tables and show that the victim was traumatized by other sexual conduct in her past. This trend conflicts with recent rape shield laws designed to protect victims from intrusion into their sexual history. For a discussion of this relatively new issue, see Faigman et al. (2002b, §13-1.5).

REFERENCES

American Psychiatric Association. (1980). *Diagnostic and statistical manual of mental disorders* (3rd ed.). Washington, DC: Author.

American Psychiatric Association. (1986). *Diagnostic and statistical manual of mental disorders* (3rd ed., rev.). Washington, DC: Author.

American Psychiatric Association. (1994). *Diagnostic and statistical manual of mental disorders* (4th ed.). Washington, DC: Author.

American Psychiatric Association. (2000). *Diagnostic and statistical manual of mental disorders* (4th ed., text rev.). Washington, DC: Author.

Anderson, M. J. (1998). Reviving resistance in rape law. *University of Illinois Law Review, 1998,* 953–1005.

Blackstone, W. (1983). *Commentaries on the laws of England.* Birmingham, AL: Gryphon Editions.

Boeschen, L., Sales, B., & Koss, M. (1998). Special theme: Sex offenders: Scientific, legal, and policy perspective: Evidentiary and remedial issue: Rape trauma experts in the courtroom. *Psychology, Public Policy and Law, 4,* 414–432.

Bracton, H. (1968). *On the laws and customs of England.* Cambridge, MA: Harvard University Press.

Brownmiller, S. (1975). *Against our will: Men, women, and rape.* New York: Bantam Books.

Brundage, J. A. (1982). Rape and seduction in the medieval canon law. In V. L. Bullough & J. A. Brundage, *Sexual practices and the medieval church* (pp. 141–148). Buffalo, NY: Prometheus Books.

Brundage, J. A. (1987). *Law, sex, and Christian society in medieval Europe.* Chicago: University of Chicago Press.

Burgess, A. (1983). Rape trauma syndrome. *Behavioral Sciences and the Law 1*(3), 97–113.

Burgess, A., & Holmstrom, L. (1974). Rape trauma syndrome. *American Journal of Psychiatry, 131,* 981–986.

Burgess, A., & Holmstrom, L. (1976). Coping behavior of the rape victim. *American Journal of Psychiatry, 133,* 413–418.

Burgess-Jackson, K. (1999). *A most detestable crime: New philosophical essays on rape.* New York: Oxford University Press.

Cling, B. J. (1988). Rape trauma syndrome: Medical evidence of non-consent. *Women's Rights Law Reporter, 10,* 243–259.

Dershowitz, A. M. (1994). *The abuse excuse: And other cop-outs, sob stories, and evasions of responsibility.* Boston: Little, Brown.

Ellis, P. B. (1995). *Celtic women: Women in Celtic society and literature.* Grand Rapids, MI: Eerdmans.

Faigman, D. L., Kaye, D. H., Saks, M. J., & Sanders, J. (2002a). Admissibility of scientific evidence. In D. L. Faigman, D. H. Kaye, M. J. Saks, & J. Sanders (Eds.), *Modern scientific evidence: The law and science of expert testimony* (2nd ed., Vol. 1, pp. 2–68). Saint Paul, MN: West Group.

Faigman, D. L., Kaye, D. H., Saks, M. J., & Sanders, J. (2002b). Rape trauma syndrome: Legal issues. In D. L. Faigman, D. H. Kaye, M. J. Saks, & J. Sanders (Eds.), *Modern scientific evidence: The law and science of expert testimony* (2nd ed., Vol. 2, pp. 103–117). Saint Paul, MN: West Group.

Frazier, P., & Borgida, E. (1988). Juror common understanding and the admissibility of rape trauma syndrome evidence in court. *Law and Human Behavior, 12*(2), 101–122.

Frazier, P., & Borgida, E. (1992). Rape trauma syndrome: A review of case law and psychological research. *Law and Human Behavior, 16*(3), 293–311.

Frazier, P. (2002). Rape trauma syndrome: The scientific status of research on rape trauma syndrome. In D. L. Faigman, D. H. Kaye, M. J. Saks, & J. Sanders

(Eds.), *Modern scientific evidence: The law and science of expert testimony* (2nd ed., Vol. 2, pp. 117–143). Saint Paul, MN: West Group.

Fried, J. M. (1996) Forcing the issue: An analysis of the various standards of forcible compulsion in rape. *Pepperdine Law Review, 23,* 1277–1315.

Harper, R. F. (1994). *The Code of Hammurabi King of Babylon: About 2250 B.C.* Holmes Beach, FL: Gaunt.

Kempe, C. (1962). The battered child syndrome. *Journal of the American Medical Association, 181*(1), 17–24.

Morse, S. J. (1998). Excusing and the new excuse defenses: A legal and conceptual review. In M. Tonry (Ed.), *Crime and justice: An annual review of research* (Vol. 23, pp. 329–406). Chicago: University of Chicago Press.

Shapo, H. S. (1975). Recent statutory developments in the definition of forcible rape. *Virginia Law Review, 61,* 1500–1543.

Soshnick, A. Z. (1987). Comment, the rape shield paradox: Complainant protection amidst oscillating trends of state judicial interpretation. *Journal of Criminal Law and Criminology, 78,* 644–695.

Taslitz, A. (1999). Gender and race in evidence policy: What feminism has to offer evidence law. *Southwest University Law Review, 28,* 171–219.

Walker, L., & Monahan, J. (1987). Social frameworks: A new use of social science in law. *Virginia Law Review, 73,* 559–597.

APPENDIX 2.1. Admission of Expert Witness Testimony on Rape Trauma
Syndrome as Evidence of Nonconsent

Expert testimony on RTS allowed as evidence of nonconsent	
Arizona (1983)	*State v. Huey*, 145 Ariz. 59, 699 P.2d 1290 (1985).
	State v. Radjenovich, 138 Ariz. 270, 674 P.2d 333 (Ariz. Ct. App. 1983).
	Logerquist v. McVey, 196 Ariz. 470, 1 P.3d 113 (2000).
Arkansas (1985)	*Hall v. State*, 15 Ark. App. 309, 692 S.W.2d 769 (Ark. Ct. App. 1985).
Florida (1995)	*Clark v. State*, 654 So. 2d 984 (Fla. Dist. Ct. App. 1995).
Georgia (1994)	*Edmonson v. State*, 212 Ga. App. 449, 442 S.E.2d 300 (Ga. Ct. App. 1994).
Illinois (1990)	*People v. Harp*, 193 Ill. App. 3d 838, 550 N.E.2d 1163 (Ill. Ct. App. 1990).
Indiana (1989, 1991)	*Henson v. State*, 535 N.E.2d 1189 (Ind. 1989). (The court concluded that when defense used RTS to show that the victim was not raped it was error to exclude RTS as evidence, when the court had previously recognized the admissability of such evidence.)
	Goodwin v. State, 573 N.E.2d 895 (Ind. Ct. App. 1991). (It was permissible to introduce expert testimony that a victim's behavior (victim age 13) was consistent with PTSD as bearing upon whether a rape had occurred.)
Iowa (1989)	*State v. Gettier*, 438 N.W.2d 1 (Iowa Sup. Ct. 1989).
Kansas (1986)	*State v. McQuillen*, 239 Kan. 590, 721 P.2d 740 (1986).
Maryland (1986)	*State v. Allewalt*, 308 Md. 89, 517 A.2d 741 (1986).
Mississippi (2002)	*Kolberg v. State*, 829 So. 2d 29 (Miss. 2002).
Montana (2001)	*State v. Detonancour*, 306 Mont. 389, 34 P.3d 487 (2001).
New Mexico (1993)	*State v. Alberico*, 116 N.M. 156, 861 P.2d 192 (1993).
North Carolina (1990)	*State v. Strickland*, 96 N.C. App. 642, 387 S.E.2d 62 (N.C. Ct. App. 1990).
Ohio (1993)	*State v. Martens*, 90 Ohio App. 3d 338, 629 N.E.2d 462 (Ohio Ct. App. 1993).
South Carolina (2003)	*State v. Schumpert*, 312 S.C. 502, 435 S.E.2d 859 (1993).
Texas (1985)	*Brown v. State*, 692 S.W.2d 146 (Tex. Ct. App. 1985).
Vermont (2000)	*State v. Kinney*, 171 Vt. 239, 762 A.2d 833 (2000).
West Virginia (1988)	*State v. McCoy*, 179 W. Va. 223, 366 S.E.2d 731 (1988).

Wisconsin (1996) *State v. Perkins,* No. 95-1353-CR, 1996 Wisc. App. LEXIS 1015, at *1 (Wisc. Ct. App. August 7, 1996).

Wyoming (1987) *Scadden v. State,* 732 P.2d 1036 (Wyo. 1987).

Expert testimony on RTS not allowed as evidence of nonconsent

California (1984) *People v. Bledsoe,* 36 Cal.3d 236, 681 P.2d 291 (1984).

Colorado (1987) *People v. Hampton,* 746 P.2d 947 (Colo. 1987).

Louisiana (2002) *State v. Chauvin,* 846 So. 2d 697 (La. 2002).

Minnesota (1982) *State v. Saldana,* 324 N.W.2d 227 (Minn. 1982).

State v. McGee, 324 N.W.2d 232 (Minn. 1982).

Missouri (1984) *State v. Taylor,* 663 S.W.2d 235 (Mo. 1984).

State v. Edwards, 785 S.W.2d 703 (Mo. Ct. App. 1990).

New Jersey (1997) *State v. Scherzer,* 301 N.J. Super. 363, 694 A.2d 196 (N.J. Super. Ct. 1997).

New York (1990) *People v. Taylor,* 75 N.Y.2d 277, 552 N.E.2d 131 (1990).

People v. Story, 176 A.D.2d 1080, 575 N.Y.S.2d 589 (N.Y. App. Div. 1991).

Pennsylvania (1988) *Commonwealth v. Zamarripa,* 379 Pa. Super. 208, 549 A.2d 980 (Pa. Super. Ct. 1988).

Tennessee (1993) *State vs. Ashburn,* 914 S.W.2d 108 (Tenn. Crim. App. 1995).

State v. Ballard, 855 S.W.2d 557 (Tenn. 1993).

Washington (1987) *State v. Black,* 109 Wash.2d 336, 745 P.2d 12 (Wash. 1987).

Unclear if expert testimony on RTS allowed or not allowed as evidence of nonconsent

Alabama (1988) *Sexton v. State,* 529 So. 2d 1041 (Ala. Crim. App. 1988). (Regarding rape of a 5-year-old, expert testified that victim's symptoms were consistent with child sexual abuse syndrome.)

Alaska (1988) *Hilburn v. State,* 765 P.2d 1382 (Alaska Ct. App. 1988). (The expert in a rape case testified that the complainant's withdrawn behavior was consistent with her having undergone a traumatic experience, but there was no mention of rape or RTS.)

Connecticut (1995) *State v. Ali,* 233 Conn. 403, 660 A.2d 337 (1995). (Expert allowed to testify in direct examination about RTS in general to explain victim's delay in reporting.)

Delaware (1987) *Wheat v. State,* 527 A.2d 269 (Del. 1987). (Refused to comment on RTS evidence though referred to cases that have not allowed RTS to be used as evidence of consent.)

District of
Columbia (1992)

Street v. United States, 602 A.2d 141 (D.C. Ct. App. 1992).
(Refused to comment on RTS as evidence.)

Idaho (1992)

State v. Roles, 122 Idaho 138, 832 P.2d 311 (Idaho Ct. App.
1992). (The court, although sympathetic to admission of
expert testimony on RTS as evidence of nonconsent, simply
held that expert testimony on PTSD is admissable if it is used
to show, in rebuttal, that the victim's behavior was consistent
with someone who had been traumatized.)

Massachusetts
(1990)

Commonwealth v. Mamay, 407 Mass. 412, 553 N.E.2d 945
(1990). (Admissible to explain complainant's postrape
behavior, that is, waiting to report the crime. Unclear if
offered as rebuttal evidence.)

Oregon (1983)

State v. Middleton, 294 Or. 427, 657 P.2d 1215 (1983).
(In the case of rape of a child by the father, it is permissible to
testify that victim's behavior was consistent with trauma, but
only applies to familial sexual abuse of a child.)

Virginia (2002)

Ward v. Commonwealth, 264 Va. 648, 570 S.E.2d 827 (2002).
(The expert was allowed to testify that the victim was
suffering from PTSD but could not testify as to what caused
the PTSD since this would be testifying to the ultimate issue of
fact.)

No cases for expert testimony allowed on RTS as evidence of nonconsent

Arkansas, Hawaii, Kentucky, Maine, Michigan, Nebraska, Nevada, New
Hampshire, North Dakota, Oklahoma, Rhode Island, South Dakota, Utah,
United States (Federal)

APPENDIX 2.2. Standards for Expert Witness Testimony

Accept essential principles of *Daubert*

Conneticut (1997)	*State v. Porter*, 241 Conn. 57, 694 A.2d 1262 (Conn. 1997).
Delaware (1993)	*Nelson v. State*, 628 A.2d 69 (Del. 1993).
Georgia (1995)	*Jordan v. Georgia Power Company*, 219 Ga.App. 690, 466 S.E.2d 601(Ga. App. 1995).
Idaho (1996)	*State v. Parkinson*, 128 Idaho 29, 909 P.2d 647 (Idaho App.1996).
Indiana (1995)	*Steward v. State*, 652 N.E.2d 490 (Ind. 1995).
Iowa (1994)	*Hutchison v. American Family Mutual Insurance Co.*, 514 N.W.2d 882 (Iowa 1994).
Kentucky (1995)	*Mitchell v. Commonwealth*, 908 S.W.2d 100 (Ky. 1995).
Louisiana (1993)	*State v. Foret*, 628 So. 2d 1116 (La. 1993).
Maine (1996)	*Green v. Cesna Aircraft Co.*, 673 A.2d 215 (Me. 1996).
Massachusetts (1994)	*Commonwealth v. Lanigan*, 419 Mass. 15, 641 N.E.2d 1342 (Mass. 1994).
Montana (1995)	*State v. Weeks*, 270 Mont. 63, 891 P.2d 477 (Mont. 1995).
Nebraska (2001)	*Schafersman v. Agland Coop*, 262 Neb. 215, 631 N.W.2d 862 (2001).
New Hampshire (1995)	*State v. Cavaliere*, 140 N.H. 108, 663 A.2d 96 (N.H. 1995).
North Carolina (1995)	*State v. Goode*, 341 N.C. 513, 461 S.E.2d 631(N.C. 1995).
Oklahoma (1995)	*Taylor v. State*, 889 P.2d 319 (Okla. Crim. App. 1995).
Oregon (1995)	*State v. O'Key*, 321 Or. 285, 899 P.2d 663 (Or. 1995).
South Dakota (1995)	*State v. Schweitzer*, 533 N.W.2d 156 (S.D. 1995).
Texas (1995)	*E. I. Du Pont de Nemours & Co., Inc. v. Robinson*, 923 S.W.2d 549 (Tex. 1995).
Vermont (1995)	*State v. Streich*, 163 Vt. 331, 658 A.2d 38 (Vt. 1995).
West Virginia (1993)	*Wilt v. Buracker*, 191 W.Va. 39, 443 S.E.2d 196 (W. Va.1993).
Wyoming (1993)	*Springfield v. State*, 860 P.2d 435 (Wyo. 1993).

State their openness to reconsidering the rule they apply

Alaska (1994)	*Mattox v. State Dept. of Revenue*, Child Support Enforcement Div., 875 P.2d 763 (Alaska 1994).
Colorado (1995)	*Lindsey v. People*, 892 P.2d 281(Colo. 1995).

Illinois (1995)   *Dotto v. Okan*, 269 Ill. App. 3d 808, 207 Ill. Dec. 190, 646
                         N.E.2d 1277 (Ill. App. 1995).

Minnesota (1995)   *Fairview Hospital and Health Care Services v. St. Paul Fire
                         & Marine Insurance Co.*, 535 N.W.2d 337 (Minn. 1995).

New Jersey (1995)   *Ripa v. Owens-Corning Fiberglass Corp.*, 282 N.J. Super.
                         373, 660 A.2d 521(N.J. Super. 1995).

Pennsylvania (1994)   *Commonwealth v. Crews*, 536 Pa. 508, 640 A.2d 395 (Pa.
                         1994).

Washington (1994)   *State v. Russell*, 125 Wash. 2d 24, 882 P.2d 747 (Wash.
                         1994).

Reject the *Daubert* standard, at least for time being, and used *Frye* or an alternative

Arizona (1993)   *State v. Bible*, 175 Ariz. 549, 858 P.2d 11522 (Ariz. 1993).

California (1994)   *People v. Leahy*, 8 Cal. 4th 587, 34 Cal. Rptr. 2d 663, 882
                         P.2d 321 (Cal. 1994).

Florida (1993)   *Flanagan v. State*, 625 So. 2d 827(Fla.1993).

Kansas (1995)   *State v. Haddock*, 257 Kan. 964, 897 P.2d 152 (Kan. 1995).

Maryland (1995)   *Schultz v. State*, 106 Md. Appl 145, 664 A.2d 60 (Md. App.
                         1995).

Michigan (1995)   *People v. Peterson*, 450 Mich. 349, 537 N.W.2d 857 (Mich.
                         1995). Amended 450 Mich. 1212, 548 N.W.2d 625 (1995).

Mississippi (2001)   *Kansas City Southern Railway Co. v. J.C. Johnson*, 2001 WL
                         107864*7 (Miss. 2001).

Missouri (1993)   *Callahan v. Cardinal Glennon Hospital*, 863 S.W.2d 852
                         (Mo. 1993).

New York (1994)   *People v. Wesley*, 83 N.Y.2d 417, 611 N.Y.S.2d 97, 633
                         N.E.2d 451 (N.Y. 1994).

North Dakota   *City of Fargo v. McLaughlin*, 512 N.W.2d 700 (N.D. 1994).
(1994)

Follow their own state version

Arkansas (1996)   *Moore v. Sate*, 323 Ark. 529, 915 S.W.2d 284 (Ark. 1996).

District of Columbia *Taylor v. United States*, 661 A.2d 636 (D.C. 1995).
(1995)

Hawaii (1995)   *State v. Maelega*, 80 Hawaii 172, 907 P.2d 758 (Hawaii
                         1995).

New Mexico   *State v. Anderson*, 118 N.M. 284, 881 P.2d 29 (N.M. 1994).
(1994)

Ohio (1995)   *State v. Clark*, 101 Ohio App. 3d 389, 655 N.E.2d 795
                         (Ohio. App. 1995).

South Carolina (1999)	*State v. Council*, 335 S.C. 1, 515 S.E.2d 508 (S.C. 1999).
Utah (1996)	*State v. Crosby*, 927 P.2d 638 (Utah 1996).
Wisconsin (1995)	*State v. Peters*, 192 Wis. 2d 674, 534 N.W.2d 867 (Wis. App. 1995).

Undecided (combination of *Frye* and *Daubert*)

Alabama (2000)	*Courtaulds Fibers, Inc. v. Long*, 779 So. 2d 198 (Ala. 2000).
Nevada (1998)	*Dow Chemical Co. v. Mahlum*, 114 Nev. 1468, 970 P.2d 98 (Nev. 1998).
Rhode Island (1993)	*Soares v. Vestal*, M.D., 632 A.2d 647 (R.I. 1993).
Tennessee (1994)	*State v. Smith*, 1994 WL 361851 (Tenn. Crim. App.1994).
Virginia (1994)	*Cotton v. Commonwealth*, 19 Va. App. 306, 451 S.E.2d 673 (Va. App. 1994).

Note. Adapted from Faigman, Kaye, Saks, and Sanders (2002a). Copyright 2002 by West Group. Adapted by permission.

3 Battered Woman Syndrome

Clinical Features, Evaluation, and Expert Testimony

NANCY KASER-BOYD

THE BATTERING RELATIONSHIP: COMMON PATTERNS

Although obtaining accurate statistics on woman battering is complicated by underreporting, experts say that about one-quarter of women in relationships will be physically abused during the course of a relationship (Eigenberg, 2001).[1] One study found that among 600 applicants for divorce, 37% of the wives cited physical abuse as one of their complaints (Levinger, 1966). According to the California Attorney General's Office, battering is the single major cause of physical injury to women, and one-third of all women killed are killed by spouses (Levy, 1984). Moreover, 50% of the battered women who leave their batterers continue to be harassed (Moore, 1979).

From the outside, the violent family may look relatively normal. When formal study of these relationships first began in the 1970s researchers were surprised to learn that spousal battery occurred in all socioeconomic groups. Battered women were not necessarily without job skills; some had professional degrees and good incomes. Batterers do not

41

necessarily collect guns. They are not necessarily violent outside of the relationship.

Walker (1979) noted that overt violence in a battering relationship is not constant; it occurs in cycles, with peaks of violence and periods of calm. A battered woman, therefore, is not under constant threat of physical assault. Instead, because the abuse is dependant on the batterer's moods, the abuse is episodic and unpredictable, and it alternates with normal or even loving behavior. Walker described three stages in the typical battering relationship: stage 1, where small incidents lead to a general sense of mounting tension; stage 2, the violent outburst; and stage 3, a period of calm after the "storm," where apologies and promises may be made and the battered woman may struggle to deny the seriousness of the pathology. This is not a universal pattern. In some cases there are long periods between violent incidents (Dutton, 1992). Individuals who have lived in violent families report that violence can erupt at any time, often over extremely small things. They describe feeling like they are "walking on eggshells." They develop the feeling that the batterer should never be displeased because this will result in anger, name calling, threats, or actual physical assault. Verbal abuse is more than simply demeaning; it contains threats and other cues that serve to remind the woman of the batterer's power and reinforce his dominance even in the absence of physical assault.

For a number of reasons, battered women often go to great lengths to minimize or deny their abuse. Probably the most frequently cited reason is fear of the batterer's anger and accusations of betrayal. Another often cited reason is shame. Battered women often blame themselves for the violence, particularly in the beginning of the relationship. The batterer uses failure messages to berate her, and she does not want her family, neighbors, coworkers, or others to see her as a failure, too. Battered women also say they kept their abuse secret because of love and loyalty. Especially in the early years of the relationship, they saw their batterer as a vulnerable individual who wanted to change and they felt compelled to help him. For these reasons, the abuse may go unreported. The battered woman may tell no one, even close friends and relatives. She may not seek medical attention or call police. On the other hand, she may have tried to get help for herself or her spouse and found that the social service and police response was confusing, frightening, or ineffective. She may have tried calling a shelter and found that there was a waiting list, or that the shelter was overcrowded and felt dangerous because of the mix of ethnic and socioeconomic groups.

Although services for battered women are generally better than when Walker first described the patterns in domestic violence—and this includes the creation and expansion of a network of battered woman's shelters, clearer spousal assault laws, and assistance filing restraining orders—escaping from or stopping the violence is still a daunting endeavor for many battered women. For example, battered women report that there was little cost to the batterer of violating restraining orders.

SEVERITY OF BATTERING

Battered women are subjected to a huge range of violent acts.[2] Almost every relationship with domestic violence also included a high level of psychological abuse. At the lower end, there is name calling ("stupid bitch," "cunt," "whore," "fat pig," "ugly," "worthless," etc.). Battered women say that these felt more damaging than hits and punches because they communicated worthlessness. Fear, however, was caused by the batterer's verbal threats, such as "If you leave me, I will tell people you are crazy," "I'll get the kids," "I will find you and hurt you," "I will hurt everyone you love." Then there is sexual abuse. In 1985, I began collecting formal data, on a case-by-case basis, on battered women referred for killing the batterer. The sample size is now 52. Most of the cases where a battered woman killed her batterer included frequent, unwanted, forced, and painful sexual activity that caused the woman to feel she could not even control her own body. Browne (1987) made a similar finding. She compared severity levels in relationships where battered women did and did not kill the batterer. Relationships where the woman killed contained more substance abuse, more severe violence, more frequent violence, more sexual abuse, more injuries, and more batterer's threats to kill.

Because battering exists on a continuum of severity, in evaluations of battered women it is important to understand the level of severity of violence experienced. This is crucial to forming an opinion about the degree of danger in a relationship, and it is also closely related to the severity of symptoms that arise from battering. "Battering" is defined as physical abuse, sexual abuse, and/or psychological abuse. How should we rate severity? In my early evaluations of battered women, I did not find existing methods (e.g., the Conflict Tactics Scale) helpful. I also decided that what mattered was not how I or other clinicians or researchers defined severity but how battered women rate various acts that they had experienced. In a sample of 40 consecutively referred battered women, I employed a Q-sort technique with cards describing a wide range of violent acts, including psychological abuse, and asked the women to sort them from "least frightening" to "most frightening." There was a surprising amount of agreement among these independent ratings. The result was a 10-point scale, the Spousal Assault Violent Acts scale (Appendix 3.1), which allows a rapid assessment of severity of the violence. Acts that individual battered women have experienced that are not on the scale can be rated in the evaluation process. The application of the severity rating to an assessment of a battered woman's state of mind (e.g., mental state at the time of a killing) will be discussed later in this chapter.

HISTORY AND TERMINOLOGY

The term "battered woman syndrome" was coined by Lenore Walker (1979) when she first described the now well-known patterns of domestic violence. For roughly a decade, this term captured the commonly observed effects of battering and helped to communicate and dispel myths about battered women. In the mid-1980s, a parallel process was occurring for those who suffered other kinds of trauma. van der Kolk (1987) and his Harvard colleagues began to publish and speak about posttraumatic stress disorder. By the early 1990s it became apparent that the psychological effects of battering were not greatly different than the effects of repeated trauma of other types, and that the experience of high levels of fear, helplessness, and physical and emotional trauma is highly similar across all types of trauma such as child abuse, rape, torture, and civilian disaster (Herman, 1992). Battered woman syndrome was then subsumed under the more general category of "posttraumatic stress disorder" (PTSD). This, however, seemed to pathologize battered women. Many clinicians objected to placing battered women within the categories of "mental disorder" of the diagnostic manual.[3] A correct understanding of the diagnosis PTSD should dispel this belief, since *any previously healthy individual exposed to a trauma* can develop PTSD. However, in the courtroom, words and impressions can change the entire outcome of a trial, and so the alternative term "effects of battering" has been proposed.

A report by the U.S. Department of Health and Human Services (National Institute of Justice, 1996), resulting from a survey of judges and attorneys, concluded that the term "battered woman syndrome" does not adequately reflect the breadth or nature of the empirical knowledge about battering and its effects and that it portrays a stereotypical image of battered women as helpless, passive, or psychologically impaired and battering relationships as matching a single pattern. The knowledge pertaining to battering and its effects does not rest on a singular construct, as the term "battered woman syndrome" implies. As for the diagnosis of PTSD, Dutton and Goodman (1994) note that between 31 and 84% of battered women are reported to have the symptoms of PTSD, and these may be helpful in understanding a woman's mental state at the time of an alleged criminal act, but the diagnosis of PTSD is not necessary to establish the relevance of previous battering to a woman's experience of fear or threat at the time of a criminal act.

An internal academic struggle over exact terminology may be difficult to explain in the courtroom. In some states the term "battered woman syndrome" has already been incorporated in the law.[4] Perhaps it would be best to say that battered woman syndrome is a shorthand term describing the effects of battering, which are now understood to be cognitive, emotional, physiological, and behavioral. I now describe findings about batterers, battered women, and the effects of battering.

THE BATTERER

Men who are violent with their partners are not necessarily easy to identify as pathological, even to the clinician. A battering spouse can have an adequate work history or a community image as a stable individual or family man. He may not have a drinking or substance abuse problem, although he often does. One of the surprising findings in the early stages of clinical research with batterers was their ability to achieve "normal limits" test profiles, for example, on the Minnesota Multiphasic Personality Inventory (MMPI). This is not the case, however, when they are tested with psychological tests that are more sensitive to personality pathology (Hamberger & Hastings, 1991), such as the Millon Clinical Multiaxial Inventory (MCMI).

Batterers have a frequently noted set of personality traits. This description is compiled from hundreds of interviews with battered women. Batterers seem to have a strong *need for control*. They feel they must make all of the family decisions and they expect their spouse to comply. Differences in opinion are belittled or, worse, lead to festering resentments or explosions of rage. Family resources such as money, food, cars, the telephone, the computer, and so on, are controlled by the batterer. At the extreme, the batterer does not allow his spouse to make decisions about her own body. Fundamental decisions like when to have sex and when to have children are made by the batterer.

Batterers are unusually *egocentric*. Family life is set up to revolve around their needs and when their needs are frustrated, anger results. Their needs take precedence over the needs of other family members. They feel *entitled*; they believe that they are entitled to more of their spouse's time, entitled to spend family money for their own needs while other family members go wanting, entitled to have their sexual needs met whenever they want, and entitled to break social, legal, or moral rules.

Batterers have *poor control of emotion and poor frustration toler-*

ance. They may be chronically angry, with outbursts of intense anger, or they may vacillate between overcontrol and undercontrol of anger, but when strong emotion is experienced, their controls are weak. Rage is not uncommon in these men. Some battered women describe a look that comes over the batterer's face that suggests dissociative qualities ("He was hitting me and hitting me and I looked in his eyes and it was like he wasn't there").

Batterers often *externalize blame*. If things don't go well, it's not *their* fault, it's their spouse's fault. They commonly blame their periods of loss of control on their wife: "If you hadn't _____, I wouldn't have hit you." The strong tendency to externalize blame is an aspect of a paranoid personality style. Batterers, in fact, often seem paranoid. They are often *profoundly jealous*. They accuse their spouses of infidelities that a frightened woman would not dare indulge. This probably reflects the defense mechanism of *projection*, where pathology is denied and projected onto another. Batterers, in fact, see the world as a hostile place. They project their hostility onto others, insisting that others treat them badly, not the reverse. They become adept at bending and distorting reality to match their own worldview and often lecture and prod the battered woman so much that she takes on his worldview.

Batterers often *lack empathy*. They look at most human transactions in terms of how they feel rather than how their actions make others feel. They seem unaware of the pain they inflict on the woman they claim to love. Some batterers are even sexually aroused by causing pain in their partner or gaining power in a battering incident.

Dutton (1988; 1995), in his work on profiling wife assaulters, asserts that batterers have borderline personality disorder. Clinical descriptions of batterers indicate traits of other DSM-IV cluster B disorders[5] as well, especially narcissism. Formal assessment research with batterers (mostly with the MCMI), have found test elevations on scales Aggressive/Sadistic, Narcissistic, Dependent, and Antisocial (Hamberger & Hastings, 1991). Violence between partners can be the result of other disorders, too. For example, individuals with brain damage (men and women) have poor control over anger and a somewhat paranoid stance toward others. Individuals in the manic phase of a bipolar disorder can be violent at times, and any disorder with psychotic features can embody violence in close relationships.

Research studies conducted on batterers commonly find that the batterer's childhood home was violent (Walker, 1984, found that 80% of the batterers in her sample of 390 violent relationships had grown up in violent homes). By itself, this does not clarify whether violent and coercive interpersonal behavior is *learned*, that is, from a violent role model, or whether it exists for more complex reasons. Sociologists often note that violence against women and male dominance are culturally sanctioned and reinforced. It seems possible and even likely that batterers have impaired emotional control and object relations as survivors of child abuse (i.e., they may have complex PTSD).[6] The proclivity to batter close others, in reality, is probably caused by some combination of these factors.

THE BATTERED WOMAN

Battered women come from all walks of life. The image of the poor, dependent woman with no skills or education is a myth. Any woman can become a battered woman. The crucial variable is the amount of violence and threat to which she has been subjected. The process of becoming a battered woman is not different than that of becoming a prisoner of war. What is required is the formation of a relationship with someone who is willing to use extreme force and psychological coercion to keep control. It is clear, however, that many battered women were victims of abuse in childhood. Walker (1979), in her National Institute of Mental Health (NIMH) study of battered women, found that about one-half of battered women had been sexually abused in childhood; about 25% had been physically abused; 44% had seen their mother physically abused; some had experienced all three traumatic stressors. It is generally accepted that childhood creates a template for adult relationships, so growing up with a mother who was a battered women would provide little information about healthy men or assertive, self-protective women. A number of researchers have followed women abused physically or sexually in childhood, especially those abused by a close family member, and found they have a greater likelihood of being "revictimized" (Herman, 1992; Roth et. al., 1997). This may be because they have had their sense of self damaged by abusive treatment. It might be because they have not been exposed to healthy relationships and do not object quickly to bad treatment. A particular danger in discussing revictimization is developing the misconception that battered women are "masochistic," that is, that they seek abusive relationships. It is important to note that revictimization occurs in male victims of child physical or sexual abuse as well. Its occurrence in both sexes goes part of the way to clarify that battered women are not simply women who have a need to be punished.

The early research on battered women was conducted in the early and mid-1970s, and a majority of the couples were married and lived together. By the 1990s it seemed clear that some of the early descriptions of battered woman did not apply to the contemporary population, especially in urban and minority areas. In Los Angeles, for example, many of the women I have worked with were battered by a man who did not live with her but who was able to threaten and intimidate her at will. The man sometimes had the same relationship with another woman at the same time and treated the second woman the same way. In many of these cases, the man was a gang member who called on members of his gang to watch and control the woman when he went to jail. Some of the women I evaluated feared their battering partner even after he had been sent to prison because of the ability of prisoners to put "hits" out for people on the outside.

The influx of immigrants from countries where women have few rights also changed the contemporary picture of domestic violence in the United States. In countries such as China, Egypt, Somalia, India, Mexico, and parts of Latin America, reporting domestic violence outside the family was unheard of, and women were expected to stay with and accept violence. These women received pressure and approbation from family—often her family *and* the batterer's family. If they attempted to get outside help, they faced total rejection by the families and certain economic hardship. In such women, the dynamics originally described by Walker and others are worse; that is, there is more shame, more denial, and more fear of leaving the relationship.

Battered women are not necessarily "shrinking violets," nor do they always appear to the casual observer to be helpless or passive. Battered women do sometimes fight back, verbally or physically. Bowker (1986) surveyed battered women to learn what strategies they used to interrupt the violence or protect themselves, and about 25% reported they fought back. This was often a strategy that they used in the early stages of the violence; many reported that this "only made him madder," and they changed strategies to minimize the violence and protect themselves. A battered woman has often tried a number of ways to reduce the family conflict or get help. She may have tried calling the police, getting a restraining order, or going to a shelter and found these to have their own sets of complications. Battered women may completely avoid getting medical care for their injuries. I have interviewed women who suffered broken bones and stab wounds without getting medical assistance, and the reason they give is fear—fear that the domestic violence will be reported by medical personnel, a move that is now mandatory in public hospitals in California.

A battered woman becomes hypersensitive to the moods of her batterer. This is a survival technique. She has often learned things that help to modulate the batterer's bad moods, but she may actually have little control over when the violence occurs or how severe it becomes. She must also develop the psychological means to cope with overwhelming levels of anxiety and emotional arousal. There are more effects of battering, and these are explained in the next section.

THE CLINICAL EFFECTS OF BATTERING

Living in a violent relationship creates strong emotions (e.g., fear, intense ambivalence) and methods of coping (avoidance, denial, emotional numbing, substance abuse) that may be difficult for the layperson to understand. Battering creates a distinct set of behavioral (i.e., observable) and psychological (not so observable) effects or symptoms. In the behavioral realm, battered women have been observed to hide or minimize the violence, fail to follow through on criminal charges, leave and return to the relationship, become more passive or immobilized, and develop low self-esteem. These responses are observed in women from a variety of backgrounds. Symptoms not readily observable by the layperson embody the biological and psychological changes associated with trauma and include symptoms such as a heightened sense of danger, biological and psychological hyperarousal and hypervigilance, flooding (reexperiencing the intense emotions of fear, vulnerability, threat, or anger), and emotional constriction (manifested by emotional "numbing," denial, dissociation or "self-medicating" with drugs or alcohol). Battered women often develop sleep disorders and physical symptoms related to stress, such as migraine headaches and lower back pain. The high levels of anxiety and unpredictable quality of their lives is associated with chronic fatigue and with impaired immune system function.

Some of the symptoms or effects of battering have been greatly misunderstood and require further explanation. Battered women are frequently reported to use "denial" about the violence and coercion to which they are subjected. In the courtroom, "denial" is often interpreted concretely to mean denying the battering or recanting the report she made at the time of the battering. Battered women do deny the battering to others, including police and the courts, usually because of fear. They may "make up" causes for the bruises or minimize the seriousness of the assault, but "denial" actually has a broader meaning. Denial is a psychological defense mechanism that may be at least partly unconscious, and it protects the person from the painful reality of the pathology of battering: the hurt, the fear, the shame, the confusion, and the anger. Denial can also be understood as one of the PTSD "Avoidance" symptoms— that is, in the space between batterings, a battered woman may avoid painful reminders and emotionally constrict so that she can carry out her daily functions. Battered women, when interviewed, use words like "I just tried not to think about it," "I wanted to believe it would never happen again," or "I just blocked it out of my mind." The blocking or numbing may be so extreme that the memories and feelings are "dissociated" or "split off" from conscious awareness. New research on the brain's response to fear ("Fear," 2003) indicates that memories laid down during a time of fear are recorded in a different part of the brain (the amygdala rather than the frontal cortex). They can be "triggered" by new signals of danger. This is a breakthrough in understanding dissociation and the sudden surge of fear and terror that a battered woman can experience when violence starts to erupt.

It should be obvious that when "blocking" occurs, memory for an event might be poor. Battered women report that they work hard to "forget" painful memories. This is actually a universal phenomenon in individuals who have experienced trauma (including men). It protects the trauma survivor from being constantly "flooded" with painful memories and the emotions that are associated. Poor memory and a wish to avoid remembering can make clinical interviews with battered women challenging. Time sequences are often unclear and histories fragmented. These interviews take more time and patience and an understanding that inconsistencies do not mean that the woman is uncooperative.

Sometimes battered women use drugs or alcohol to help them quell their anxiety and the other strong emotions that come from being battered. Walker (1984), in her eight-state NIMH-funded survey found that 20% of battered women used alcohol in the time span of the serious batterings and 7% used street or prescription drugs.

The more extreme the physical and psychological abuse, the more severe the effects of battering. This means more fear and hypervigilance to danger, more desperation and helplessness, more exhaustion, and more extreme psychological defense mechanisms (denial, dissociation). It is not common but it is not inconceivable that a badly battered woman would develop psychotic symptoms. These are usually secondary to a profound clinical depression (major depressive episode) and are considered "mood-congruent." An example of this type of "psychotic" symptom is hearing a voice that tells her to kill herself, or to kill herself and the children. Women who have experienced terrifying assaults and severe injury may also have severe trauma symptoms, including dissociative flashbacks that resemble hallucinations or psychotic symptoms.

It is important to note in discussing the effects of battering that the list of effects or symptoms is not a checklist. A battered woman may have some but not all of the effects or symptoms. She may be so emotionally constricted that the effects of battering are hidden. She may have symptoms or behaviors that are not discussed here but that are unique to the violence she has endured; for example, an Egyptian-American woman who had been genitally mutilated as a 7 year old, then badly sexually abused and battered by her husband, killed him in self-defense during a battering and sexual assault, then cut off his genitals. His abuse of her triggered her memories of abuse and triggered a dissociative episode where she carried out acts that were symbolic of her own genital mutilation.

FORENSIC EVALUATION OF BATTERED WOMEN

The forensic evaluation of a battered woman may vary somewhat depending on the forensic arena for expert testimony about the effects of battering. The arena may be family court, involving child custody; it may be criminal or federal court, involving a defense of a battered woman who has fought back and is charged with spousal assault, a battered woman who has killed her batterer in self-defense, or a battered woman who is charged as a codefendant in a crime her battering partner committed. Less common but equally important, it may be in civil court, when a battered woman sues her battering spouse for the emotional and physical damage she suffered.

In criminal court, the forensic evaluation is focused on identifying the effects of battering and their severity, ruling out malingering[7], and tying the effects of battering to the woman's mental state. In family court, the evaluation is usually focused on the battered woman's parenting lapses, and the evaluator needs to identify and measure the effects of battering, evaluate credibility, explain how the effects of battering were the cause of parenting problems, and discuss how battered women *recover* from the effects of battering. In civil court, the focus is on the clinical symptoms, their severity, the woman's credibility, and establishing that the battering was the *proximate cause* of her symptoms. This chapter cannot substitute for careful forensic training and experience in evaluating and presenting cases in each of these arenas.

The forensic evaluation always begins with a review of background documents. These are fundamental to forming questions for the clinical interviews because they provide perspectives other than the battered woman's and alert the evaluator to "facts" that may be presented in court. In the typical case of a battered woman killing her batterer, background materials may include the following:

- Any videotapes or audiotapes that were collected at the time.
- Statements of the defendant (written).
- The police investigation.
- Witness statements.
- The autopsy report and other reports of the physical evidence.

- Preliminary hearing transcripts.
- Police reports from past incidents of domestic violence.
- Mental health records, if any.
- Any other pertinent health records.
- Diaries, journals, or letters that reveal the client's mental state or the nature of the relationship.

The clinical interview of a woman can take from 6 to 20 hours. Battered women often cannot easily relate their stories. Memory difficulties in traumatized individuals have been well documented in the literature. Accurate memories may not be encoded during times of extraordinary anxiety. Alternatively, the emotional constriction and numbing of PTSD may have established a pattern of avoiding memories or thoughts of past incidents, making them vague or jumbled as to time sequence. This means that the interviewer needs more patience to reconstruct the battering history and the details of the more serious assaults. Battered women are also frequently described as scattered in their interviews. This is very likely a result of their extraordinary anxiety and the fragmenting effect of trauma. To assist in pulling together the data, it can be helpful to use a semistructured interview, or interview techniques that help to organize the history. For example, Walker suggested that an interviewer ask about the first incident, the second incident, the *worst* incident, and the last incident. It is also important to ask about the woman's response to each of these. For example, did she call the police? Receive medical treatment? File a restraining order? Go to a shelter? Leave and return? In a murder trial, the unsophisticated juror or prosecutor might insist, "She could have left him, she didn't have to kill him," but most battered women have tried a number of different strategies to escape or stop the violence, and the killing is a sudden response to injury or death that seems *inescapable*. The Spousal Assault Violent Acts scale (Appendix 3.1) can be used to jog the woman's memory as well as to help the evaluator establish an overall violence severity rating.

Every battered woman should also receive a careful interview about her early life (childhood/adolescence), since earlier traumas can combine with battering, "kindling" more serious trauma symptoms (van der Kolk, 1987). Battered woman often experience shame when asked to tell their stories. They often blame themselves for their situation, even when they have defended themselves against imminent danger. This means they may leave out important aspects of the abuse. The most common area of omission in my interviews with over 50 battered women who killed their batterer was in the sexual domain. One woman who had assaulted her boyfriend with a baseball bat was interviewed for over 30 hours across 6 months before she disclosed that her boyfriend had been forcibly sodomizing her. After careful interviewing, which may span many hours, with breaks to keep the client from being overwhelmed, the forensic evaluator should consider whether to conduct any formal psychological testing. This is discussed in greater detail next.

PSYCHOLOGICAL TESTING
AND THE EFFECTS OF BATTERING

There are some differences in attitudes about the use of psychological tests with battered women. Some specialists in the effects of battering are not trained or educated to conduct psychological testing and make their conclusions based on their experience in conducting hundreds of clinical interviews, reading the literature, attending conferences, and so forth. When psychologists serve as experts in the effects of battering, it is reasonable to assume that they will use the tools of their trade to identify and measure symptoms. Psychological testing has the additional advantage of assessing credibility, since several of the objective personality tests have validity scales that can rule out malingering.

There is a small but important literature about battered women and traditional tests such as the MMPI and MMPI-2 (the revision of the MMPI) and the Rorschach. Rosewater and Walker (1985) pointed out, early in the history of discussion about battered women, that they may be elevated on MMPI scales that are elevated in Paranoid Schizophrenia (Scales 6 and 8). She noted it was not surprising that women who had been battered would be *fearful* or feel threatened (Scale 6) or that they would have some disruptions in their boundaries or their reality testing (Scale 8), because of the destabilizing and fragmenting effect of trauma. A newer and experimentally sophisticated study (Kahn, Welch, & Zillmer, 1993) had similar findings. Battered women were again found elevated on Scales 6 and 8. They were also elevated on Scale 4, a scale elevation that would cause a poorly trained psychologist to diagnose antisocial traits without knowing that this scale also is elevated in those with a high level of family discord. Rhodes (1992) compared the MMPIs of 46 battered women with a control group of 46 nonbattered women. She found that the battered women were significantly elevated on Scale 4 and also on the Harris and Lingoes (1968, cited in Graham, 1990) subscale of Family Discord.[8]

There are many other MMPI studies with individuals with PTSD from other types of trauma, and these are fairly consistent in their finding of elevations on Scales 2, 4, 6, 7, and 8. Wilson and Walker (1990) have explained how PTSD is captured by these particular MMPI-2 scales; for example, Scale 2 may capture the PTSD symptom of emotional numbing; Scale 4 may capture the emotional detachment, alienation, or anger seen in cases of interpersonal violence; Scale 6 measures the hypervigilance to danger; and Scale 8 may reflect intrusive reminders of the trauma, or profound vulnerability and fragmentation.

The MCMI is also widely used in forensic settings, and it has been used with battered woman. The MCMI has three validity scales that permit an assessment of test-taking "set." In the early 1980s I began to use the MCMI-II with battered women referred by dependency court (allegations of child abuse or neglect) and in the criminal evaluations I conducted. I chose the MCMI-II because its scales had the potential to capture some of Walker's descriptions of battered women as well as some of the DSM-IV criteria for PTSD. The MCMI-II Avoidant scale, in particular, had items that reflected internal numbness, flashbacks, and the conflict between a desire for and fear of closeness. Millon has now published a third edition of the test and has included a PTSD scale. In my clinical work with battered women, I found they were commonly elevated on the scales Avoidant, Dependent, Self-Defeating, Anxiety, and Dysthymia. To learn more about battered women and battered women who killed a battering spouse, I conducted a research study (Kaser-Boyd, 1992) that compared two groups of battered women. One study question was "Is the MCMI-II sensitive to the symptoms of battered woman syndrome?" Another question was "Can battered women be distinguished from women in a clinical sample?" A third question was "Do battered women in different circumstances look different on this test?" In this study I compared 20 battered women who were on trial for killing their battering spouses with 25 battered women who were referred by the dependency court (i.e., family court) for exposing children to domestic violence and 23 women referred by the Dependency court for other reasons. Women were included in Groups 1 and 2 if they had experienced two or more incidents of physical assault by a spouse and met DSM-IV criteria for PTSD.

There were no significant differences between Groups 1, 2, and 3 in age, ethnicity, religion, or education. The two groups of battered women were significantly elevated on scales Dependent, Avoidant, and Self-Defeating. They also had higher mean elevations on scales measuring anxiety and chronic depression. Battered women who had killed their batterer were higher overall in their elevations, suggesting a more severe form of battered woman syndrome. They also had a significantly greater mean elevation on the scale Schizoid, which captures the emotional numbness and constriction that is seen in severe states of PTSD.

The Rorschachs of battered woman, especially when the battering has been more severe and prolonged, resemble the Rorschachs of other individuals with PTSD (Kaser-Boyd, 1993). When women are tested shortly after leaving a battering relationship or shortly after killing their batterer, they deliver Rorschach protocols flooded with images of harm and danger, with formal Rorschach scores that suggest helplessness and a preoccupation with morbid and aggressive content. When time has elapsed (e.g, some months later), Rorschach protocols are more constricted—they are shorter records that are more form-based and seem to avoid seeing or mentioning morbid or aggressive percepts. This type of record is associated with the immobilization of reasoning and problem solving and with impaired psychological defenses. The Rorschach has been regarded by many leading trauma researchers as one of the best psychological tests for assessing the effects of trauma because it often captures vivid trauma imagery. Many of the battered woman on trial in my sample responded immediately to the red color of the blots, which first appears on Card II, with memories of the homicide; for example, one woman who shot her husband in the family living room said "This card reminds me (*long pause, getting tearful*) of the blood on the wall . . . it splattered behind him." Rorschach data bases indicate it is rare for women to identify sexual percepts on the Rorschach, yet battered women who have been sexually abused often give one morbid percept with sexual content; for example, one woman said "It reminds me of my vagina after he hurt me . . . he tore me up inside, and I was bleeding and hurting, and he didn't care."

Overall, psychological tests can be very useful in identifying and measuring the severity of the effects of battering. These can by organized by symptoms, for example, feeling profoundly fearful, feeling overwhelmed or helpless, feeling worthless, being exhausted, feeling shame, and so on, with a summary of test signs that support each symptom or effect.

CAN BATTERED WOMAN SYNDROME OR THE EFFECTS OF BATTERING BE FAKED?

The high stakes of criminal and child custody matters require experts in battered woman syndrome to specify a methodology to rule out malingering. Clinical interviews and structured, standardized interviews yield a substantial amount of clinical data but do not have validity scales that assist the evaluator in identifying exaggeration or malingering. While there is some merit to an argument that "clinical judgment" or the experience of interviewing many battered women was used to rule out malingering, this determination is enhanced by the use of more formal measures. Battered woman syndrome is a subtype of PTSD (or Complex PTSD), and this means there is a body of test literature with which to compare a given battered woman's profile. In so doing, it is important to remember that trauma syndromes are phasic.[9] It is also important to remember that not every battered woman has every symptom in the generally recognized list of the effects of battering.

In my research with the MCMI-II and battered women, I wondered whether a woman who learned about battered women from television or books could "fake" the effects of battering. Using the MCMI-II finding with the two samples of battered women described earlier, I set out to test whether an *informed faker* could take the MCMI-II and generate a profile that would be accepted by a psychologist as a valid one. I created a pool of *informed fakers* by recruiting graduate students from my class on assessment. I taught the students about the effects of battering; they had also received lectures on the MCMI-II. They were asked to answer the MCMI-II questions *as if* they suffered from the effects of battering. These sophisticated subjects were given written information about battered woman syndrome, a case vignette, and the DSM-IV criteria for PTSD. They were asked to assume that they "were in jail as a result of killing their spouse" and that it would be to their legal advantage to exhibit symptoms of battered woman syndrome.

Nineteen graduate students in clinical psychology completed the study. Their mean MCMI-II elevations were computed and compared to Group 1 from Study 1, battered women who killed their batterer. "Malingerers" were significantly higher than battered women on the scales Debasement, Schizoid, Avoidant, Dependent, Self-Defeating, Borderline, Anxiety, Somatoform, Dysthymia, and Major Depression. "Fakers" achieved elevations on the scales previously found elevated in battered women as well as other scales that assess acute distress and emotional instability, but their elevations were much higher than the real battered women. In general, the "malingerers" endorsed most of the items about emotional distress and therefore obtained profiles that were considerably more elevated than real battered women.

The data were further analyzed to determine whether validity scale cutting scores could maximize accurate classification as "battered" or "faking." The Disclosure scale was not significantly elevated in "fakers." The Debasement scale, on the other hand, was significantly different between groups. A cutting score of base rate 85 correctly classified 75% of "fakers" and 85% of battered women. A cutting score of bate rate 92 identified the same number of fakers while improving the hit rate for battered women to 95%—only one "real" battered woman was misclassified. This means that the Debasement scale could be used to rule out malingering.

Of course, in a real evaluation for criminal court, a woman would not be judged a "malingerer" based on one psychological test. The MMPI-2 has a standard set of validity scales (L, F, and K, plus TRIN, and VRIN) to evaluate test-taking stance, and there is a substantial literature on individuals who have experienced trauma (see Armstrong &

Kaser-Boyd, 2003), in addition to the excellent study, cited earlier, by Kahn et al. (1993) highlighting battered women's elevations on Scale F. There have been malingering studies with the Rorschach, but unfortunately they have been methodologically flawed. There is no current data to suggest that it would be easy to "fake" the symptoms of trauma on the Rorschach, especially since some of the symptoms of trauma are illustrated in the formal scores, which are obscure to the untrained.

DEFENDING BATTERED WOMEN

Battered woman syndrome is relevant in a variety of ways in criminal matters, both state and federal, and it is relevant in dependency court and family court. The current discussion will focus on criminal matters. The effects of battering are highly relevant when a woman kills her batterer. They are also relevant when she commits a crime because she is afraid of the batterer—crimes such as bank robbery, transporting or selling drugs, or felony child abuse.

When a woman kills her batterer, there are two crucial aspects of battered woman syndrome: fear and the perception that escape is not possible. Fear is a normal response to physical injury and threats of injury. In my research sample of battered women who killed, all of the women had experienced battering at a level of "9" on the Spousal Assault Violent Acts scale (Appendix 3.1). Most had been subjected to violent sex, and most had been threatened with death on a prior occasion or occasions. Many had been previously choked into unconsciousness or threatened with weapons. Many had their parents threatened. Battered women in the NIMH-funded Rocky Mountain study (Walker, 1984) believed that the batterer would or could kill them. Forty-eight percent said they believed he could kill them, and when asked, "If someone had to die during a battering incident, who would it be?", 87% said "me." In Browne's (1987) sample of 42 battered women who killed, the sense of threat for battered women who killed their batterer was enhanced by the frequency of battering incidents, the severity of their injuries, the batterer's threats to kill them or commit suicide, the severity of the man's substance abuse, and his forced sexual acts.

The perception that escape is not possible is usually developed over time and is a direct by-product of the battering and coercive relationship. Dutton (1988) has described batterers' fears of abandonment. Whatever the reason, batterers often say things like "If you leave, I'll find you and hurt/kill you," "Don't think you can hide from me," or "If you leave, I'll find you and make you look so bad, no one will want you." A battered woman *realistically* believes these threats. She knows what kinds of acts her spouse is capable of. There is no question that these relationships can be lethal. Women in California are more likely to be killed by a spouse than a stranger. Leaving the relationship does not diminish the potential lethality. In a Florida study (Bernard, Vera, Vera, & Newman, 1982) of the lethal assaults by men on their wives, 57% of the women had been trying to separate. Battered women also say they stay because of love. They say they continued to hope that their spouse would get help. In these cases, the woman has not faced the true dangerousness of her situation, and this may not become real for her until the immediate time frame of the homicide, when she suddenly feels in imminent danger.

SELF-DEFENSE AND IMPERFECT SELF-DEFENSE

At the time of the killing[10] of a battering husband, many battered women are experiencing overwhelming fear and anticipating imminent harm. The majority of the spousal killings in my Los Angeles research sample occurred in the midst of a battering episode or shortly after a threat to kill the woman—a threat she believed. A *reasonable* person who has been previously assaulted, with injury, will likely feel the threat of great bodily injury of death if that same person again becomes angry, makes threats, or begins physically menacing behavior. A battered woman has become hypervigilant to the cues of her spouse's impending violent assault. Because of her past relationship with the batterer, she knows his pattern, as well as the unique circumstances of the incident at hand. For example, a woman who had been trying to separate from her violent husband was kidnapped and held prisoner in their apartment, where she was raped repeatedly at gunpoint. Her husband began to talk about dying "the way Romeo and Juliet died." She became convinced that he was going to kill her and commit suicide because of this statement and because he did not use a condom during sex, abandoning his previous concern about having children. Other women describe "a look in his eye" or a new sense of desperation in the batterer's mood.

In California, where I see the majority of cases, the level of education about the effects of battering has been good enough, at least in the major urban centers, that district attorneys may not file cases where self-defense is obvious, that is, where the batterer was clearly in the midst of an assault, was shot or stabbed in a face-to-face position (rather than in the side or back), or where the woman has injuries (from strangling or battering). More complicated cases where the threat or its imminence is not as clear will probably be filed, for example, where the battered woman kills the batterer while he is sleeping, where the wounds are to the batterer's back, where the body is defaced, or where the woman goes to lengths to hide the killing. Expert testimony is usually required to show how the batterer's patterns of violence led the battered woman to perceive imminent threat and how she *reasonably perceived* the killing to be necessary to protect herself from imminent injury or death. Expert testimony would also help explain unusual acts, for example, when a badly sexually abused woman who killed in the midst of a battering and sexual assault cuts off the genitals of the corpse. For self-defense in California, the woman's belief must be *honest and reasonable*. This is usually taken to mean "objectively reasonable," that is, anyone would have found the threat to be imminent. If the woman's belief is *honest* but subjective, there is support for what California terms "imperfect" self-defense, which can reduce the crime to voluntary manslaughter. Hempel (see Chapter 4, this volume) reviews the relevant legal standards in other states.

Sometimes the level of fear is so great that the battered woman enters a dissociative state. "Dissociation" often comes during periods of intense anxiety or physical pain, usually in individuals with a history of severe trauma with terror or great physical pain. Dissociation involves an altered state of consciousness, a split between the normally integrated mental functions. It is a mental state where thought, emotion, and behavior are "split off" from conscious awareness. This is explained in different ways by different people—for example, as an "out of body" experience, feeling like one is watching a movie, seeing oneself injured but feeling no pain, or having no memory for the terrifying event. Dissociation is seen in the more extreme cases of battering and sexual abuse. New research on brain functioning during high levels of fear ("Fear," 2003) provides a biological model that explains the phenomenon of dissociation. Dissociation can be simple and brief (i.e., for moments), or it can be prolonged and include complex behaviors that are outside of conscious control. If there is clinical evidence that a battered woman was in a dissociative state, other legal defenses may apply.

California has the defense of "unconsciousness," and the jury instructions state: "This rule applies to persons who are not conscious of acting but who perform acts while asleep or while suffering from a delirium of fever, or because of an attack of epilepsy, a blow on the head, the involuntary taking of drugs, or the involuntary consumption of liquor, or any similar cause. Unconsciousness does not require that a person be incapable of movement." Diagnosing a dissociative state requires training and experience beyond that usually obtained by a doctoral-level psychologist or by a psychiatrist, that is, it requires specialty training in trauma. Although dissociation is more difficult to explain and defend in court, a successful unconsciousness defense results in complete acquittal.

In states where there is no unconsciousness defense, a dissociative state can also be described as a psychotic state, since dissociative flashbacks cause an individual to *reexperience* or remember, vividly, past incidents, and react honestly but unrealistically to the current situation. In such cases, the woman is usually so overwhelmed with fear (based on her past experiences) that she experiences clearly psychotic thinking. In some cases, the overwhelming stress of battering does cause psychotic symptoms. The word "psychotic" needs to be applied carefully and only in the rare case, since the average battered woman who has a high level of fear is *realistically* perceiving danger. The general procedures for diagnosing psychotic thinking should be used. As noted earlier, psychotic thoughts, when present in battered women, tend to be mood-congruent psychotic thoughts associated with a severe clinical depression (major depressive episode). A "not guilty by reason of insanity"[11] defense is less desirable, since it would typically result in a period of detention at a mental health facility until "sanity" is restored, and because it conveys the message that the battered woman is not reacting like any other person who has been traumatized and is in fear for his or her life. The ultimate defense strategy has to be the best fit for the facts and the laws of the jurisdiction where the case is tried.

OTHER CRIMINAL ACTS

Women involved with batterers may become involved in criminal activity for reasons other than their own; that is, they may not have formed the intent to commit the crime. They may not have been involved in the crime charged if they had not been in a relationship with the batterer and afraid to resist him. These crimes can be as serious as kidnapping or murder. In these cases, the legal defense might be *duress*. "Duress" in California requires that the defendant has a reasonable belief that her life would be in danger if she did not engage in the criminal conduct, and that this danger is imminent. This defense was successfully used in *People v. Yolanda Garcia*, a California Superior Court case in which I served as an expert witness. In this case, an undocumented Hispanic woman began living with a man she met in her family home. One week after she moved in with him, he began to beat her. The beatings were severe and life threatening (beating around the head, causing brain injury, choking, electrocution, etc.), and, in addition, he subjected her to a number of conditions more typically associated with prisoners of war: imprisonment in a small car or locked in a motel room, deprivation of food and sleep, constant threats of death toward her and her family, and discussions about others he had killed. He even forced her to observe his murder of her son and another woman. When he began to kidnap and torture additional victims, she did not resist, nor did she attempt to escape. In fact, to subsequent victims her apparent cooperation with the man caused her to be charged as a co-conspirator to kidnap, rape, and a number of other serious felonies. In presenting the duress defense, it was important to use expert testimony about battered woman syndrome, combined with testimony about the psychological functioning of prisoners of war and torture victims, to explain why (1) she did not escape; (2) why she reasonably perceived her life and the lives of her family to be in danger; and (3) why she believed this threat to be imminent. California has new case law that clarifies that duress is no longer a defense to murder.[12]

Offenses where duress may apply are commonly federal charges, crimes such as income tax evasion, sale of illegal drugs, or bank robbery. What is critical to understanding a battered woman's involvement in even these crimes is the extreme coerciveness of the battering relationship. Simply put, a battered woman is more than likely *afraid* to defy her batterer. She often considers the threat of arrest and conviction *less frightening* than her batterer's threats.

Family courts (also called dependency courts) have also been inclined to charge battered women with Failure to Protect either when the batterer has physically or sexually abused the child, or when domestic violence has occurred in the presence of the child. With all of the published work in psychology, law, and social work journals, it still seems to require an expert to explain why a battered woman may have been *unable* to protect the minor, why she may have been too fearful to interrupt the battering of the child, why she may have been too fearful or overwhelmed to seek medical treatment for the child (or herself), or too fearful to leave the situation.

TESTIFYING FOR THE PROSECUTION

Much of this chapter has focused on uses of testimony to defend battered women. Testimony about battered women can also be used by the prosecution in cases of domestic violence. It is often the case that the prosecutor is the first to come in contact with a battered woman, and therefore it is the prosecutor who is in the best position to intervene in cases of domestic violence when the violence is still in its early stages. Vigorous prosecution of these cases communicates a no-tolerance policy that has the potential to decrease battering before the violence reaches a lethal level.

The clinical descriptions in this chapter of the batterer and the battered woman can be used to educate the jury or the court, to dispel myths about battered women: for example, why a given woman might have returned to her battering husband on previous occasions; why such a competent woman did not take effective steps to protect herself; why a battered woman recanted a statement made earlier to police, and so forth. The prosecution often puts on the stand a generic expert on battered woman syndrome to talk generally about battering and battered woman's syndrome, then the prosecution may ask a series of hypothetical questions to illustrate the common dynamics of domestic violence and the effects of battering. Hypothetical questions must typically be based on the facts of the case, but are designed for testimony from an expert who has not actually evaluated the woman. The testimony is often offered to buttress the testimony of the woman, who may come under scrutiny for having recanted, for a delay in reporting, for being inconsistent in her account, or for any of the other commonly reported problems with testimony from battered women. Many of the questions in Appendix 3.2 can be adapted for this purpose.

EXPERT TESTIMONY

Expert testimony is essential in legal matters involving battered women because many of the findings about battered women defy common sense—for example, why would a woman stay with a man who hurts her? Why would she leave and return? Why would a woman with no criminal history go along with a serious criminal act? Why wouldn't she anticipate that her children might be in danger? Expert testimony is probably best when it is specifically crafted to the language of the jurisdiction and to the facts of the case. Every case has unique aspects that make a canned or textbook approach to questions and testimony inadequate. Long and more generic testimony often leaves a juror confused about how it relates to the jury instructions or awash in all of the details and clinical language. There are essential points to make that depend on the arena. For example, in criminal court, the most fundamental issue is fear. The expert needs to explain how the fear developed, increased over time, and was an expected result of the amount of threat to her safety. When a woman kills her batterer, the expert needs also to be skilled at identifying the various attempts the woman made to leave or change the relationship. The same prosecutor's office that supports the battered woman when the batterer is on trial for spousal assault turns alarmingly adversarial when the battered woman kills her batterer, with questions such as the following: "She could have gone to a shelter, couldn't she?" "She had the ability to work and live independently from the victim, didn't she?" "She left her previous husband who battered her, didn't she?" "She called 911 on the victim previously, didn't she?" A good expert can explain why on *this* day, *given all of her previous experience with the batterer*, she reasonably felt a high level of fear for her safety and did not perceive an escape.

As noted earlier, there will be different issues in family court, or in civil court. Many experts will work primarily to explain battered woman syndrome in courtrooms where batterers are being prosecuted. A list of generic direct examination questions that can be adapted to specific court settings appears in Appendix 3.2.

Expert testimony should establish that the woman is a battered woman, that she clearly has common symptoms that result from battering (effects of battering); that these symptoms may make her seem less credible but they are common effects and she does appear to give a credible account of the violence; that she does not appear to be malingering; and that there is a nexus between the crime (e.g., murder) or the legal issue (e.g, parenting) and the experience of battering.

NOTES

1. This prevalence rate is slightly higher in Canada and Australia and in Japan (Eigenberg, 2001).
2. Walker's (1980) research project listed the following: push, shove, punch, slap, hit, burn, claw, scratch, hit with object, use knife, hurt with motor vehicle, kick, throw bodily, use gun, wrestle, try to drown, strangle. This should not be considered an all-inclusive list.
3. The American Psychiatric Association's *Diagnostic and Statistical Manual of Mental Disorders*, now in a text revision of its fourth edition (DSM-IV-TR).
4. The following states use the term "battered woman syndrome" or "battered spouse syndrome" in statutes: California, Maryland, Missouri, Ohio, South Carolina, and Wyoming. Only the following states make no use of this term in annotation or black-letter law: Alabama, Delaware, Idaho, Maine, Minnesota, Mississippi, Nebraska, Utah, and Vermont.
5. Cluster B disorders include antisocial personality disorder, borderline personality disorder, histrionic personality disorder, and narcissistic personality disorder. These are generally considered to be more pathological, especially in interpersonal relationships.
6. Defined by Roth, Newman, Pelcovitz, van der Kolk, and Mandel (1997) as a group of symptoms that result from chronic exposure to trauma. Symptoms include alterations in the regulation of emotion and impulses, alterations in perceptions of self and others, and alterations in consciousness. They indicate that these individuals hold distorted beliefs about others, they swing between idealizing and devaluing others, they have an inability to trust, and they may be preoccupied with hurting those who have hurt them.
7. "Malingering" is a term that usually refers to simulating or faking a disorder, or exaggerating the severity of a disorder.
8. Battered women also scored higher than controls on the Harris and Lingoes subscales "Social Alienation" and "Self-Alienation." Individuals who elevate on "Social Alienation" feel isolated, misunderstood, unloved, and unhappy. Those who elevate on "Self-Alienation" are unhappy, have difficulty concentrating, and report many feelings of regret and guilt. It is not surprising that these types of items would be endorsed by a

battered woman. MMPI Scale 8 can be analyzed using the Harris and Lingoes scales as well. When this is done, it is clear that there are many items on this scale that measure feelings of profound helplessness (in the language of the MMPI, "lack of ego mastery").

9. Both PTSD and battered woman syndrome are considered phasic disorders. The symptoms are worse during and shortly after the traumatic experiences. A state of being "flooded" with symptoms such as nightmares, flashbacks, fear, and the like alternates with emotional constriction, where there is a considerable conscious and unconscious attempt to "avoid" the memories and feelings associated with traumatic events. These phases are clear from a reading of the "B" and "C" criteria of DSM-IV under PTSD.

10. A killing is not necessarily a "murder." This is a legal conclusion. In California, "murder" is in the first degree (with the requirement of premeditation and deliberation) or the second degree (with the requirement of malice aforethought). If the proof falls short of these standards, the conviction could be for voluntary manslaughter or even involuntary manslaughter. A killing could also be justified, as in self-defense.

11. States vary in their criteria for the insanity defense. California uses the McNaughten standard which is essentially a cognitive test: Was the defendant laboring under such a defect of reason, from disease of the mind, that she did not know the nature and quality of her act, nor that it was wrong? Consider a case where the battered woman had come to believe that her battering husband was part of a conspiracy that included her parents, her minister, and several other family members, who she believed were out to steal her child. These beliefs were a result of her fear that she would lose custody of her child to the batterer, but her overwhelming level of fear had taken these beliefs to a psychotic proportion. She heard voices that told her she must kill her husband to protect her child and she was unable to consider the ultimate wrongfulness of killing her husband.

12. In *People v. Anderson*, 28 Cal.4th 767, 770, 50 P.3d 368, 369-370 (2002), the California Supreme Court said: "We conclude that, as in Blackstone's England, so today in California: fear for one's own life does not justify killing an innocent person. Duress is not a defense to murder. We also conclude that duress cannot reduce murder to manslaughter. Although one may debate whether a killing under duress should be manslaughter rather than murder, if a new form of manslaughter is to be created, the Legislature, not this court, should do it."

REFERENCES

Armstrong, J., & Kaser-Boyd, N. (2003). Projective assessment of trauma. In M. Hilsenroth & D. Segal (Eds.), Objective and projective assessment of personality and psychopathology. In M. Hersen (Ed.-in-Chief), *Comprehensive handbook of psychological assessment* (Vol. 2). New York: Wiley.

Bernard, G. W., Vera, H., Vera, M., & Newman, G. (1982). "Till death do us part": A study of spouse murder. *Bulletin of the American Academy of Psychiatry and Law, 19*(4), 271–280.

Bowker, L. H. (1986). *A guidebook based on the experiences of 1,000 battered wives.* Holmes Beach, FL: Learning Publications.

Browne, A. (1987). *When battered women kill.* New York: Free Press.

Dutton, D. G. (1988). Profiling of wife assaulters: Preliminary evidence for a trimodel analysis. *Violence and Victims, 3*(1), 5–25.

Dutton, D. G. (1995). *The domestic assault of women*. Vancouver: University of British Columbia Press.

Dutton, M. A. (1992). Understanding women's responses to domestic violence: A redefinition of battered woman syndrome. *Hofstra Law Review, 21*(4), 1191–1242.

Dutton, M.A., & Goodman, L. (1994). Posttraumatic stress disorder among battered women: Analysis of legal implications. *Behavioral Sciences and the Law, 12*, 215–234.

Eigenberg, H. M. (2001). *Woman battering in the United States: Till death do us part*. Prospect Heights, IL: Waveland Press.

Fear: The brain plus emotions. (2003, March) *Discover Magazine*, pp. 33–39.

Graham, J. (1990). MMPI-2: *Assessing personality and psychopathology*. New York: Oxford University Press.

Hamberger, K. L., & Hastings, K. E. (1991). Personality correlates of men who batter and non-violent men: Some continuities and discontinuities. *Journal of Family Violence, 6*(2), 131–147.

Herman, J. L. (1992). Complex post traumatic stress disorder: A syndrome in survivors of prolonged and repeated trauma. *Journal of Traumatic Stress, 5*(3), 377–389.

Kahn, F. I., Welch, T. L., & Zillmer, E. A. (1993). MMPI-2 profiles of battered women in transition. *Journal of Personality Assessment, 60*(1), 100–111.

Kaser-Boyd, N. (1992). *Faking battered woman syndrome: An MCMI-II study*. Paper presented at the annual meeting of the Society for Personality Assessment, Washington, DC.

Kaser-Boyd, N. (1993). Rorschachs of women who commit homicide. *Journal of Personality Assessment, 60*(3), 458–470.

Levinger, G. (1966). Sources of marital dissatisfaction among applicants for divorce. *American Journal of Orthopsychiatry, 89*, 804–806.

Levy, B. (1984). *Skills for violence-free relationships*. Santa Monica, CA: Southern California Coalition on Battered Women.

Moore, D. M. (1979). *Battered women*. Beverly Hills, CA: Sage.

National Institute of Justice. (1996). *The validity and use of evidence concerning battering and its effects in criminal trials: Report responding to Section 40507 of the Violence Against Women Act*. Washington, DC: Author.

Rhodes, N. R. (1992). Comparison of MMPI psychopathic deviate scores of battered and non-battered women. *Journal of Family Violence, 7*(4), 297–307.

Rosewater, L. B., & Walker, L. E. A. (Eds.). (1985). *Handbook of feminist therapy: Women's issues in psychotherapy*. New York: Springer.

Roth, S., Newman, E., Pelcovitz, D., van der Kolk, B., & Mandel, F. S. (1997). Complex PTSD in victims exposed to sexual and physical abuse: Results from the DSM-IV field trial for posttraumatic stress disorder. *Journal of Traumatic Stress, 10, 539–555*.

van der Kolk, B. A. (1987). *Psychological trauma*. Washington, DC: American Psychiatric Press.

Walker, L. (1979). *The battered woman*. New York: Harper & Row.

Walker, L. (1984). *The battered woman syndrome*. New York: Springer.

Wilson, J. P., & Walker, A. J. (1990). Toward an MMPI trauma profile. *Journal of Traumatic Stress, 3*(1), 151–168.

APPENDIX 3.1. Spousal Assault Violent Acts Scale

Name: _____ Date: _____

Time period of ratings (e.g, 10 years, all of relationship, etc.): _____

Are you still in the relationship? _____

Please underline the specific behavior of your spouse. After your underline, write in a number to indicate how many times you think this happened. This information will serve as a basis for your interview.

Severity rating	Type of abuse
0	None
1	Put-downs/insults (e.g., called "stupid," "can't do anything right.") Blaming/accusations (e.g., "You caused me to _____.")
2	Called cruel names ("bitch," "whore," etc.) Sexual and physical put-downs (e.g., "You're a fat pig.") Withdrawal (giving you the "silent treatment," sleeping elsewhere)
3	Pushed, shoved, physically restrained Accusations of infidelity Monitoring your activities Destroyed objects
4	Slapped Controlled conception Inspected body for signs of infidelity Disrupted your work or school
5	Punched, kicked Kept you from sleeping Threatened to leave you
6	Beat you (defined as multiple hits, punches, kicks) but you did not think you needed hospitalization Coercive sex (made you perform sex acts that you didn't want to) Threatened your pet
7	Battered your children Threatened to take your children from you Threatened to have you declared "mentally ill"
8	Beat you and you required hospitalization (even if you didn't go) Threatened you with a gun, knife, or other lethal weapon Sexually molested your child/children Stalked you
9	Burned you, cut you, or attempted to drown you Choked you Raped you (violent sexual assault, with or without an object) Made verbal threats to kill you or a loved one
10	Shot you Strangled you to unconsciousness Attempted to kill you (may include acts under "9" but includes your perception that you were going to die)

APPENDIX 3.2. Sample Direct Examination Questions

Foundation:

1. What is your current occupation?

2. What formal education, training, and experience do you have that qualifies you to be a clinical psychologist?

3. You are also a forensic psychologist? What does that mean?

4. Do you have any specialty within the field of clinical psychology?

5. How long have you had your doctorate?

6. How many years have you been working in the field of domestic violence?

7. Have you had an opportunity to speak to many people who have been abused by their spouses?

8. About how many people would you say you have come into contact with who have been battered by spouses or partners?

9. You are a general clinical psychologist, is that correct? Does that mean that you see people with all types of psychological disorders? Schizophrenia? Depression? Organic brain syndromes? Substance abuse disorders? You also see children? Give us an idea of how many children you have seen in the 20 years of your professional career.

10. Do you give training to other professionals?

11. What kind of training have you given?

12. On what kind of issues or topics do you train?

13. You have lectured and written about battered woman syndrome. Is that a syndrome that generally describes the common effects of living in a battering relationship?

14. Are the phrase "battered woman syndrome" and the phrase "effects of battering" referring to more or less the same thing?

15. You also mentioned posttraumatic stress disorder. What is that? Is that the same thing as battered woman syndrome?

16. Have you written or lectured on posttraumatic stress disorder?

17. How do you come across patients with posttraumatic stress disorder? How many have you evaluated or seen clinically?

18. What is malingering?

19. Have you written or lectured on malingering?

20. How many conferences or presentations have you given on battered woman syndrome or the effects of battering? To whom are those given?

21. How many conferences or presentations have you given on posttraumatic stress disorder? To whom are those given?

22. And have you given presentations on malingering as well?

23. You teach at (name of university), is that correct? What have you taught and what do you teach?

24. Do you have an academic appointment?

25. Have you taught at other academic institutions?

26. Do you conduct research?

27. Do you also keep up on research being developed and that has been developed in this area?

28. Have you testified in court as an expert on previous occasions?

29. How many times have you testified before today regarding the effects of battering or battered woman syndrome? How many times have you testified about posttraumatic stress disorder?

30. What kind of courts have you testified in?

31. Have you testified for both prosecution and defense?

32. Now I want to clarify some things that you've said: battered woman syndrome is the same as or different than posttraumatic stress disorder?

33. How does a person get posttraumatic stress disorder?

34. What does a patient have to exhibit in order to get this diagnosis?

35. Would an adult woman who's been raped have these same symptoms?

36. How about a soldier who served in Desert Storm and saw combat?

37. How about a victim of a strong-arm robbery?

38. Are the symptoms of posttraumatic stress disorder constant over time? I mean, are they the same right after a traumatic incident as they are 1 year later? Do people recover?

39. What are flashbacks?

40. What is an altered state of consciousness?

41. What is dissociation? What is a dissociative episode?

42. So, battered women can also have posttraumatic stress disorder?

43. How does a woman get battered woman syndrome?

44. What is battering?

45. Is forced sex considered battering?

46. Does "battering" exist on a spectrum of violence?

47. Are symptoms worse if the degree of violence suffered is worse?

48. Does every woman who is battered get battered woman syndrome?

49. What clinical effects does battering cause?

50. Are there other characteristics of women with battered woman syndrome?

51. Do battered women receive other mental health diagnoses when seen by mental health professionals?

52. In violent marriages, is the violence constant?

53. What types of things typically provoke a battering?

54. What kinds of injuries are common among battered women?

55. Are there typical personality traits of a batterer?

56. What are they?

57. Is it the case that women are sometimes battered while pregnant? Is this common?

58. Are batterers often jealous?

59. Does alcohol or drug use play a role in battering?

60. Are there usually witnesses to the battering?

61. Is it typical for a woman to be battered and injured and not seek medical attention?

62. Is it reasonable to expect there will be police reports for every battering?

63. You said that a woman who has experienced serious violence will typically develop posttraumatic stress disorder. Does this mean that she will have flashbacks?

64. In order to be called a flashback, does she have to feel that she is actually back in the previous violent situation?

65. Is it common for battered women to experience dissociative episodes?

66. Does a battered woman always act helpless?

67. I want to turn now to the area of psychological tests. Why do psychologists use psychological tests to assess individuals?

68. Are psychological tests commonly used in forensic evaluations? Why?

69. I want to take each of the tests you administered or relied on and have you describe what it is and what kind of data you get from it.

70. Is it possible to fake battered woman syndrome or posttraumatic stress disorder?

Questions Regarding the Client

1. Were you asked to conduct an assessment of _____?

2. Did you conduct an evaluation of her?

3. And what did you do to accomplish that?

4. Do you speak Spanish?

5. When you communicated with _____, did you use an interpreter?

6. What have you reviewed in the form of discovery that has been presented to the defense in this case?

7. How long did you personally spend with _____?

8. What was the purpose of the tests that you administered?

9. Did you review the content of the interview with the defendant by Officer _____?

10. Were you able to arrive at an opinion as to whether _____ has any psychological problems?

11. What is your opinion?

12. You found that she had posttraumatic stress disorder? What was that from?

13. You also found her to exhibit many of the effects of spousal battering? You opined that she had battered woman syndrome? What life experiences with her husband, in your opinion, caused her to get battered woman syndrome? What symptoms did she display?

14. Did you reach the opinion that _____ was afraid of her husband throughout the course of the marriage?

15. Did _____ discuss with you the false accusations that her husband would make against her regarding fidelity to him?

16. Is this a common theme in the disorder?

17. Could she have left her husband?

18. Why didn't she leave?

19. Of the types of abuse present in this marriage, which type or types were the most debilitating or damaging to her?

20. Why would sexual abuse be the most debilitating?

21. If she finished college during her marriage to her husband, does this mean that she wasn't helpless?

22. If she confronted some of her husband's other women, does this mean that she didn't feel helpless?

23. Would the cruel names—bitch, whore, slut—be more or less abusive for a Mexican woman like _____?

24. Is it consistent with battered woman syndrome that she would have periods of time in her relationship with her husband when things were good or when she was not being battered?

25. Where does she fit on the scale of severity of abuse?

26. If she suffered battering at the extreme ends of the spectrum, does this mean that her symptoms are at the extreme end of the spectrum?

27. Do you have the ability to describe the condition(s) from which she suffered at the time of the killing?

28. What was that?

29. What was her psychological condition after the killing? Why did she hide and then deface the body?

30. I'd like to turn now to the psychological tests. What do they add to your understanding of her psychological state?

31. What is the prognosis for someone such as her if she does receive treatment?

32. Do you consider that, or do any of your tests indicate that, she is a violent person?

33. If a woman is suffering from the prolonged effects of battering and the batterer is no longer alive, does she still suffer from the condition?

34. Do you consider there to be any chance at all of a repeat of this killing?

Note. These questions are adapted from a case with early sexual trauma and spousal violence. They can be further adapted to address the particular issues in a battered woman's case.

4 Battered Women Who Strike Back

Using Expert Testimony on Battering and Its Effects in Homicide Trials

CARRIE L. HEMPEL

By the time Jodie was convicted for the murder of her batterer in 1987, she had suffered a lifetime of abuse from virtually every important man in her life. The abuse began with her father and ended with her trial attorney. Her father repeatedly sexually assaulted her beginning at age 9, and raped her at 12. During her teenage years, he beat her. When she was a young adult, he fired a gun in her direction several times. One night he fired blanks directly at her, and she moved out.

Not long after moving out of her father's house, Jodie entered her first physically abusive romantic relationship. She married a man who battered her. The relationship ended when her husband was sentenced to prison. She then became romantically involved in another abusive relationship that lasted about a year. During this second relationship, she began to use alcohol. When she finally checked herself into a recovery program for her alcoholism approximately 10 years later, her substance abuse counselor asked her on a date as soon as she moved back home. He moved in with her a month or so later. She ended this relationship when he sexually abused both her and her two children.

When Jodie met Mark, however, he initially seemed different than these men. She thought she had finally found her "knight in shining armor." He was quiet, polite, and respected her sobriety. He was protective of her, and much bigger physically, 6 inches taller and 60 pounds heavier.

Six months after their first date, they began living together. Soon after, his protectiveness turned to irrational jealousy. He told Jodie she was fat, ugly, and a tramp. He encouraged her to drink again, and she did. The first time he physically assaulted her, she suffered a fractured tailbone. Over the course of the next 4 years, his jealousy and violence toward her escalated. He pointed a gun at her and then hit her in the head with it. Another time, he stabbed her in the leg with a buck knife. He burned her with a curling iron, pushed her hand through a window, hit her with a chair, punched her, and held her head under water in a swimming pool. He choked her several times, knowing that because she suffered from asthma, choking was particularly terrifying. Jodie sometimes would fight back, or suggest that they break up. Mark told her that if he could not have her, no one would. He threatened to kill himself if she left him. She once told him that she was raped to avoid a confrontation when she did not arrive home at the time by which he told her to return.

Finally, Jodie found the courage to make plans to leave. The day before he died, Mark found out about them. The next evening, he confronted her outside their home with a shotgun in his hand. He told her that he knew of her plans, talked about killing himself and then about killing her. She ran away from him, but he followed her, pushed her to the ground and choked her, putting his knees on her throat and chest. He then let her get up, pushing the gun at her and telling her to kill him or he would kill her. He came charging toward her and she shot him.

She remained with Mark's body through the night. The next morning, two people found her there. They contacted the police. Initially, Jodie told the police that someone else shot Mark, and then that she shot him by mistake. When homicide detectives arrived, she was talking in an incoherent manner. Eventually, she explained that she shot Mark after he threatened to kill her.

Although her trial attorney knew that evidence of battering and its effects had been used successfully in other homicide trials, he had never used such evidence and chose not to investigate the potential use of it to support Jodie's self-defense claim. He would not even discuss her history of abuse by Mark or others, but asked her to describe in detail her sexual practices with Mark. At trial, he described Jodie as "pond scum" in a conversation with the judge and prosecutor. He thoroughly misunderstood his client, adopting many negative stereotypes that an understanding of battering and its effects would have dispelled.

Moreover, the prosecution also effectively employed many of these same stereotypes in its case against Jodie. Police witnesses testified that

Jodie had initially given incorrect and incoherent versions of the shooting. One witness testified that the violence in the relationship appeared to be mutual combat. In his closing argument, the prosecutor argued that the facts that Jodie did not leave the relationship and testified that she loved Mark indicated that she had not been battered. He also damaged her overall credibility by portraying Jody as a habitual liar, because of her false initial statements to the police and her claim of being raped. The prosecutor characterized her as the aggressor in the relationship because she was a drug user and fought back. The jury convicted Jodie of second-degree murder.

Fortunately, in California today battered women such as Jodie, who killed a batterer prior to 1992 and did not have expert testimony on battering and its effects introduced at trial, have a statutory right to have their conviction overturned and be granted a new trial.[1] In any state today, a battered woman who kills her abuser in a confrontational situation such as Jodie's should be permitted to present such expert testimony to support a self-defense claim. This information is presented to the trier of fact through the testimony of an expert witness, usually a mental health professional with specialized knowledge on the effects of battering. Kaser-Boyd (Chapter 3, this volume) sets forth the various psychological effects that may result from being battered, and the ways in which a battering experience may shape the perceptions of a woman who kills her abuser. This chapter discusses the current legal standards for the presentation of expert testimony on battering and its effects in a homicide trial, to assist a battered woman in presenting a claim of self-defense.

The first section of the chapter presents statistical information about the incidence of battering in the United States, to give the reader a better understanding of the magnitude of the problem of abuse by intimate partners, including the number of women killed by an abuser. The section discusses the lack of available resources to assist victims of abuse, one of the many reasons why a battered woman may not leave a battering relationship. Also presented are statistics on the number of women who kill an intimate partner, demonstrating that it is overwhelmingly women who are the victims when a death occurs. The section concludes by noting that most women who kill their abusers do so in confrontational settings. In such situations, the use of expert testimony on battering and its effects has been particularly helpful.

The second section of this chapter discusses how expert evidence on battering and its effects is used in a criminal trial to assist an intimate violence victim in proving that she killed her batterer in self-defense. The section first corrects two common misconceptions about the use of such expert testimony: that all such testimony concerns a static condition known as "battered woman syndrome," and that the testimony is used to support a special, freestanding "battered woman defense," rather than as additional evidence to support a self-defense claim. This portion of the chapter also sets out the usual elements of the defense of self-defense, and explains what a judge will first require a defendant to demonstrate in order to obtain a ruling that battering evidence may be introduced at trial. The remainder of the section discusses the various ways in which expert testimony on battering and its effects is used to strengthen a defense of self-defense, and for what purposes such evidence may be admitted. The discussion includes illustrations of how expert testimony would have helped support the self-defense claim in Jodie's criminal trial (the case example provided earlier). It should be kept in mind, however, that jurisdictions vary as to what a defendant must first show in order for the court to permit the introduction of such testimony, and as to the permissible scope and relevancy of the testimony. This section relies extensively on Parrish's (1996) comprehensive 50 state and federal court survey on the uses of expert testimony on battering and its effects. Parrish's article built upon Maguigan's earlier seminal work on this topic (Maguigan, 1991).

Finally, this chapter concludes by suggesting that courts should, in appropriate cases, generally allow battered women to introduce evidence of battering and its effects to support another traditionally recognized defense to a murder charge, known as a "heat of passion" or "provocation" defense. Traditionally, male criminal defendants have successfully used a provocation defense in situations where they killed another male during a physical fight, or killed their wife or her paramour after discovering her in the act of adultery. Criminal law has deemed it reasonable that a man could lose self-control in such situations, and thus has determined that he should be punished less harshly than those who kill without such passion. This chapter argues that it seems equally, if not more, reasonable that a woman who has been battered could lose her self-control and strike back, killing her batterer. Expert testimony on the effects of battering could help convince a jury that such loss of self-control occurred and was reasonable given the circumstances.

INTIMATE VIOLENCE IN THE UNITED STATES AND THE LACK OF RESOURCES AVAILABLE TO VICTIMS

Violence between intimate partners is a very serious problem in the United States, and women are overwhelmingly the victims of such violence. The exact magnitude of the problem is difficult for researchers to determine, however, because of the widely accepted belief that the incidence of such abuse is seriously underreported (Mahoney, Williams, & West, 2001). Nonetheless, several studies have concluded that at least

1.3 million women are severely beaten by their intimate partners each year in the United States, and about one-quarter of all women in this country will experience intimate violence at some time in their lives (Mahoney et al., 2001). In far too many instances, the violence ultimately becomes lethal.

Statistics on the percentage of female victims killed by an intimate partner vary greatly, at least in part due to a lack of police documentation as to the nature of the relationship between the victim and the perpetrator. One review of available statistics indicated that 30 to 64% of such homicides were the culmination of a pattern of intimate violence (Mahoney et al., 2001). In the United States in 2000, at least 1,247 women were killed by an intimate partner, according to a Department of Justice survey (*www.ojp.usdoj.gov/bjs/abstract/ipv01.htm*).[2]

Society does not provide adequate community-based resources to help women who have experienced intimate violence. Prior to 1976, community services for battered women were practically nonexistent. The first services developed out of the feminist movement of the 1970s, when community activists and formerly battered women began organizing to define and address the problem that came to be called domestic violence. Over the past 28 years, the battered women's shelter movement has been somewhat successful in educating the public and increasing the services available to victims of intimate violence. Nevertheless, although the number of assistance programs for battered women has increased dramatically since the first shelters were opened, shelter care is still available for only a small percentage of those who seek this assistance, and for a relatively short period of time. The National Coalition Against Domestic Violence estimates that shelter space currently is available for only one in four women who seek it (Sullivan & Gillum, 2001).

The lack of adequate legal protection for women who are suffering from violence at the hands of an intimate partner compounds the problem. In most jurisdictions today a victim of intimate violence has two options: to seek a civil restraining or protective order, or report the violence to criminal justice officials in the hope that the perpetrator will be prosecuted. Neither option results in protection from further violence in the majority of cases.

Civil restraining orders, on their face, prohibit the abuser from having further contact with his victim. Every state and the District of Colombia now provide for the issuance of civil restraining orders. Nonetheless, most restraining orders are violated. In one recent nationwide survey, more than two-thirds of the restraining orders obtained by women against intimates who raped or stalked them were violated, and approximately one-half of the orders obtained by women against intimates who physically assaulted them were violated (Tjaden & Thoennes, 2000). A study of women in Massachusetts who obtained restraining orders produced similar results (Klein, 1996). Whether or not civil restraining orders are deterring some re-abuse, such orders are not sufficiently effective at protecting the women who obtain them.

Likewise, the few studies conducted thus far with respect to the effect of criminal prosecutions consistently conclude that there is no reliable evidence that prosecution makes a difference in the recidivism rate in intimate violence cases (Iovanni & Miller, 2001).

In sum, because community services for the majority of victims of intimate violence are not available and the legal avenues created to protect such women are still substantially ineffective at preventing re-abuse, it is understandable that some battered women eventually resort to using violence to defend themselves. In their efforts to stop the abuse, some of these women kill their batterers. Despite perceptions to the contrary, according to a seminal study on the subject, as many as 90% of battered women who kill their batterers do so when faced with either an ongoing attack or an imminent threat of death or serious bodily injury (Maguigan, 1991, 2000).

THE USE OF EXPERT TESTIMONY ON THE EFFECTS OF BATTERING TO ASSIST A CLAIM OF SELF-DEFENSE

A battered woman who kills her abuser in response to the batterer's violent behavior toward her or other family members may be charged with a homicide offense of murder or voluntary manslaughter. If the woman can meet certain preliminary requirements, her trial judge may admit expert evidence that she was battered by the deceased, and that as a result of the battering experience she had different perceptions of and reactions to her interactions with him. This evidence is admitted to support her defense to the criminal charge, generally the traditionally recognized defense of self-defense. Such expert testimony on battering and its effects is now admissible to support a self-defense claim, at least to some degree, in every state and the District of Colombia (Parrish, 1996).[3] Before discussing in detail how such evidence may provide support to a battered woman's claim of self-defense, however, it is important to point out two popular, but inaccurate, beliefs about the uses of this testimony.

Misconceptions about Expert Testimony on Battering and Its Effects

Two commonly held misconceptions about the use of expert testimony on battering and its effects are that (1) all such testimony concerns a condition properly referred to as "battered woman syndrome," and (2) the testimony is used to support a special or freestanding defense to criminal behavior, or a "battered woman's defense" (Dutton, 1996; Parrish, 1996).

Although it is true that many mental health professionals, lawyers, and judges initially used the phrase "battered woman syndrome" when discussing the admission of expert evidence on battering and its effects, the use of the term has increasingly become disfavored, particularly among legal scholars and some experts (Dutton, 1996; Maguigan, 1998; Parrish, 1996). A significant number of state legislatures, however, have incorporated this term into statutes that address the use of expert testimony on the effects of battering at trial. Acknowledging this reality, some courts, such as the California Supreme Court, have continued to use the phrase "battered woman syndrome" in their written opinions, while recognizing that its continued use is disfavored for the following reasons.[4]

Legal scholars and mental health experts on battering who recommend that the use of the phrase "battered woman syndrome" be discontinued do so for several reasons. First, the word "syndrome" carries implications of pathology or disease, or that the person to whom the term is applied necessarily suffers from some mental illness or defect as a result of the battering. The phrase also suggests to some that the defendant is entitled to use this kind of evidence because she had a disease or defect that predisposed her to being in a battering relationship. In many if not most cases, these assumptions are not accurate. The phrase "battered woman syndrome" also has been criticized for failing to adequately convey the breadth or nature of the scientific knowledge available about battering and its effects, and suggests a single pattern of response to battering. As is discussed in detail by Kaser-Boyd (Chapter 3, this volume), the effects of battering experiences vary widely.

For the preceding reasons, legal scholars, mental health experts, and attorneys who represent battered women generally should use the phrase "expert testimony on battering and its effects" rather than "battered woman syndrome" testimony because the former language more accurately conveys the nature and breadth of such evidence and is less likely to convey a narrow concept of who is entitled to the benefit of the testimony. At the same time, if the term "battered woman syndrome" is currently incorporated into a particular jurisdiction's statutes and/or published case law, it is important for attorneys and experts to be mindful of this reality and discuss the evolution of the language used when doing so will assist the understanding of the jurors or judges making decisions in a given case.

Although some legal professionals have referred to the use of a "battered woman defense" as a special or freestanding defense to a homicide, this characterization also is incorrect. As stated earlier, evidence on battering and its effects has been admitted at trial primarily because it is deemed to be relevant to a self-defense claim, and no state has recognized a "battered woman defense" (Dutton, 1996; Maguigan, 2000; Parrish, 1996).

Definition of Self-Defense

Although each state has its own statutes that define the elements of all crimes and defenses, most modern statutory schemes use the same general criteria to determine when a person who has killed another has done so under conditions that the law recognizes as a justified use of force in self-defense. Generally, a defendant must prove that she *honestly* and *reasonably* believed that (1) she was in imminent or immediate danger of unlawful bodily harm; (2) her use of force was necessary to save her life or prevent serious bodily injury; and (3) the force used was not excessive in relation to the threatened force. She must also demonstrate that she did not initiate the violence in the encounter (LaFave, 2003). If the defendant is able to demonstrate all of these elements, she will have established a *perfect* self-defense claim and will be found innocent of any crime as the result of killing another. If the defendant is able to prove only that she *honestly* (but not reasonably) believed that (1) she was in imminent or immediate danger of unlawful bodily harm, and (2) her use of force was necessary to save her life or prevent serious bodily injury, she will have established what is known in the law as an *imperfect*, or *partial* self-defense claim. Her actions will be *partially* excused under criminal law, and as a result, she will be found guilty of the less serious crime of voluntary manslaughter (LaFave, 2003).

State statutes typically have the same general definition of self-defense, but differ somewhat in how they interpret various terms in this definition. These differences are important to battered women because they may determine whether a defendant is able to use expert testimony on battering and its effects, and the extent to which such testimony may be used. It is beyond the scope of this chapter to provide a comprehensive survey of these differences. Rather, the following paragraphs provide an overview of the nature of the differences that do exist, and how such differences may impact the use of expert testimony in a given jurisdiction.

First, states differ with respect to which, if any, particular characteristics of the defendant may be considered in addressing the reasonableness of the belief in the need for the force used. Traditionally, the standard of reasonableness was defined in terms of the supposedly objective "reasonable man" or "reasonable person." The trier of fact, usually a jury, was not instructed to take into account any consideration of the particular characteristics of the defendant. Today, however, most jurisdictions permit a jury to consider the physical characteristics of the defendant, such as her age, sex, physical disabilities, or physical size relative to the defendant. Many states, such as California, permit the jury to consider whether a defendant's actions were reasonable from the point of view of a reasonable person "in a similar situation and with similar knowledge as the defendant."[5] A few states have even endorsed a special standard of reasonableness when the defendant is a battered woman.[6] The use of expert testimony on battering and its effects will be more helpful to a defendant in a case in which a jury is permitted to consider the particular situation of, and information known to, the defendant than in one in which the jury is not.

States also differ in the way they define the requirement of the temporal proximity of the danger facing the defendant (Maguigan, 2000). Most statutes require that the impending harm be "imminent," which suggests that it be during an ongoing confrontation, although some statutes use language that suggests a greater period of time, such as that the defensive force must be against an unlawful attack "on the present occasion," or that the defendant must believe she is "about to be injured" (LaFave, 2003). Other statutes state that the force must be "immediately necessary" (LaFave, 2003). Regardless of the language used, however, most states have interpreted the requirement to be broader than the particular instant of the defendant's action and to include its context—the circumstances surrounding the action, including past events (Maguigan, 1991, 2000). Significantly, more than 10 states have allowed the use of testimony on the effects of battering to support a self-defense claim in nonconfrontational settings, such as while the batterer is sleeping.[7] Such rulings suggest a much broader interpretation of the definition of imminent harm than that the force was immediately necessary.

With respect to the amount of force that may be used to meet the threatened harm, no jurisdiction has a per se rule prohibiting the use of a weapon against an unarmed attacker. The proportionality of the force is measured on a case-by-case basis, taking into consideration the relative sizes, ages, and physical conditions of the decedent and the defendant, as well as the history of violence between them (Maguigan, 1991, 2000).

A small number of states generally require a person to retreat before using deadly force if she can do so with safety (LaFave, 2003).[8] Of the states with this requirement, some do not require a person to retreat if she is in her place of work or residence, unless the aggressor also works or lives in the same place.[9]

With these self-defense concepts in mind, we can look at how an expert on battering and its effects may be crucial to the investigation and preparation of a defense of self-defense, and an effective presentation of the defense at trial.

The Use of an Expert Prior to Trial: Investigation and Preparation of a Case

As the outcome of Jodie's trial demonstrates, early consultation with an expert on battering and its effects may be essential to the success of a battered woman's self-defense claim. A defense lawyer who obtains the assistance of an expert on battering and its effects immediately after learning of the deceased's abuse of her client will hopefully avoid making the highly prejudicial mistakes made by Jodie's lawyer. Immediate employment of the expert may help the lawyer develop an awareness of the extent to which he or she shares common misconceptions about battered women, and the risk that those misconceptions will taint early analysis of the case (Maguigan, 2000). A person who has been battered and who has just killed an intimate partner may suffer from symptoms of post-traumatic stress disorder such as memory lapse, and/or may distrust men, attorneys, or any person in a position of authority as a result of her prior experiences with the batterer, police, or others who were unable or unwilling to assist the defendant in her efforts to stop the abuse. An expert can help the attorney to recognize such a lack of trust, and to determine what steps to take to overcome this barrier to effective communication. In this respect, the expert can assist the attorney by suggesting appropriate interviewing techniques and topics for inquiry in the initial and subsequent interviews with the defendant (Maguigan, 2000).

An expert also may be helpful to the attorney in determining how to approach and interview witnesses to the abuse. Such witnesses may be crucial to the outcome of the case.

In certain instances, and if resources permit, the use of two experts on battering and its effects may be desirable. One expert then could be retained to assist with the investigation and preparation of the defense strategy, and another could be retained to testify at trial. An advantage of using two experts is that an attorney may provide the investigation expert with more complete information about the case, without having to be concerned with the possibility of introducing any information that could be harmful or prejudicial to the client at the trial.

Threshold for Admission of Expert Testimony on Battering and Its Effects

Amount of Evidence That Must Be Introduced before a Judge Will Admit Expert Testimony

States vary in the standards that they require a judge to use to determine whether expert testimony on battering and its effects will be admitted in a particular case. Generally, a defendant must, at minimum, tell the judge that she is going to present a self-defense claim before the evidence will be admitted (Parrish, 1996).[10] Other states require the defendant to present what is termed a *prima facie* case of self-defense, or enough evidence to establish the defense if her evidence were uncontested by the prosecution, before expert testimony can be introduced (Parrish, 1996).[11] Additionally, some states require some evidence that "battered woman syndrome" is accepted in the scientific community (Parrish, 1996).[12] Other states have specifically ruled that no such general acceptance evidence need be presented, concluding that it is beyond question that the existence of battered woman syndrome is commonly accepted in the scientific community.[13] Finally, some states require that the defendant present sufficient evidence to demonstrate that she is a battered woman before expert testimony on battering and its effects may be introduced (Parrish, 1996).[14] Once the threshold requirements of the state have been met, the defendant's lawyer must then establish that the chosen expert is qualified to testify on battering and its effects.

Establishing Qualifications of Expert to Testify

The establishment of the qualifications of a proposed expert is a procedure whereby the defense attorney, by questioning the expert on the stand, establishes that the proposed witness has a special expertise in the area about which he or she intends to testify. In many instances, the question of qualification is resolved prior to trial through the defense and prosecution attorneys stipulating that a proposed witness or witnesses are qualified.

Scope of Expert Testimony

Once a witness has been qualified, the extent of his or her testimony also depends on the state in which he or she is testifying. Significant consensus exists among states as to the issues on which expert testimony on battering and its effects is admissible, although differences do exist (Parrish, 1996). The various matters to which an expert is permitted to testify are outlined in the next section.

General Testimony about the Effects of Battering

Most states permit the introduction of general testimony on battering and its effects without reference to the specific defendant (Parrish, 1996; Maguigan, 2000). At least two-thirds of states permit an expert, in his or her initial testimony to the jury, to address the question of why a battered woman might not leave a battering relationship (Maguigan, 2000; Parrish, 1996).[15] One-third of states have explicitly noted that such testimony is admissible to rebut common myths and misconceptions about battered women (Parrish, 1996).[16] Such testimony might include the following information, depending on its relevance to the particular case:

- That many battered women were victims of abuse in childhood.
- That battered women often self-medicate with alcohol or drugs in an attempt to lessen their suffering.
- That a common reaction to severe trauma is memory loss, particularly surrounding an event such as the death of the abuser.
- That battered women may develop assaultive behaviors as defense mechanisms.
- That a battered woman may lie to the batterer and others protect herself from further abuse at the hands of her abuser.
- Why a battered woman may not seek medical care for injuries inflicted by a batterer.
- Why she may have inappropriate boundaries in personal relationships.
- Why she may lie about the existence of the abuse, or fail to reveal it to others.
- Why she may not immediately report the true facts about the killing of her batterer to authorities.
- Why she may still love the batterer in spite of the abuse.
- Why she may be unable to leave the relationship.
- Why, at the time of an offense, a battered woman may have the perception that escape is not possible.

The admission of such general testimony may greatly enhance the credibility of the defendant in the eyes of jurors, who might otherwise find her testimony about the relationship and circumstances surrounding the killing unbelievable. Additionally, such general testimony may have a rehabilitative effect on a prosecutor's specific efforts to undermine the defendant's credibility. Prosecutors often rely, in their cross-examination of a defendant, and in their closing arguments, on common myths and misconceptions about battered women. These include myths such as that a truly battered woman would have left the relationship, would never fight back, and would not still love her abuser. They include the possible misconception that a battered woman's stated inability to recall the details or even occurrence of certain events is actually dishonesty, rather than memory loss due to the trauma of the events. General testimony on the effects of battering can counteract such efforts on the part of the prosecution, by providing the jury with an alternative explanation for a battered woman's perceptions and behavior.

For example, in Jodie's case, general testimony about the facts of battering would have helped the jury to understand the reasons for many of her actions toward the defendant and others. It would have provided an explanation as to why she continued to live with the deceased after repeated incidents of abuse, and maintain that she loved him even at the time of his death. It would have given the jury an explanation as to why she used alcohol and drugs during much of her relationship with the batterer, did not obtain medical assistance when Mark stabbed her in the leg and inflicted other serious injuries, and lied to Mark and others about being raped. An expert's testimony that battered women sometimes fight back in response to attacks would have assisted the jury in determining whether the battering incidents should be viewed as "mutual combat." Testimony about the potential for memory loss as a result of the trauma of killing a batterer would have assisted a jury in evaluating Jodie's behavior after killing her batterer, when she initially lied to the police. Finally, general testimony about how the cumulative effects of battering impact a battered woman's perception of the imminence of the harm would have assisted the jury in evaluating Jodie's testimony that she was in fear of her life at the time she shot her batterer.

The Veracity of the Defendant's Claim That She Suffers from the Effects of Battering

Most states also allow the introduction of expert testimony to prove that the defendant is a battered woman or that she suffered from "battered woman syndrome" at the time of the offense (Parrish, 1996).[17] Prior to trial, the expert would interview the defendant about her relationship with the deceased, and with respect to other prior relationships in which she may have been abused. The expert would also review any other available evidence of battering, such as statements of witnesses to the abuse, police reports, and/or health records of the defendant and the deceased.[18] The expert would then be qualified to testify as to his or her opinion of whether the defendant was abused by the deceased.

In Jodie's case, an expert's opinion that she was in fact suffering from the effects of battering at the time of the offense would have added credibility to her testimony that she was battered by the decedent. It would also have supported the veracity of her stated reasons for many of her behaviors prior to and at the time of the killing of her batterer.

Testimony as to Whether the Defendant Believed That She Was in Immediate Danger of Death or Serious Bodily Harm at the Time She Killed Her Batterer

Several states explicitly permit an expert on battering and its effects to testify as to his or her opinion of whether the defendant believed that she was in imminent danger of death or serious bodily harm at the time she killed her abuser.[19] This issue is considered an ultimate issue in the case, because if the jury finds the issue to be true, the defendant cannot be convicted of murder (although she can still be convicted of manslaughter if the jury finds that her belief in such danger was unreasonable). Some states do *not* permit expert opinion testimony on ultimate issues of fact in a criminal trial, such as the honesty of the defendant's belief in the need to use deadly force.[20] Because expert witnesses generally have a high degree of credibility with a jury, such evidence would likely enhance the credibility of a defendant's testimony that she feared for her life.

Testimony by an expert that it is her opinion that Jodie was in fear of imminent death or serious bodily harm at the time she shot Mark would have substantially supported her own testimony that she was in fear of imminent bodily harm at that moment. [21]

If a jury, with the benefit of expert testimony, were to find that Jodie honestly believed that she was in imminent danger, she could not be found guilty of murder. She would, at most, be convicted of voluntary manslaughter because she would have met the requirements for an imperfect self-defense claim.[22]

Testimony as to Whether the Defendant's Belief as to the Danger Was Reasonable

A significant minority of states have found that an expert also can give his or her opinion as to whether the defendant's belief in the need to use force was reasonable (Maguigan, 2000; Parrish, 1996).[23] This issue is also an ultimate question in a claim of self-defense. As such, the majority of jurisdictions have determined that the answer to the question of reasonableness is a matter for the jury to determine without an expert opinion directly addressing the issue. Testimony by an expert witness that it was reasonable for Jodie to be in imminent fear of serious bodily harm or death at the time she shot Mark likely would have been helpful to Jodie in persuading the jury to find her belief reasonable.

Statutory Codification of Admissibility of Expert Testimony on Battering and Its Effects

At least 11 states have statutes that specifically provide for the admissibility of expert testimony on battering and its effects.[24] For example, in 1991, California enacted a statute titled "Expert Testimony on Battered Women's Syndrome in Criminal Actions." The law states that "expert testimony is admissible by . . . the defense regarding battered women's syndrome, including the physical, emotional, or mental effects upon the

beliefs, perceptions, or behavior of victims of domestic violence. . . ."
The statute also provides that such evidence shall be admitted if the defendant establishes its relevancy and the proper qualifications of the expert witness, and that "expert opinion testimony shall not be considered
a new scientific technique whose reliability is unproven."[25] Wyoming's
statute, titled "Battered Woman Syndrome" and enacted in 1993, defines battered woman syndrome as "a subset under the diagnosis of
Post-Traumatic Stress Disorder established in the "Diagnostic and Statistical Manual of Mental Disorders III" and states that "if a person is
charged with a crime involving the use of force against another, and the
person raises the affirmative defense of self-defense, the person may introduce expert testimony that the person suffered from the syndrome, to
establish the necessary requisite belief of an imminent danger of death or
great bodily harm as a element of the affirmative defense, to justify the
person's use of force."[26] Such statutes are obviously very helpful to battered women who have been charged with murder and seek to introduce
expert testimony on the effects of battering, because they eliminate any
ambiguity as to the legitimacy of introducing such expert testimony in
an appropriate case.

Use of Expert Testimony Subjects Defendant to Adverse Psychological Examination

Generally, when an expert testifies on behalf of a defendant concerning
the defendant's mental state at the time of the crime, courts permit the
prosecution to call its own expert to testify about the defendant's mental
state. Accordingly, the few states that have addressed this issue have held
that offering expert testimony on battering subjects a defendant to an
adverse psychological examination by the prosecution's expert (Parrish,
1996).[27]

USE OF EXPERT TESTIMONY ON BATTERING AND ITS EFFECTS TO SUPPORT A PROVOCATION DEFENSE

As noted in the earlier section "Intimate Violence in the United States
and the Lack of Resources Available to Victims," a seminal study concluded that most battered women who kill their batterers do so when
faced with an imminent threat of serious physical injury (Maguigan,
1991). In such circumstances, the best defense would usually be that of
self-defense, a claim that the defendant killed as a result of her reasonable belief that she was in imminent danger of death or serious bodily injury. A defendant charged with murder who succeeds in her self-defense

claim is completely absolved of criminal responsibility. In some situations, however, a battered woman may kill her batterer under circumstances in which she will be unable to convince a jury that she had a fear of *imminent* death or serious bodily harm, such as when a battered woman kills her batterer while he is sleeping. In such a situation, a battered woman charged with the murder of her batterer still might be able to successfully prove a provocation defense, or that she killed the batterer as a result of a provocation that would cause a reasonable person to lose normal self-control. A defendant charged with murder who succeeds in a provocation defense would be convicted of manslaughter, a less serious crime than murder. Depending on the circumstances in a given case, an attorney might decide to present both a claim of self-defense and a provocation defense to the jury. As in the context of self-defense, the use of expert testimony on battering and its effects could provide substantial support to a battered woman's defense of adequate provocation.

The remainder of this section sets forth the typical requirements for a provocation defense and the potential value of the use of expert testimony on battering and its effects in support of this defense. Although each state has its own statute that defines the elements of a provocation defense, most modern statutory schemes use the same general criteria to define the defense. Only a few published opinions have mentioned the use of a provocation defense in a case where a battered woman has been charged with murder as result of killing her batterer.[28] Therefore, it is not possible, on the basis of a review of current published case law, to analyze the scope of admissibility of expert testimony on the effects of battering to support a provocation defense. Thus, the following paragraphs discuss the various ways in which such testimony *potentially* could be helpful to a battered woman asserting this defense, depending on the admissibility of the testimony in her jurisdiction.

As is discussed in more detail in the earlier subsection "Threshold for Admission of Expert Testimony on Battering and Its Effects," in the context of a self-defense claim a defendant seeking to introduce expert testimony in support of a provocation defense would first need to satisfy whatever threshold standards exist for the admission of expert testimony in the relevant jurisdiction. Likewise, a defendant would need to establish the qualifications of the particular expert in accordance with the standards of the jurisdiction in which she is being tried.[29]

Definition of a Provocation Defense

A defendant may prove a defense to murder if she can show that her killing was in response to extenuating circumstances that the law defines as reasonable, or "adequate" provocation. The typical elements of a provocation defense are (1) the existence of a reasonable provocation; (2) that the defendant was in fact provoked; (3) that a reasonable person so provoked would not have cooled off in the interval of time between the provocation and the fatal act; and (4) that the defendant did not in fact cool off during that interval (LaFave, 2003). If a defendant can prove that these four circumstances existed at the time of the killing, an intentional killing that would otherwise be murder will be reduced to the lesser crime of voluntary manslaughter. Some jurisdictions do not require that a defendant demonstrate that a reasonable person so provoked would not have cooled off in the interval of time between the provocation and the fatal blow (requirement 3 in the preceding list). In such jurisdictions, if a defendant has demonstrated that she was reasonably and actually provoked, and that she had not cooled off at the time she killed another person (requirements 1, 2, and 4 above), the defendant's crime is manslaughter rather than murder (LaFave, 2003).

Although states differ in what constitutes a "reasonable provocation," it is typically defined as a provocation that would cause a "reasonable person" to lose normal self-control. The loss of self-control can be expressed in any intense emotion, though usually is expressed as anger, rage, or fear. Traditionally, only two circumstances were considered to be a reasonable provocation: a man witnessing his wife in the act of adultery, and a physical altercation—that is, a physical fight between two men. Eventually, courts permitted the use of the defense by women as well as men, and have expanded the circumstances that may constitute reasonable provocation. Under current law, the following circumstances typically will constitute reasonable provocation: a violent, painful physical attack on the defendant by the deceased, mutual combat between the defendant and the deceased, conduct by the deceased that causes injury to a close relative of the defendant's, and a defendant's reasonable belief that his or her deceased spouse has committed adultery (LaFave, 2003).

A substantial minority of state criminal codes have adopted a version of the Model Penal Code (MPC) test for provocation manslaughter.[30] This test introduces some subjectivity into its definition of what constitutes a reasonable provocation. The MPC states that a homicide that would otherwise constitute murder is manslaughter if "committed under the influence of extreme mental or emotional disturbance for which there is a reasonable explanation or excuse," the reasonableness of which is to be "determined from the viewpoint of a person in the actor's situation under the circumstances as he believes them to be."[31] The MPC suggests that the definition should take into account certain physical disabilities such as "blindness, shock from traumatic injury, and extreme grief," but not a defendant's "idiosyncratic moral values."[32] Additionally, the MPC definition does not include any requirement with respect to whether a reasonable person would have cooled off in the interval of time between the provocation and the killing.

States also differ in their definitions of what constitutes a reasonable time to cool off. The traditional heat-of-passion manslaughter case is one in which a specific event, such as a physical battery or the witnessing of an adulterous act, immediately produces a rage in the defendant. Some jurisdictions now take a more modern approach, finding that a reasonable provocation can be produced by a series of events occurring over a considerable span of time. In those jurisdictions, the measurement of the cooling time commences with the last provoking event (LaFave, 2003).[33] In any event, what constitutes a reasonable cooling time in a particular case depends on the kind of provocation and the circumstances surrounding its occurrence, and the decision will usually be left to the jury, except in extreme circumstances (LaFave, 2003).[34]

The typical circumstances in which a battered woman kills her batterer would often satisfy the elements of a provocation defense. A battered woman, by definition, has been subjected to two or more violent, painful physical attacks at the hands of her batterer, circumstances that typically constitute reasonable provocation, the first element of the defense. A battered woman usually kills her batterer at a time when she is in a state of extreme fear, satisfying the second element that she was in fact provoked at the time of the killing, and the fourth requirement, that she had not "cooled off" (Kaser-Boyd, Chapter 3, this volume).

Typically, a battered woman who kills her batterer does so in response to a triggering event that occurs shortly before the fatal act (Kaser-Boyd, Chapter 3, this volume). If the event was another violent physical attack, the third requirement (that a reasonable person so provoked would not have cooled off in the interval of time between the provocation and the fatal act) also would likely be satisfied, even in jurisdictions that continue to take a more traditional approach to this element. In jurisdictions that take the more modern approach that a reasonable provocation can be produced by a series of events occurring over a considerable span of time, the last provoking event could be something less than another violent physical attack, such as a verbal threat of injury or other actions that would reasonably cause the battered woman to experience intense fear because of her past experiences with the batterer. In those jurisdictions that have adopted the MPC or eliminated the third requirement altogether, no showing with respect to a reasonable cooling time would be necessary.

Potential Uses of Expert Testimony to Support a Provocation Defense

For a woman who kills her abuser, expert evidence on battering and its effects could be extremely helpful to the successful presentation of a provocation defense. In much the same way as described earlier in the context of a self-defense claim, an expert's general testimony about the effects of battering could greatly enhance a defendant's credibility in the eyes of jurors, who might otherwise find her testimony about the relationship, the circumstances of the provoking events, and her fear at the time she killed her batterer unbelievable. Also as in the context of a self-defense claim, general testimony about the effects of battering could help to rebut common myths and misconceptions about a battered woman, such as the misconception that a woman who was truly battered would leave the relationship. In order for a battered woman to demonstrate reasonable provocation, it would be imperative for the jury to believe that her testimony concerning the abuse, which would constitute provoking events, was truthful. General testimony about the increasing level of fear a battered woman experiences as her battering experiences accumulate could also provide support for a defendant's claim that she was in fear at the time she killed her batterer.

Expert testimony could also assist a defendant claiming adequate provocation by rehabilitating her credibility after an attack by a prosecutor. An expert's testimony that memory loss is a common reaction to severe trauma could be helpful to proving a provocation defense as well as self-defense. An expert's testimony that the inability of a battered woman to recall all of the details of the death of her abuser, or other battering incidents, is a common effect of battering could support a defendant who has trouble recalling all of the details of prior physical attacks. An expert's general testimony that a battered woman may experience emotional constriction, or a shutting down of emotions, to avoid the painful memories of the battering could also assist a defendant who was experiencing emotional constriction at the time of an interrogation by police, or at the time of trial (Kaser-Boyd, Chapter 3, this volume). Without expert testimony, such emotional flatness likely could be interpreted by a jury uninformed of the effects of battering as inconsistent with the idea of a woman who was not in control of her emotions at the time of the killing.

Expert testimony also could be used to support the veracity of the defendant's claim that she was in fact battered by the deceased and that, as a result, she suffers from the effects of that battering. This kind of testimony also would assist the defendant in proving the existence of a reasonable provocation, that is, repeated physical and/or sexual assaults by the deceased. Testimony supporting the history of assaults would be particularly helpful in jurisdictions that have adopted the position that reasonable provocation can be created by a series of events occurring over a period of time.

CONCLUSION

The recognition of the importance of the use of expert testimony on battering and its effects to assist battered women in defending homicide charges has greatly increased since Jodie's murder trial in 1987. Today, courts in every state in the United States have held that such testimony is, in certain cases, admissible for the purpose of assisting a battered woman's self-defense claim. In a number of jurisdictions, state legislatures have codified the admissibility of this evidence. The California legislature has even passed a statute that permits battered women who were convicted of a homicide before such evidence was generally admitted to challenge their convictions and receive a new trial. Courts and legislatures should continue to consider additional ways in which the use of expert testimony on battering and its effects will create a more equitable criminal justice system. As discussed in this chapter, one use that should be permitted is the admission of such evidence to support a provocation defense.

ACKNOWLEDGMENTS

My thanks to research assistants Nick Peterson, Emilie Morin, and Christina Moore, and to my editor, B. J. Cling, who encouraged me to write about my experiences representing battered women who killed their abusers.

NOTES

1. Cal. Pen. Code §1473.5, enacted in 2001, permits a battered woman who (1) was convicted prior to January 1, 1992 of a homicide of her batterer and (2) did not have expert evidence on the effects of battering introduced at trial to seek a reversal of her conviction. The state may choose to retry a woman whose conviction is overturned pursuant to this statute, but if retried she would have the opportunity to present expert testimony on battering and its effects in support of her defense claim.
2. According to statistics compiled by the United States Department of Justice, in 1998 alone, "persons age 12 or older experienced about 1,043,670 violent crimes by a current or former spouse, boyfriend or girlfriend." The vast majority of these incidents

involve a male abusing his female partner. In 1998, females experienced 876,340 (85%) such violent victimizations, whereas males experienced 157,330 (15%).

3. As discussed above, my surveys of the status of the law in various states benefited greatly from the 1996 work of Janet Parrish, published in "Trend Analysis: Expert Testimony on Battering and Its Effects in Criminal Cases." In some instances, Parrish's work provides a more comprehensive list of cases adopting a particular rule than that provided in the notes to this chapter. Additionally, where appropriate, I have included additional case citations not cited in the Parrish article to reflect changes in the law since the article's publication.

4. See, for example, *People v. Humphrey*, 13 Cal. 4th 1073, 1083 note 3 (1996); *Smith v. State*, 268 Ga. 196, 199 (1997).

5. *People v. Humphrey*, 13 Cal. 4th at 1083; see also *State v. Wanrow*, 559 P.2d 548, 555 (Wash. 1997) ("The justification of self-defense is to be evaluated in light of all the facts and circumstances known to the defendant, including those known substantially before the killing.")

6. See, for example, *Bechtel v. State*, 840 P.2d 1, 26-27 (Okl. Crim. App. 1992) (In battered woman syndrome cases, reasonable person instruction should be replaced with instruction stating "self-defense is a defense, although the danger to life or personal security may not have been real, if a person, in the circumstances and from the viewpoint of the defendant, would reasonably have believed that she was in imminent danger of death or great bodily harm."); *State v. Stewart*, 763 P.2d 572, 577 (Kan. 1988) ("In cases involving battered spouses, 'the objective test is how a reasonably prudent battered wife would perceive [the aggressor's] demeanor' " (citations omitted)).

7. States that allow expert testimony on battering and its effects in "sleeping man" cases include Alabama (*Ex Parte Hill*, 507 So. 2d 558 (Ala. 1987)); California (*People v. Aris*, 215 Cal. App. 3d 1178, 1185 (Cal. Ct. App. 1989)); Georgia (*State v. Chapman*, 367 S.E.2d 541, 543 (Ga. 1988) (finding that a lapse in time between a husband's last abusive act and a wife's homicide does not preclude the use of expert testimony on battery and its effects, specifically in a case where a husband is shot while bathing)); Kansas (*Stewart*, 763 P.2d at 573); Michigan (*People v. Wilson*, 487 N.W.2d 822, 825 (Mich. Ct. App. 1992)); Minnesota (*State v. Hennum*, 441 N.W.2d 793, 798 (Minn. 1989) (en banc)); New Hampshire (*State v. Briand*, 547 A.2d 235, 236 (N.H. 1988)); North Carolina (*State v. Norman*, 378 S.E.2d 8, 11 (N.C. 1989)); North Dakota (*State v. Leidholm*, 334 N.W.2d 811, 819 (N.D. 1983)); Ohio (*State v. Manning*, 598 N.E.2d 25, 28 (Ohio App. Ct. 1991), *reh'g denied*, 580 N.E.2d 786 (1991), *cert. denied*, 112 S. Ct. 1961 (1992)); South Carolina (*Robinson v. State*, 417 S.E.2d 88, 90 (S.C. 1992), *reh'g denied* (6/3/92)); Tennessee (*State v. Aucoin*, 756 S.W.2d 705, 713 (Tenn. Crim. App. Apr. 12, 1989)); Wisconsin (*State v. Landis*, 406 N.W.2d 171, 172 (Wis. Ct. App. 1987), *review denied*, 415 N.W.2d 162 (1987), *State v. Felton*, 329 N.W.2d 161, 162 (Wis. 1983)). Several states have permitted such testimony in "hire to kill" cases: Alabama (*Ex Parte Haney*, 603 So.2d 412, 413 (Ala. 1992), *reh'g denied* (8/28/92), *cert. denied*, 113 S.Ct. 1297 (1993)); Colorado (*People v. Yaklich*, 833 P.2d 758, 759 (Colo. Ct. App. 1991), *reh'g denied* (1/9/92), *cert. denied*, (8/10/92)); Massachusetts (*Commonwealth v. Grimshaw*, 590 N.E.2d 681 (Mass. 1992)); North Carolina (*State v. Clark*, 377 S.E.2d 54, 62 (N.C. 1989)); Ohio (*State v. Lampkin*, 1990 Ohio App. LEXIS 4315 (Ohio Ct. App. Oct. 3, 1990), *cause dismissed*, 573 N.E.2d 674 (1991)); Tennessee (*State v. Leaphart*, 673 S.W.2d 870 (Tenn. Crim. App. 1983)); Texas (*Ortiz v. State*, 834 S.W.2d 343, 344 (Tex. Crim. App. 1992)); Washington (*State v. Hutcheson*, 813 P.2d 1283 (Wash. Ct. App. 1991), *recon. denied* (9/30/91), *review denied*, 827 P.2d 1012 (Wash. 1992)).

8. LaFave, in note 69 on page 547, lists the following cases as examples of states that ad-

here to this rule: *King v. State*, 233 Ala. 198, 171 So. 254 (1936); *State v. Marish*, 198 Iowa 602, 200 N.W.5 (1924); *State v. Cox*, 138 Me. 151, 23 A.2d 634 (1941); *Sydnor v. State*, 365 Md. 205, 776 A.2d 669 (2001); *State v. Austin*, 332 N.W.2d 21 (Minn. 1983); *State v. Davis*, 214 S.C. 34, 51 S.E.2d 8 (1948). The following additional cases are also useful illustrations of how the rule is applied: *Conner v. State*, 361 So. 2d 774 (Fla Dist. Ct. App. 1978), *reh. denied*, (1978); *State v. Grierson*, 69 A.2d 851, 854 (N.H. 1949); *State v. Pontery*, 117 A.2d 473 (N.J. 1955).

9. See, for example, *State v. Bobbitt*, 415 So. 2d 724, 726 (Fla. 1982); *Carter v. State*, 469 So. 2d 194, 195 (Fla. Dist. Ct. App. 1985); *State v. Shaw*, 441 A.2d 561, 565-66 (Conn. 1981); *State v. Pontery*, 117 A.2d 473, 482 (N.J. 1955); *State v. Grierson*, 69 A.2d 851, 854 (N.H. 1949) (all cases held that the privilege not to retreat in one's dwelling does not apply when the attacker is a co-occupant of the dwelling). Additionally, *State v. Gartland*, 694 A.2d 564, 569-71 (N.J. 1997) (upholding application of New Jersey's minority rule, noting burden imposed on battered women defendants, and urging legislature to reconsider the current statutory imposition of a duty to retreat when attacked in the home by a cohabitant); *Hennum*, 428 N.W.2d 866-67 (defendant had a duty to retreat in her own home); *State v. James*, 734 A.2d 1012, 1018 (Conn. App. 1999) (dwelling exception to the duty to retreat does not apply if the actor is threatened by another person who also dwells, or is usually lodged, in the same place); *Weiand*, 732 So. 2d at 1049 (Fla. 1999) (recognizing a limited duty to retreat within the residence to the extent reasonably possible when threatened by a cohabitant); *State v. Thomas*, 673 N.E.2d 1339, 1347 (Ohio 1997) (Pfeifer, J., dissenting) (rejecting the court's holding that a cohabitant need not retreat before resorting to lethal force in self-defense against another cohabitant).

10. Parrish lists the following states as having this requirement: Florida (*Terry v. State*, 467 So. 2d 761, 763-64 (Fla. Dist. Ct. App. 1985) (holding that expert testimony on battered woman syndrome is admissible to support a claim of self-defense)); Georgia (*Pruitt v. State*, 296 S.E.2d 795 (Ga. Ct. App. 1982)); Illinois (*People v. Jackson*, 535 N.E.2d 1086 (Ill. App. Ct. 1989) (upholding trial court's decision not to admit expert testimony on battered woman syndrome because defendant did not plead self-defense)); Kansas (*State v. Dunn*, 758 P.2d 718 (Kan. 1988); *Stewart*, 763 P.2d 572 (where self-defense claim is asserted, expert evidence on battered woman syndrome is admissible as evidence of deceased's long-term cruelty and violence toward defendant); *State v. Meyer*, No. 59, 213, slip op. (Kan. Ct. App. Dec. 4, 1986)); Louisiana (*State v. Burton*, 464 So. 2d 421 (La. Ct. App. 1985) (in the absence of evidence of an overt act by the victim at the time of the shooting, defendant was not permitted to present evidence of the violent relationship between the two)); Maryland (*Boyd v. State*, 581 A.2d 1 (Md. 1990) (testimony on battered woman syndrome not allowed where the evidence was insufficient to generate an issue of self-defense)); Massachusetts (*Commonwealth v. Rodriguez*, 633 N.E.2d 1039 (Mass. 1994) (exclusion of evidence that defendant had suffered a long history of physical abuse by victim was reversible error where a claim of self-defense is at issue)); Mississippi (*Lentz v. State*, 604 So. 2d 243 (Miss. 1992)); Missouri (*State v. Williams*, 787 S.W.2d 308 (Mo. Ct. App. 1990); *State v. Clay*, 779 S.W.2d 673 (Mo. Ct. App. 1989)); New Mexico (*State v. Branchal*, 684 P.2d 1163 (N.M. Ct. App. 1984)); Ohio (*State v. Lundgren*, 1994 Ohio App. LEXIS 1722 (Ohio Ct. App. Apr. 22, 1994); *State v. Dowd*, 1994 Ohio App. LEXIS 132 (Ohio Ct. App. Jan. 19, 1994), *dismissed*, 634 N.E.2d 1023 (1994); *State v. Calvin Redding*, 1992 Ohio App. LEXIS 972 (Ohio Ct. App. Mar. 5, 1992); *State v. Marcia Redding*, 1992 Ohio App. LEXIS 972 (Ohio Ct. App. Mar. 5, 1992); *State v. Pargeon*, 582 N.E.2d 665 (Ohio Ct. App. 1991) (expert testimony as to the battered woman syndrome can only be admitted when the issue of self-defense has

been raised); *State v. Poling*, 1991 Ohio App. LEXIS 2294 (Ohio Ct. App. May 17, 1991), *dismissed*, 579 N.E.2d 212 (1991)); *State v. Koss*, 551 N.E.2d 970 (Ohio 1990); *Bechtel*, 840 P.2d 1); South Carolina (*Hill*, 339 S.E.2d 121); Texas (*Fielder v. State*, 756 S.W.2d 809 (Tex. Crim. App. 1988); *Ortiz*, 834 S.W.2d 343); Utah (*State v. Hazel*, No. 931400263, 4th Judicial District Court for County of Utah, State of Utah (Memorandum Decision 9/7/93)); Washington (*State v. Hanson*, 793 P.2d 1001 (Wash. Ct. App. 1990), *recon. denied* (8/31/90), *review denied*, 803 P.2d 325 (1990)); Wisconsin (*State v. Balke*, 498 N.W.2d 913, slip op. (Wis. Ct. App. 1992), *review denied*, 501 N.W.2d 458 (Wis. 1993)); Wyoming (Jahnke v. State, 682 P.2d 991 (Wyo. 1984)).

11. Parrish lists the following states as having this requirement: Indiana (*Fultz v. State*, 439 N.E. 2d 659 (Ind. Ct. App. 1982); Missouri (*State v. Anderson*, 785 S.W.2d 596 (Mo. Ct. App. 1990), *denial of habeas corpus aff'd by Anderson v. Goeke*, 44 F.3d 675 (8th Cir. 1995), *reh'g denied* (12/15/95)); Ohio (*Lundgren*, 1994 Ohio App. LEXIS 1722).

12. Parrish lists the following states as having this requirement: Alaska (*Haakanson v. State*, 760 P.2d 1030 (Alaska Ct. App. 1988)); District of Columbia (*Ibn-Tamas v. U.S.* , 407 A.2d 626 (D.C. 1979); *Ibn-Tamas v. U.S.* , 455 A.2d 893 (D.C. 1983)); Florida (*Hawthorne v. State*, 470 So. 2d 770 (Fla. Dist. Ct. App. 1985); *Terry*, 467 So. 2d 761)); Georgia (*State v. Chapman*, trial transcript from unidentified case no. (Ga. 1987) (*voir dire* and testimony of Cheryl Christian)); Kansas (*State v. Hodges*, 716 P.2d 563 (1986), *overruled on other grounds; State v. Meyer*, No. 59,213, slip op. (Kan. Ct. App. Dec. 4, 1986)); Kentucky (*Dyer v. Commonwealth*, 816 S.W.2d 647 (Ky. 1991); *Brandenburg v. Commonwealth*, No. 86-CA-1834-M (Ky. Ct. App. Aug. 5, 1988) (unpub. op.); *Commonwealth v. Rose*, 725 S.W.2d 588 (Ky. 1987), *cert. denied*, 484 U.S. 838 (1987), *overruled by Commonwealth v. Craig*, 783 S.W.2d 387 (Ky. 1990)); Massachusetts (*Commonwealth v. Moore*, 514 N.E.2d 1342 (Mass. App. Ct. 1987); Minnesota (*State v. Borchardt*, 478 N.W.2d 757 (Minn. 1991)); New Jersey (*State v. Kelly*, 478 A.2d 364 (N.J. 1984)); New Mexico (*State v. Gallegos*, 719 P.2d 1268 (N.M. Ct. App. 1986)); Ohio (*Koss*, 551 N.E.2d 970); Oregon (*State v. Milbradt*, 756 P.2d 620 (Or. 1988)); Washington (*State v. Riker*, 869 P.2d 43 (1994)); Wyoming (*Frenzel v. State*, 849 P.2d 741 (Wyo. 1993); *Buhrle v. State*, 627 P.2d 1374 (Wyo. 1981); *Jahnke*, 682 P.2d 991).

13. Courts in at least ten states have noted that it is beyond question that "battered woman syndrome" is commonly accepted in the scientific community, and therefore no showing need be made: California (*Humphrey*, 13 Cal. 4th 1073); Connecticut (*State v. Borrelli*, 629 A.2d 1105 (Conn. 1993)); Florida (*Rogers v. State*, 616 So. 2d 1098 (Fla. Dist. Ct. App. 1993), *reh'g denied* (5/4/93), *approved in part, quashed in part*, 630 So. 2d 177 (Fla. 1993), *State v. Hickson*, 630 So. 2d 172 (Fla. 1993), *State v. Stiles*, No. 92-16173, slip op. (Fla. Cir. Ct., Hillsborough County Ct. June 1993)); Illinois (*People v. Minnis*, 455 N.E.2d 209 (Ill. App. Ct. 1983)); Minnesota (*Hennum*, 441 N.W.2d 793); Missouri (*Williams*, 787 S.W.2d 308); New York (*People v. Torres*, 488 N.Y.S.2d 358 (N.Y. Crim. Ct. 1985)); Ohio (*State v. Flowers*, No. 89 CR 463, App. No. 90 T 4452 (Ohio Ct. of Common Pleas, Trumbull County Ct. 6/1/90) (testimony of Stan Palumbo)); Utah (*State v. Hazel*, No. 931400263, 4th Judicial District Court for County of Utah, State of Utah (Memorandum Decision 9/7/93)); Washington (*Hanson*, 793 P.2d 1001).

14. Parrish lists the following states as having this requirement: Florida (*Stiles*, No. 92-16173, slip op.); Georgia (*Pruitt*, 296 S.E.2d 795); Maine (*State v. Anaya*, 438 A.2d 892 (Me. 1981)); Massachusetts (*Rodriguez*, 633 N.E.2d 1039); Ohio (*State v. Daws*, 1994 Ohio App. LEXIS 3295 (Ohio Ct. App. July 7, 1994), appeal allowed by 641

N.E.2d 203 (1994); *State v. Roquemore*, 620 N.E.2d 110 (Ohio Ct. App. 1993); *State v. Coulter*, 598 N.E.2d 1324 (Ohio Ct. App. 1992), *denial of post-conviction relief aff'd*, 1992 WL 193658 (Ohio Ct. App. Aug. 10, 1992); *State v. Rice*, 1991 Ohio App. LEXIS 2731 (Ohio Ct. App. June 6, 1991), dismissed, 579 N.E.2d 1392 (1991); *Pargeon*, 582 N.E.2d 665; *Poling*, 1991 Ohio App. LEXIS 2294; *Koss*, 551 N.E.2d 970; *State v. Seymour*, 1993 Ohio App. LEXIS 5387 (Ohio Ct. App. 1993), *dismissed*, 632 N.E.2d 519 (1994), *recon. denied*, 638 N.E.2d 1041 (1994)); Oklahoma (*Bechtel*, 840 P.2d 1); Pennsylvania (*Commonwealth v. Dillon*, 598 A.2d 963 (Pa. 1991); *Commonwealth v. Stonehouse*, 555 A.2d 772 (Pa. 1989); *Commonwealth v. Tyson*, 635 A.2d 623 (Pa. 1993)); Washington (*State v. Allery*, 682 P.2de 312 (Wash. 1984)); Wisconsin (*State v. Balke*, 498 N.W.2d 913, slip op. (there is some question whether this code applies to this case)); Wyoming (*Griffin v. State*, 749 P.2d 246 (Wyo. 1988) (there is some question whether this code applies to this case)).

15. Parrish lists the following states as permitting this testimony: Alaska (*State v. Pabst*, No. 3LN-87-764CR (Alaska Super. Ct., 3rd Jud. Dist. at Kenai 1988); California (*People v. Day*, 2 Cal App. 4th 405 (Ca. Ct. App. 1992)); Colorado (*Yaklich*, 833 P.2d 758); Connecticut (*Borrelli*, 629 A.2d 1105); District of Columbia (*Ibn-Tamas*, 407 A.2d 626; *Ibn-Tamas*, 455 A.2d 893); Florida (*Hawthorne v. State*, 470 So. 2d 770 (Fla. Dist. Ct. App. 1985); *Terry*, 467 So. 2d 761); Georgia (*Thompson*, 203 Ga. App. 339); Illinois (*Minnis*, 455 N.E. 2d 209); Indiana (*Dausch v. State*, 616 N.E. 2d 13 (1993)); Iowa (*State v. Jones*, Crim. No. D7X107208 (Iowa 1st Jud. Dist., Black Hawk County Ct. 1989)); Kansas (*Hodges*, 716 P.2d 563); Kentucky (*Commonwealth v. Jones*, Indictment No. 92-CR-00006 Ky. Circ. Ct., Rockcastle County Ct. (11/10/93)); Louisiana (*Laughlin v. Breaux*, 515 So. 2d 480 (La. Ct. App. 1987)); Maine (*Anaya*, 456 A.2d 1255); Massachusetts (*Rodriguez*, 633 N.E. 2d 1039); Michigan (*People v. Wilson*, 194 Mich. App. 599 (Mich. Ct. App. 1992)); Missouri (*Hunziger v. Noellsch*, No. CV591-cc, slip op. (Mo. Cir. Ct., Holt County Ct. March 2, 1994)); New Hampshire (*State v. Masters*, No. 85-S-220 (N.H. Super. Ct. Concord 1987) (*voir dire* and testimony of Sheila Stanley)); New Jersey (*Kelly*, 478 A.2d 364); New Mexico (*State v. Vigil*, 110 N.M. 254 (1990)); New York (*Torres*, 128 Misc. 2d 129); North Carolina (*Norman*, 324 N.C. 253); Ohio (*Koss*, 551 N.E.2d 970); Oklahoma (*McDonald v. State*, 674 P.2d 1154 (Okla. Crim. Appp. 1984)); Pennsylvania (*Stonehouse*, 555 A.2d 772); Rhode Island (*McNaugh v. State*, 612 A.2d 725 (R.I. 1992)); South Carolina (*Doe v. Greenville Hospital System*, 448 S.E.2d 564 (S.C. Ct. App. 1994)); Texas (*Pierini v. State*, 804 S.W.2d 258 (Tex. Crim. App. 1991)); Vermont (*State v. Verrinder*, 161 Vt. 250 (1993)); Virginia (*Commonwealth v. Plantz*, No. CR90-1176 (Va. Cir. Ct. Virginia Beach 1990)); Washington (*State v. Ciskie*, 110 Wash. 2d 263 (1998)); Wisconsin (*State v. Slade*, 168 Wis. 2d 358 (Wis. Ct. App. 1992), *review denied*, 490 N.W. 2d 23 (Wis. 1992)); West Virginia (*State v. Steele*, 178 W. Va. 330 (1987)); Wyoming (*Frenzel*, 849 P.2d 741).

16. Parrish lists the following states as permitting this testimony: California (*Day*, 2 Cal App. 4th 4050; Connecticut (*Borrelli*, 227 Conn. 153); District of Columbia (*Ibn-Tamas*, 407 A.2d 626; *Ibn-Tamas*, 455 A.2d 893); Kansas (*Hodges*, 716 P.2d 563); Michigan (*Wilson*, 194 Mich. App. 599); Minnesota (*Hennum*, 441 N.W.2d 798); New Hampshire (*Masters*, No. 85-S-220 (*voir dire* and testimony of Sheila Stanley)); New Jersey (*Kelly*, 478 A.2d 364); New Mexico (*State v. Vigil*, 110 N.M. 254 (1990)); New York (*Torres*, 128. Misc. 2d 129; Ohio (*Koss*, 551 N.E.2d 970); Oklahoma (*Bechtel*, 840 P.2d 1); Pennsylvania (*Dillon*, 598 A.2d 963); Utah (*Hazel*, No. 931400263, 4th Judicial District Court for County of Utah, State of Utah); Vermont (*Blair v. Blair*, 154 Vt. 201 (1990)); Wyoming (*Frenzel*, 849 P.2d 741).

17. Parrish lists the following states as permitting such testimony: Alaska (*State v. Charliaga*, Alaska Super.Ct. at Kodiak 10/91) (information in National Coalition for

the Defense of Battered Women files)); Alabama (*Haney*, 603 So. 2d 412); California (*Aris*, 215 Cal. App. 3d 1178); Colorado (*Yaklich*, 833 P.2d 758); Connecticut (*Knock v. Knock*, 224 Conn. 776 (1993)); District of Columbia (*Ibn-Tamas*, 407 A.2d 626; *Ibn-Tamas*, 455 A.2d 893); Deleware (*State v. McBride*, Criminal Action Nos. IK-80-05-0058, IK-80-05-0059, IK-80-05-0027(Del. Super. Ct., Kent County Ct. 1982)); Florida (*Jackson*, 648 So. 2d 85); Georgia (*Thompson*, 203 Ga. App. 339); Idaho (*Curtis v. Firth*, 123 Idaho 598 (1993)); Illinois (*People v. Sheila Smith*, 241 Ill. App. 3d 446 (1993)); Indiana (*Dausch*, 616 N.E.2d 13); Kansas (*State v. Cramer*, 17 Kan. App. 2d 623 (1992)); (*Hodges*, 716 P.2d 563); Kentucky (*Jones*, Indictment No. 92-CR-00006); Louisiana (*Laughlin*, 515 So. 2d 480); Maine (*Anaya*, 456 A.2d 1255); Maryland (*State v. Evelyn Smith*, Crim Trial 91-2547TX (Md. Cir. Ct., Prince Georges County Ct. 1992)); Massachusetts (*Rodriguez*, 418 Mass. 1); Minnesota (*State v. Mick*, No. K-84-497 (Minn. Dist. Ct., 8th Jud. Ct., Kandiyohi County Ct. 1984)); Missouri (*Hunziger*, No. CV591-5CC, slip. op.); Montana (*State v. Hess*, 252 Mont. 205 (1992), *reh'g denied*, (3/31/92)); Nebraska (*In re Interest of C.P.* , 235 Neb. 276 (1990)); New Hampshire (*Briand*, 130 N.H. 650); New Mexico (*State v. Swavola*, 114.N.M. 472(1992), *cert. denied*, 114 N.M. 501(1992)); New York (*People v. Barrett*, 189 A.D.2d 879 (1993)); North Carolina (*Clark*, 324 N.C. 146); North Dakota (*Leidholm*, 334 N.W.2d 811); Ohio (*State v. Higgs*, 1992 Ohio App. LEXIS 2731 (Ohio Ct. App. Oct. 7, 1992)); Oklahoma (*McDonald*, 674 P.2d 1154); Oregon (*State v. Bockorny*, 124 Or. App. 585 (Or. Ct. App. 1993, *review denied*, 318 Or. 351(1994)); Pennsylvania (*Dillon*, 528 Pa. 41); Rhode Island (*McNaugh*, 612 A.2d 725); South Carolina (*State v. Wilkins*, 305 S.C. 272 (S.C. Ct. of Appeal 1991)); Tennessee (*State v. Furlough*, 797 S.W.2d 631 (Tenn. Crim. App. 1990)); Texas (*Hayward v. State*, 1993 Tex. App. LEXIS 945 (Tex. Ct. App. Apr. 1, 1993)); Virginia (*Wilmoth v. Commonwealth*, 10 Va. App. 169 (Va. Ct. App. 1990)); Washington (*Kelly*, 102 Wash. 2d 188 (1984)); West Virginia (*Steele*, 178 W. Va. 330). Additionally, Wyoming has found this testimony admissible (*Witt v. State*, 892 P.2d 132 (Wyo. 1995)).

18. See Kaser-Boyd (Chapter 3, this volume) for a more comprehensive discussion of relevant background materials and witness preparation.

19. The following states have allowed, or held that it permissible for, an expert to testify as to whether the defendant had an honest belief that she was in imminent danger: Alabama (*Harrington v. State*, 2002 Ala. Crim. App. LEXIS 230 (Ala. Ct. of Appeals, Oct. 25, 2002)); Colorado (*State v. Darbe*, 62 P.3d 1006 (Colo. Ct. App. 2002)); Florida (*Weiand*, 732 So. 2d 1044); Illinois (*State v. Fleming*, 507 N.E.2d 954 (Ill. App. Ct. 1987)); Missouri (*State v. Edwards*, 60 S.W.3d 602 (Mo. Ct. App. 2001)); New Mexico (*Gallegos*, 719 P.2d 1268); New York (*People v. Emick*, 481 N.Y.S.2d 552 (N.Y. App. Div. 1984)); North Carolina (*Norman*, 378 S.E.2d 8); South Carolina (*State v. Wilkins*, 407 S.E.2d 670); Tennessee (*Furlough*, 797 S.W.2d 631); Texas (*Fielder v. State*, 756 S.W.2d 809 (Tex. Crim. App. 1988)); West Virginia (*Steele*, 359 S.E.2d 558).

20. California (*People v. Erickson*, 57 Cal App. 4th 1391,1401 (1997)); Iowa (*State v. Griffin*, 564 N.W.2d 370 (Iowa 1997)); Kentucky (*Commonwealth v. Rose*, 725 S.W.2d 588 (Ky. 1987)); Louisiana (*State v. Necaise*, 466 So. 2d 660 (La. Ct. App. 1985)); Oklahoma (*Bechtel v. State*, 840 P.2d 1); Wisconsin (*State v. Richardson*, 525 N.W.2d 378 (Wis. Ct. App. 1994)); Wyoming (*Witt*, 829 P.2d 132).

21. Because Jodie killed her abuser in California, opinion testimony as to whether she was actually in fear at the time of the killing would not be permitted. See *People v. Erickson*, 57 Cal. App 4th 1391, 1401 (1997). (Pursuant to California Penal Code § 29, "an expert is not permitted to testify as to the expert's opinion that she *actually perceived* that she was in danger and needed to defend herself.")

22. See discussion of imperfect self-defense in the earlier Section "Definition of Self-Defense."

23. Parrish lists the following states as permitting testimony on the reasonableness of the defendant's actions: Alaska (*Pabst*, No. 3LN-87-764CR); Florida (*State v. Soubielle*, No. 87-508-CFA (Fla Cir. Ct., Crim. Div., Seminole County Ct. 1988)); Georgia (*Smith v. State*, 247 Ga. 612 (1981)); Kansas (*State v. Dunn*, No. 85-CR-59T (Kan. Dist. Ct., Shawnee County Ct. 1992)); Maine (*Anaya*, 438 A.2d 892); New Hampshire (*Masters*, No. 85-S-220); New Mexico (*Gallegos*, 104 N.M. 247); New York (*People v. Ciervo*, 123 A.D.2d 393 (1986)); North Carolina (*Norman*, 324 N.C. 253); Oregon (*Bockorny*, 124 Or. App. 585; *State v. Moore*, 695 P.2d 985 (Or. Ct. App. 1985)); South Carolina (*Wilkins*, 305 S.C. 272); Tennessee (*Furlough*, 797 S.W.2d 261); Texas (*State v. King*, Trial Ct. Cause No. 461,560 (Tex. 351st Dist. Ct. Harris Co. 1987)); Virginia (*Pancoast v. Commonwealth*, 2 Va. App. 28 (Va. Ct. App. 1986)).
24. The states are: California (Cal. Evid. Code §1107 (West 1991)); Georgia (Ga. Code Ann., §16-3-21(d) (Michie 1994)); Louisiana (La Code Evid. Ann. art. 404 (A) (2) (West 1989)); Maryland (Md. Cts & Jud. Proc. Code Ann. §10-916) (1991); Massachusetts (Mass. Gen. Laws Ann. Ch 233 §23F (West 1994)); Missouri (Mo. Ann. Stat. §563.033 (Vernon 1991)); Nevada (Nev. Rev. Stat. § 48.061 (1993)); Ohio (Ohio Rev. Code Ann. §§ 2901.06 & 2945.392 (Anderson 1990)); Oklahoma (Okla. Stat. Ann. tit. 22, §40.7 (West 1992)); South Carolina (S.C. Code Ann. §17-23-170 (Law Co-op. 1995)); Wyoming (Wyo. Stat. §6-1-203 (1993)).
25. See Cal. Evid. Code § 1107.
26. See Wyo. Stat. Ann. § 6-1-203. Maryland and Ohio have similar statutes; see Ohio Rev. Code Ann. § 2901.06; Md. Cts. & Jud. Pro. § 10-916 (West 2003).
27. See, for example, *People v. Seeley*, 720 N.Y.S.2d 315 (N.Y. Sup. Ct. 2000) (specifically permitting psychiatric examination of defendant by state).
28. See, for example, *Aris*, 215 Cal. App. 3d 1178; *Anaya*, 438 A.2d. 892; *Norman*, 324 N.C. 253; *Stonehouse*, 521 Pa. 41.
29. See the earlier section, "Establishing Qualifications of Expert to Testify."
30. In 1962, the American Law Institute, a group of law professors, judges, and lawyers, published a uniform criminal law code, titled the Model Penal Code. Meant to offer a comprehensive revision of the criminal law, the Model Penal Code is not law and has no binding authority. It has, however, been the model for many state criminal codes and continues to influence legislators and judges at all levels.
31. Model Penal Code § 210.3.
32. Model Penal Code § 210.3.
33. See, for example, *People v. Barry*, 18 Cal. 3d 509 (1976).
34. LaFave lists the following cases as examples of cases in which a court held, as a matter of law, the cooling time was reasonable or unreasonable: *State v. Ramirez*, 116 Ariz. 259 (1977); *People v. Pouncey*, 437 Mich. 382 (1991); In re *Fraley*, 3 Okla. Crim. 719 (1910); *State v. Williford*, 103 Wis. 2d 98 (1981).

REFERENCES

Dutton, M. A. (1996). Validity of "battered woman syndrome" in criminal cases involving battered woman. In M. Gordon (Ed.), *The validity and use of evidence concerning battery and its effects in criminal trials: Report responding to Section 40507 of the violence against women act* (pp. 17–20). Washington, DC: U.S. Department of Justice.
Iovanni, L. A., & Miller, S. L. (2001). Criminal justice system responses to domes-

tic violence: Law enforcement and the courts. In C. M. Renzetti, J. L. Edelson, & R. K. Bergen (Eds.), *Sourcebook on violence against women* (pp. 303–313). Thousand Oaks, CA: Sage.

Klein, A. R. (1996). Re-abuse in a population of court-restrained male batterers: Why restraining orders don't work. In E. S. Buzawa & C. G. Buzawa (Eds.), *Do arrests and restraining orders work?* (pp. 192–207). Thousand Oaks, CA: Sage.

LaFave, W. R. (2003). *Criminal law* (4th ed., pp. 539–546, 550, 777–779, 786–787). St. Paul, MN: West.

Maguigan, H. (1991). Battered women and self-defense: Myths and misconceptions in current reform proposals. *University of Pennsylvania Law Review, 140,* 379, 384–385, 397–401, 414–416, 419–423).

Maguigan, H. (1998). It's time to move beyond "battered woman syndrome." *Criminal Justice Ethics, 17,* 50–57.

Maguigan, H. (2000). *A defense perspective on battered women charged with homicide: The expert's role during preparation and conduct of trials.* New York: National Association of Women Judges.

Mahoney, P., Williams, L., & West, C. M. (2001). Violence against women by intimate partners. In C. M. Renzetti, J. L. Edelson, & R. K. Bergen (Eds.), *Sourcebook on violence against women* (pp. 143, 149–150, 153). Thousand Oaks, CA: Sage.

Parrish, J. (1996). Trend analysis: Expert testimony on battering and its effects in criminal cases. *Wisconsin Women's Law Journal, 11,* 75, 78, 83–87, 99–100, 112–115, 117–118, 121–123, 127, 131. Madison: University of Wisconsin Law School.

Sullivan, C. M., & Gillum, T. (2001). Shelters and other community-based services for battered women and their children. In C. M. Renzetti, J. L. Edelson, & R. K. Bergen (Eds.), *Sourcebook on violence against women* (pp. 247–248). Thousand Oaks, CA: Sage.

Tjaden, P., & Thoennes, N. (2000, July). Extent, nature and consequences of intimate partner violence. *Findings from the national violence against women survey* (p. 53). Retrieved December 1, 2003, from *http://www.ojp.usdoj.gov/nij.*

5 Stalking

BARRY ROSENFELD
B. J. CLING

Beginning with the widely publicized murder of the actress Rebecca Schaeffer at the hands of a mentally disturbed man who had been harassing her, the term "stalking" was catapulted into the contemporary lexicon. Historical references to obsessive love and repetitive harassment have existed for centuries, but this behavior had rarely been labeled criminal until the intense media attention began to reveal the magnitude of problems caused by these behaviors. Since 1990, when the first "anti-stalking" law was passed by California in response to Ms. Schaeffer's murder as well as those of several other California women who were shot by men who stalked them (Jordan, Quinn, Jordan, & Daileader, 2000), social scientists, criminologists, and legal scholars have focused on understanding, preventing, and responding to stalking behaviors. In the decade that followed California's anti-stalking law, every state in the United States, along with a handful of countries (e.g., Britain, Australia, Canada) have passed similar laws, criminalizing or increasing the applicable penalties for repetitive harassment behaviors.

Numerous definitions exist for the phenomena labeled stalking, but most share several key elements including repetitive, unwanted contact that is perceived by the victim as intrusive and/or threatening. The National Institute of Justice (1993) offers a model anti-stalking statute, wherein stalking is defined as the action of "any person who purposefully engages in a course of conduct directed at a specific person that would cause a reasonable person to fear bodily injury to himself or herself or a member of his or her immediate family . . . [and] has knowledge or should have knowledge that the specific person will be placed in reasonable fear . . . is guilty of the crime of stalking." Although all 50 states have developed their own definitions of stalking, and the elements of this crime (and their definitions) have varied somewhat across these different laws, the general themes outlined by the National Institute of Justice have been applied relatively consistently throughout most of the recent legislation.

Although the term "stalking" is itself somewhat misleading, since many individuals do not actually follow (in a stealthy manner) the target of their harassment, this term has become such an integral part of the emerging literature that it is used in this chapter for the sake of clarity and consistency. The behaviors included in most definitions of stalking range from direct contact with the victim (following him or her, waiting outside of the home or workplace, physical assault directed toward either the target or a third party) to behaviors that may never result in face-to-face contact (e.g., repeated telephone calls; sending letters, gifts, or unwanted objects; or surveillance/harassment through the Internet and e-mail[1]). Targets of stalking can include former intimate partners, family members, employer/coworkers with whom one has had either problematic interactions or romantic aspirations, and strangers (including public figures, such as celebrities, politicians, and athletes). The motives behind stalking also vary, with many individuals harboring romantic aspirations, whereas others are driven by revenge and some by a mixture of the two or other, idiosyncratic motives. Although an exhaustive review of stalking is beyond the scope of this chapter (and could easily fill an entire book itself), this chapter will provide a brief overview of the nature of stalking, characteristics of stalking perpetrators, the impact on victims, and the laws designed to protect them.

IS THERE A STALKING "EPIDEMIC"?

Despite the relatively recent identification of the crime of stalking, the frequency of this social problem has been described as an epidemic. A growing number of surveys have documented high rates of victimization, particularly among women, perpetrated by stalking offenders. The most widely cited survey of the general public was conducted by Tjaden and Theonnes (1998), who surveyed 16,000 adults (8,000 men and 8,000 women) living in the United States. They defined stalking as "a course of conduct directed at a specific person that involves repeated visual or physical proximity, nonconsensual communication, or written or implied threats, or a combination thereof, that would cause a reasonable person fear" (p. 2). They observed a lifetime prevalence rate of 8% for women and 2% for men, corresponding to roughly 1,000,000 women and nearly 370,000 men stalked annually.

Substantially higher rates of stalking were observed in the British Crime Survey (Budd & Mattinson, 2000); however, that study applied a much broader definition of stalking than the one utilized by Tjaden and Thoennes, which more closely mirrored the legal standards applied in most jurisdictions (i.e., requiring fear of harm rather than simply focusing on harassing behavior). The British Crime Survey defined stalking as having been "pestered or harassed, either by someone [you know] or by strangers." They surveyed nearly 10,000 adults living in England and Wales, finding a lifetime prevalence rate of 16% among women and 7% among men, more than double the rate observed in the United States. Similarly high levels of stalking prevalence were reported in a sample of 6,000 Australian women, with 15% reporting having been stalked (Australian Bureau of Statistics, 1996; Mullen, Pathé, & Purcell, 2000).

Rates of stalking among college students have been even higher than these large national surveys, despite the obvious fact that younger individuals have less opportunity to have been stalked. For example, in one of the first published studies of stalking among U.S. college students, Fremouw and colleagues (Fremouw, Westrup, & Pennypacker, 1997) found that 31% of women and 17% of men reported having been stalked. Other studies of college students have observed similar rates (e.g., Bjerregaard, 2000; Logan, Leukefeld, & Walker, 2000), typically observing rates between 25 and 30% for women and 10 and 15% for men. These studies, however, have often utilized small and nonrepresentative samples and vague definitions of stalking, raising questions as to the accuracy of these findings. Not surprisingly, stalking among college students has typically been of shorter duration, and more often in response to the dissolution of a romantic relationship compared to among the general public, where stalking can last for years or even decades, often when no relationship existed between the perpetrator and target.

Particularly noteworthy is the consistency with which women have reported higher rates of stalking than men across virtually all studies conducted. The ratio of female to male stalking victims has varied somewhat across studies but has typically hovered between 3:1 and 4:1. In their review of the stalking literature, Spitzberg and Cupach (2003) estimated that three of every four stalking victims are female. Perpetrators of stalking, on the other hand, are much more likely to be male, as men account for roughly 80% of all stalkers. This disproportionate gender ratio has led many researchers to presume that stalking is invariably linked to intimate relationships. In fact, some writers have suggested terms such as "obsessive relational intrusion" as preferable to "stalking" (e.g., Cupach & Spitzberg, 2000), presumably to highlight the relational nature of stalking behavior. However, empirical research has demonstrated a plethora of stalking motivations beyond the desire to initiate or regain a prior intimate relationship, including anger or revenge over perceived mistreatment, and an obsessional (but not romantic) fixation (sometimes termed "morbid infatuation"). Tjaden and Thoennes (1998) estimated that former intimate stalkers comprise roughly 60% of stalking cases in which women are the target and 33% of cases in which men are targeted, although these individuals are not necessarily motivated to resume the romantic relationship.[2] Thus, the conceptualization of stalking as a problem facing women who attempt to terminate a romantic relationship, while not uncommon, is certainly an oversimplification of the complex stalking phenomenon.

Another possible explanation for the disproportionate number of female stalking victims is that women are more likely to become afraid and complain when harassment occurs, whereas men interpret the same behaviors as being more innocuous. For example, several studies have found that a large proportion of men report feeling "flattered" when they experienced stalking or harassment behaviors.[3] Bierregaard (2000), in her study of college student stalking victims, found that women reported significantly greater fear than men did in response to comparable experiences. Several other studies have found comparable rates of stalking experiences between men and women, further supporting the possibility that some of the differences in prevalence rates may partially reflect a greater concern, and by extension, a greater likelihood of seeking legal system or mental health intervention on the part of women.

Some writers have also attributed the gender differences in reported rates of stalking victimization to differing perceptions of what constitutes stalking among men and women (Spitzberg & Cupach, 2003). Dennison and Thompson (2002), in one of the few experimental studies to focus on perceptions of stalking, found that Australian women were significantly more likely to label a vignette as stalking compared to men (86 vs. 73%). Phillips and colleagues (Phillips, Quirk, O'Connor, & Rosenfeld, 2004), however, found much more complex relationships between gender and perceived concerns. These authors conducted two studies with college student samples in which participants read a short vignette and were asked whether the behaviors reflected "stalking" and if the target of the harassment should be concerned for his or her safety (using several different questions). Gender of the characters described in the vignette (male perpetrator and female target vs. female perpetrator and male target) did not influence perceptions of stalking in these vignettes; however, women study participants were slightly (but significantly) more likely to characterize the behaviors described (regardless of the gender of the characters) as "stalking" in one of the two studies. Interestingly, prior experience with stalking did not appear to influence subject perceptions of the vignettes, contradicting the hypothesis that stalking victims may become "sensitized" to stalking due to a previous experience. On the other hand, gender of the vignette characters significantly influenced responses to questions about safety concerns in both studies. In particular, when the vignette described a male perpetrator and female target, participants were much more likely to rate the stalker as potentially violent, to discourage face-to-face contact, and to recommend contacting the authorities compared to scenarios in which a female stalker targeted a male. There were no differences in perceived safety concerns based on gender of study participant (i.e., both men and women perceived male stalkers as more worrisome than female stalkers). Thus, although women may be more likely to express fear in response to stalking behaviors (an integral aspect of most legal standards), the perception of stalking per se does not appear to be markedly influenced by gender.

WHEN DOES HARASSMENT VIOLATE THE LAW?

Although harassment has long been considered a criminal offense, the growing awareness of the problems posed by stalkers illuminated the problems in the laws that regulated harassment prior to the 1990s. For example, prior to the recent surge in anti-stalking legislation, virtually all laws prohibiting stalking labeled this behavior as a misdemeanor offense, enabling offenders to repeatedly engage in harassment with little risk of serious repercussions. But beginning with California's first anti-stalking law, a wave of legislative reform swept through the United States and many other developed countries, better defining the contours of stalking and facilitating the prosecution of offenders (Jordan, Quinn, Jordan, & Daileader, 2000). Many of these laws still consider first and/or nonviolent stalking offenses to be misdemeanors, but possible penalties increase for repeat offenses or more serious acts (e.g., stalking a minor).[4]

Anti-stalking laws share a number of common features, but also many important differences. Most of these laws, however, require several key elements in order to classify harassing behaviors as stalking, including (1) willful or intentional behavior on the part of the perpetrator, (2) the presence of either a credible threat toward the target or a third party (e.g., a family member), and (3) fear on the part of the target (Miller, 2001). Unfortunately, defining these criteria has often proven to be more difficult than many legal scholars initially anticipated. For example, proving that a perpetrator intends to engage in the course of conduct that constitutes the harassment or, in many jurisdictions, to instill fear in the target is often quite difficult. Many statutes respond to this ambiguity by requiring that the target specifically instruct the offender to stop the harassment. Threats, too, may be difficult to define, particularly when the communications are not explicit but rather imply a potential harm. Finally, determining whether a target's fear is "reasonable" rather than an exaggerated response to seemingly benign interactions requires an understanding of the normative reaction to harassment.

The issue of "intent" that is present in nearly all anti-stalking laws has different implications depending on the jurisdiction, since important distinctions exist between the concepts of general intent and specific intent. The requirement of general intent demands proof that the stalker deliberately engaged in the conduct and that the conduct itself was illegal, but not that the stalker *intended* to break the law. Specific intent, on the other hand, requires that the stalker *intended* the result of his or her actions. Thus, statutes that require specific intent on the part of the stalker must prove not only that the perpetrator deliberately engaged in the behavior, but that he or she intended to cause the fear that resulted (a much more difficult standard; Pappas, 1996).[5]

Another important element of most anti-stalking legislation pertains to the appropriateness of the target's reaction. Most jurisdictions rely on the "reasonable person" standard to make such determinations, as this criterion is widely used in many areas of the law (e.g., sexual harassment, tort law). However, reactions to stalking behaviors vary widely across individuals, and little research has focused on understanding how typical individuals react to stalking. Thus, despite the potential to apply research findings to guide determinations of the reasonableness of an individual's reaction to stalking, these decisions are typically based upon the juror's intuitive sense of reasonableness rather than empirical data about normative reactions among stalking victims.

Recent anti-stalking legislation has also been accompanied by a number of constitutional challenges (i.e., challenging the constitutionality of the laws on various legal grounds), including charges of overbreadth and vagueness. Overbreadth refers to a statute that is so broad that it prohibits behaviors that are constitutionally protected or otherwise innocent. For example, because telephoning someone or waiting outside a building is usually legal, prohibiting such behaviors through an anti-stalking statute has the unwanted effect of criminalizing otherwise reasonable behaviors. Vagueness, on the other hand, refers to the excessive ambiguity present in many anti-stalking statutes. Terms such as a "persistent course of conduct" or "reasonable fear of harm" have been challenged on the grounds that these terms are not sufficiently well defined as to enable the court (or the public) to differentiate when behaviors violate the law. In general, however, these challenges have been unsuccessful, as most courts have upheld the anti-stalking statutes (Jordan et al., 2000). Thus, despite occasional roadblocks and ambiguities, anti-stalking legislation has become increasingly accepted and utilized.

WHO ENGAGES IN STALKING?

As is often the case in new research areas, much of the early stalking research focused on descriptive analyses characterizing the nature of stalking offenders. These descriptive studies revealed a number of interesting findings, such as the disproportionate age (older), ethnicity (predominantly white), and education level (better educated) of stalkers compared to the typical criminal offender (e.g., Harmon, Rosner, & Owens, 1995; Meloy & Gothard, 1995; Schwartz-Watts et al., 1997). For example, in one of the first studies of stalking offenders, Harmon and colleagues (1995) described a sample of 48 adults referred for court-ordered psychiatric evaluations who had been charged with crimes related to stalking. They found that this subset of offenders were more likely to be female, significantly older, more often married, and better educated than the "typical" offender referred to this clinic. In addition, they found a high rate (14 of 48) of stalkers diagnosed with a delusional disorder (typically erotomanic or paranoid types), particularly compared to the less than 0.1% prevalence rate estimated by the *Diagnostic and Statistical Manual of Mental Disorders* (DSM-IV; American Psychiatric Association, 1994). Interestingly, Harmon et al. also observed a large proportion of other mental disorders such as schizophrenia and psychotic disorder not otherwise specified (15 of 48 stalking offenders) and personality disorders (9 of 48 offenders). They concluded that, despite the emphasis on erotomanic offenders that characterized the early interest in stalking, these offenders still comprise a minority of the total stalking population.

Rosemary Purcell and her colleagues (Purcell, Pathé, & Mullen, 2001) conducted the only study specifically comparing male and female stalkers, identifying a number of interesting gender differences. For example, in their sample of 190 stalking offenders, 40 of whom were female (21%), they found that women were significantly more likely to target females than male offenders were to target males (i.e., a greater proportion of same-sex stalking for women compared to men). They were also significantly *less likely* than males to have prior criminal offenses unrelated to stalking or to have a history of substance abuse. Female offenders were also significantly less likely to target strangers (5% of women compared to 21% of men) but were more likely to harass individuals with whom they had professional contact (e.g., mental health professionals, attorneys, teachers). Interestingly, there was no difference between male and female stalkers in rates of physical assault (22.5% of women vs. 36.7% of men). There was also no difference in rates of delusional disorder (30.0% of women vs. 24.7% of men), but women were more likely to be motivated by intimacy needs compared to men (45.0% vs. 29.3% of men).

More recently, investigators have focused on psychological characteristics that differentiate stalkers from comparison subjects, incorporating themes from attachment theory and cognitive psychology (e.g., Do stalkers use distinctive decision-making or problem-solving styles?) (Lewis, Fremouw, Del Ben, & Farr, 2001; Roberts, 2002; Rosenfeld & Harmon, 2002), as well as confirming early assumptions regarding the relatively high rate of erotomanic delusions (which were thought to be extremely rare prior to the emergence of the stalking literature). For example, Lewis and colleagues (2001) compared a sample of undergraduate college student stalkers (based on self-admission of repetitive intrusive behaviors) to a group of students who did not acknowledge stalking behaviors on a number of psychological characteristics. They found that stalkers had more attachment difficulties and borderline personality traits than the comparison sample although the two groups did not differ in terms of problem-solving style or empathy. Nonetheless, this pattern of findings led the authors to conclude that stalkers had a general inability to maintain appropriate interpersonal relationships. Of course, their reliance on undergraduate psychology students who admitted to having engaged in stalking behaviors obviously raises questions about the generalizability of these findings to the larger population of stalking offenders. Thus, although studies such as these provide fodder for clinicians and theorists, there is relatively little data to help distinguish which etiological models of stalking are most accurate.

Despite the relative absence of empirically supported theories of stalking, clinicians and theorists have developed a number of different typologies to describe stalking offenders, some of which are largely overlapping but others which are quite different from one another. One of the earliest typologies of stalking was offered by Zona, Sharma, and Lane (1993), based upon their review of records compiled by the Los Angeles police department. They divided stalking cases into three groups: erotomanic stalkers, whose psychosis leads them to believe that the target is actually in love with them; "love obsessional" stalkers, who hope to win the affection of their target through the use of persistent courtship or harassment behaviors; and "simple obsessional" stalkers, who typically are former intimate partners who are unable to accept the termination of the relationship.

Since Zona's early work, a number of other theorists have offered typologies (Del Ben & Fremouw, 2002; Holmes, 2001), ranging in level of theoretical complexity and empirical sophistication. However, most have identified several "types" of stalkers, including the erotomanic stalker who targets a stranger (often a celebrity or other public figure), former domestic partners who cannot accept the termination of the relationship, and revenge-motivated stalkers who target individuals whom they perceive as having "wronged" them in the past. Mullen and colleagues (Mullen, Pathé, Purcell, & Stuart, 1999) offered a somewhat more comprehensive model of stalking offenders, positing five "types" of offenders based primarily on motivation and social functioning. Based on clinical evaluations of stalking offenders referred to a psychiatric clinic, they classified offenders into one of five different categories: rejected, intimacy-seeking, incompetent, resentful, and predatory. Rejected stalkers were typically those individuals who targeted a former intimate partner, and often expressed both romantic as well as angry feelings toward the target. Intimacy-seeking stalkers, on the other hand, sought to elicit the affection of the target, often due to romantic feelings based on erotomanic delusions. Incompetent stalkers also sought an intimate relationship with the target, but, unlike the intimacy-seeking group, these individuals were aware that their affection was not reciprocated. Resentful stalkers were those offenders motivated to frighten or intimidate the target, generally in response to a perceived insult or wrong. Finally, predatory stalkers were the rarest subgroup in their sample, as they typically stalked in the context of a rape or sexual assault (and all had prior convictions for sexual assault). This typology differentiated stalkers on a number of different criteria including the type of stalking behaviors, the frequency of violence, and diagnosis.

However, despite the growing number of different typologies that have been offered, there has been relatively little attempt to empirically investigate either the validity or clinical utility of these models. Moreover, the limited research that has investigated typological classifications has often proven far less comprehensive than the models would suggest. For example, Harmon et al. (1995) and Rosenfeld (2000) have described a typology of stalkers based upon the nature of the motivation (revenge vs. amorous) and the relationship between stalker and target (real vs. fantasy). Rosenfeld hypothesized that these distinctions would correspond to differential rates of mental disorder, with particular diagnostic categories appearing in some types of stalkers and not others. However, a large-scale study of stalkers referred for court-ordered psychiatric evaluation (Rosenfeld & Harmon, 2002) did not fit these expectations, as diagnoses were distributed throughout each of the "types" of stalking hypothesized. Hence, the primary utility of these typologies has been in identifying differential risk patterns associated with the stalker types. For example, Mullen and colleagues found that rates of assault varied significantly across the five stalker types they described, suggesting that their typology may help differentiate high- versus low-risk stalkers.

Indeed, identifying violence risk factors in stalking and harassment cases has become an increasingly popular focus for researchers. Early studies of stalking-related violence focused on simple comparisons between violent and nonviolent offenders (e.g., Menzies, Federoff, Green, & Isaacson, 1995; Schwartz-Watts & Morgan, 1998). More recently, however, researchers have attempted to apply more sophisticated modeling techniques to account for the potentially complex interrelationships among stalker characteristics, stalking behaviors, and stalking-related violence. For example, Palarea, Zona, Lane, and Langhinrichsen-Rohling (1999) studied violence risk factors in the context of stalking between former intimate partners. They analyzed 223 stalking cases that had been identified by the Los Angeles Police Department's Threat Management Unit, focusing on identifying variables that distinguished violent from nonviolent stalkers. Their path analysis model revealed that threats, victim–offender relationship (former intimates were significantly more often violent than other stalkers), a history of previous violence, and level of contact between victim and offender (ranging from distant, such as only contacting the victim through phone messages or mail, to actual face-to-face contact) all influenced the likelihood of violent behaviors. However, most of the associations between these variables, although statistically significant, were relatively small, leaving much of the variance in violent behaviors unexplained. Interestingly, they did not observe significant relationships between stalking-related violence and prior psychiatric history, criminal history, prior domestic violence, or threats to property or third parties, all variables that have been theorized to predict violence in stalking cases.

More recently, Rosenfeld and Harmon (2002) analyzed predictors of violence in a sample of 204 stalking offenders referred for court-ordered psychiatric evaluations. They found a number of significant predictors of violence, including demographic, clinical, and criminological variables. They found that several demographic predictors differentiated violent and nonviolent offenders, including age (offenders under 30 were more often violent compared to older offenders), race (white offenders were less likely to be violent than non-whites), and education (lower levels of education corresponded to higher rates of violence), although other variables such as gender did not. A number of psychiatric diagnoses were also associated with violence, including the presence of a psychotic disorder (associated with a *lower* rate of violence), a history of substance abuse (associated with a higher rate of violence), and the presence of a personality disorder (also associated with a higher rate of violence). In particular, cluster B disorders such as borderline, antisocial, or narcissistic personality disorder were associated with the highest rate of violence, and when these personality disorders were considered separately, other personality disorders (e.g., dependent, obsessive–compulsive, paranoid) were no longer associated with violence. Finally, a number of criminological variables differentiated violent and nonviolent offenders, including a criminal history unrelated to stalking, the presence of threats during the course of stalking, and a prior intimate relationship between offender and victim (associated with a higher rate of violence than stalkers who targeted acquaintances, strangers, or family members). Interestingly, a history of domestic violence was not associated with stalking-related violence in these analyses. When the authors entered the various predictors of violence into a multivariate model, they found that five variables (age, education, race, presence of threats, prior intimate relationship) provided unique, significant contributions to the prediction of stalking-related violence.

Rosenfeld (2004) recently used a meta-analysis to analyze predictors of violence across the emerging stalking literature. Analyzing results from 12 studies, he identified a number of risk factors for violence in stalking cases, including the presence of threats, a prior intimate relationship between victim and offender, and the presence of a substance abuse disorder. Psychotic stalkers, on the other hand, were significantly less likely to engage in violence across a number of different studies, likely due to the relative frequency of erotomanic delusions and therefore a romantic motivation on the part of these offenders. Interestingly, a number of violence risk factors that appear in other criminal justice populations, such as a prior history of violence or prior arrests (unrelated to stalking) were not associated with stalking-related violence in the extant literature. These findings led the author to conclude that risk assessment in stalking cases must be tailored to the specific population in question rather than relying on a literature developed in other criminal justice settings.

Not only are prior intimates more likely to be violent, but they may also be the subgroup most likely to renew their harassment after an initial arrest. Although clinical lore has typically cited erotomanics as the subgroup of stalkers who are most resistant to attempts to intervene, often maintaining their pursuit of the stalking target for many years, a recent study of stalking recidivism provided contradictory evidence. In the only published study of recidivism among stalking offenders to date, Rosenfeld (2003) found that delusional stalkers (many of whom had erotomanic delusions) were actually at a relatively low risk for reoffend-ing when considered as a group. Instead, those stalkers who targeted former intimate partners, and offenders diagnosed with a personality disorder (particularly borderline, narcissistic, or antisocial personality disorders) were significantly more likely to reoffend compared to other subgroups of offenders. In fact, the combination of a personality disor-der and substance abuse proved to be particularly problematic, as virtu-ally all of these offenders reoffended, often within an exceptionally brief period of time. Thus, clinical lore aside, offenders with a primary per-sonality disorder diagnosis and those with a history of substance abuse appear to be among the most problematic subset of stalking offenders.

THE IMPACT OF STALKING
ON PSYCHOLOGICAL FUNCTIONING

There is a near-unanimous consensus among social scientists that the im-pact of stalking on victims (or targets, as they are often referred to) can be profound and extreme (Mechanic, Uhlmansiek, Weaver, & Resick, 2000; Spitzberg & Cupach, 2003). Of course, the extent to which stalk-ing disrupts the lives of victims depends on a number of factors, includ-ing the severity and intrusiveness of the stalking behavior, the resources (both psychological and material) of the victim, and the extent of supports available to the victim. Early anecdotal reports described long-term, highly intrusive stalking scenarios in which an individual was targeted and harassed for many years (e.g., Orion, 1998). Despite seem-ingly extreme measures on the part of the victim—such as changing telephone numbers, relocating to another city, or even changing names—some stalkers manage to continue their harassment for extended periods of time. Even legal system interventions, which were admittedly weak before the emergence of anti-stalking laws, had little impact on the stalk-ing behaviors, as many offenders routinely violated orders of protection, sometimes even continuing their harassment *while incarcerated* (e.g., telephoning the victim from the jail pay phone).

Systematic studies of stalking victims, however, have been relatively infrequent, and those that have appeared have often relied on relatively idiosyncratic samples. For example, Kamphius and Emmelkamp (2001) described the psychological adjustment among 201 Dutch stalking vic-tims recruited through an anti-stalking organization. They solicited par-ticipants through newspaper advertisements, requesting they complete a series of self-report questionnaires assessing overall physical and psycho-logical health as well as trauma-related symptoms in particular. They found that the vast majority (97%) reported feeling afraid for their safety as a result of the stalking experience, and that actions such as changing telephone numbers and altering daily routines were common. They also found levels of trauma-related symptoms that were comparable to samples of patients who had suffered other forms of trauma. The characterization of stalking victims as traumatized has led some writers to posit a "stalking victimization syndrome" (Collins & Wilkas, 2001), although the evidence for such phenomena (particularly if the syndrome is presumed to be distinct from a more general posttraumatic stress disorder reaction) is still lacking.

Blaauw and colleagues (Blaauw, Winkel, Arensman, Sheridan, & Freeve, 2001) also studied psychological effects of stalking in a sample of 241 Dutch stalking victims. More than half of their respondents reported having been physically assaulted by the stalker, and symptoms such as anxiety, insomnia, depression, and somatic complaints were common among stalking victims. They characterized the mental health of these stalking victims as more comparable to psychiatric outpatient samples, although this finding may have reflected the sample methodology. Nevertheless, they found that the more intrusive stalking behaviors, such as following and theft/destruction of property, were associated with higher levels of psychological distress, and that the frequency and overall number of stalking behaviors experienced were significantly associated with higher levels of psychological distress. However, they did not find any association between victim–offender relationship or violence and psychological distress, suggesting that stalking can be highly distressing even when violence has not actually occurred.

SUMMARY

During the past decade, a substantial and diverse literature has explored the phenomena of stalking from a number of different perspectives. Epidemiological surveys have documented high rates of stalking behaviors, particularly among women, although prevalence rates have clearly varied in response to study methodology. Numerous studies have also identified characteristics, both demographic and clinical, of stalking offenders in an attempt to understand what leads individuals to engage in this behavior. This literature has also bolstered the growing set of clinical interventions, such as helping to guide violence risk assessment and helping develop effective victim-service interventions.

However, despite this rapidly growing stalking literature, a careful analysis reveals substantial and important gaps in our existing knowledge base. Very few studies have employed true experimental paradigms to understand either victim perceptions or the relative efficacy of alternative interventions. Although countless anti-stalking laws have been enacted over the past few years, no research has assessed the efficacy of these laws nor analyzed which variations are most successful. Indeed, a surprising proportion of the existing literature on stalking has relied on college student samples, despite obvious concerns as to the generalizability of these studies. Hence, countless questions remain, such as what psychological characteristics lead individuals to engage in stalking and what if anything can be done to reduce the frequency or psychological consequences of these acts. Until such questions are answered, the number of stalking victims will continue to increase and intervention efforts will remain haphazard.

NOTES

1. The term "cyberstalking" has been used to describe the use of the Internet, e-mail, or other electronic communication devices for the purpose of stalking/harassment (Merschman, 2001). Cyberstalkers may threaten or harass their victims via e-mail, in chat rooms, or through news groups and on message boards. They may also incite others to harass the victims by posting online messages (Packard, 2000). Although the phenomenon of cyberstalking has become an increasingly common topic among writers and clinicians, there is virtually no empirical research into this behavior.
2. Although this is not the focus of the current chapter, Tjaden and Thoennes (1998) also reported a "strong link" between stalking and domestic violence. According to their research, "81 percent of women who were stalked by a current or former husband or cohabiting partner were also physically assaulted by that partner and 31 percent were also sexually assaulted by that partner" (p. 2). (See Kaser-Boyd, Chapter 3, this volume, for a discussion of domestic violence.)
3. It should be noted that even if men perceive stalking as threatening, and do report it to the authorities, their complaints may be disproportionately minimized and not investigated seriously due to gender stereotyping.
4. In 10 states, harassment or stalking of a minor results in enhanced felony penalties In 12 states, a first offense resulting in conviction is automatically a felony, and in 23 states a first offense may be a felony. In the other 15 states, a first offense is a misdemeanor, but a repeated stalking offense is a felony (U.S. Department of Justice, 2001).
5. There have been suggestions of how to alleviate these legal problems in the various stalking laws. Noteworthy among these are Jordan's list of helpful elements to be included in a model stalking statute (Jordan et al., 2000, pp. 576–579). She recommends an objective standard of offender conduct; a general intent standard (the offender intended to engage in the conduct); making "following" per se stalking (whereas "harassment" would require nonconsent); a broadening of the "fear" requirement to include other negative reactions and use of an objective "reasonable" fear standard (so the crime is not dependent on the resilience of the victim); a broad definition of what the victim might fear; an aggravated level of stalking (for prior offenses, possession of a weapon, etc.); protective orders against stalkers; and a civil right of the victim to sue the stalker.

REFERENCES

Australian Bureau of Statistics. (1996). *Women's safety, Australia 1996.* Canberra: Commonwealth of Australia.

Bjerregaard, B. (2000). An empirical study of stalking victimization. *Violence and Victims, 15,* 389–405.

Blaauw, E., Winkel, F. S., Arensman, E., Sheridan, L., & Freeve, A. (2001). The toll of stalking: The relationship between features of stalking and psychopathology of victims. *Journal of Interpersonal Violence, 17,* 50–62.

Budd, T., & Mattinson, J. (2000). *Stalking: Findings from the 1998 British Crime Survey* (Research Findings No. 129). London: Home Office Research.

Collins, M. J., & Wilkas, M. B. (2001). Stalking trauma syndrome and the traumatized victim. In J. A. Davis (Ed.), *Stalking crimes and victim protection: Prevention, intervention, threat assessment, and case management* (pp. 317–334). Boca Raton, FL: CRC Press.

Cupach, W. R., & Spitzberg, B. H. (2000). Obsessive relational intrusion: Incidence, perceived severity, and coping. *Violence and Victims, 15,* 1–16.

Del Ben, K., & Fremouw, W. J. (2002). Stalking: Developing an empirical typology to classify stalkers. *Journal of Forensic Sciences, 47,* 152–158.

Dennison, S., & Thomson, D. M. (2002). Identifying stalking: The relevance of intent in common sense reasoning. *Law and Human Behavior, 26* 543–561.

Fremouw, W. J., Westrup, D., & Pennypacker, J. (1997). Stalking on campus: The prevalence and strategies for coping with stalking. *Journal of Forensic Science, 42,* 666–669.

Harmon, R., Rosner, R., & Owens, H. (1995). Obsessional harassment and erotomania in a criminal court population. *Journal of Forensic Sciences, 40,* 188–196.

Holmes, R. M. (2001). Criminal stalking: An analysis of the various typologies of stalkers. In J. A. Davis (Ed.), *Stalking crimes and victim protection: Prevention, intervention, threat assessment, and case management* (pp. 387–424). Boca Raton, FL: CRC Press.

Jordan, C. E., Quinn, K., Jordan, B., & Daileader, C. R. (2000). Stalking: Cultural, clinical, and legal considerations. *University of Louisville Brandeis Law Journal, 38,* 513–575.

Kamphius, J. H., & Emmelkamp, P. M. G. (2001). Traumatic distress among support-seeking female victims of stalking. *American Journal of Psychiatry, 158,* 795–798.

Lewis, S. F., Fremouw, W. J., Del Ben, K., & Farr, C. (2001). An investigation of the psychological characteristics of stalkers: Empathy, problem-solving, attachment and borderline personality features. *Journal of Forensic Sciences, 46,* 80–84.

Logan, T. K., Leukefeld, C., & Walker, B. (2000). Stalking as a variant of intimate violence: Implications from a young adult sample. *Violence and Victims, 15,* 91–111.

Mechanic, M. B., Uhlmansiek, M. H., Weaver, T. L., & Resick, P. A. (2000). The impact of severe stalking experienced by acutely battered women: An examination of violence, psychological symptoms, and strategic responding. *Violence and Victims, 15*, 443–458.

Meloy, J. R., & Gothard, S. (1995). A demographic and clinical comparison of obsessional followers and offenders with mental disorders. *American Journal of Psychiatry, 152*, 258–163.

Menzies, R., Federoff, J. P., Green, C., & Isaacson, K. (1995). Prediction of dangerous behavior in male erotomania. *British Journal of Psychiatry, 166*, 529–536.

Merschman, J. (2001). The dark side of the Web: Cyberstalking and the need for contemporary legislation. *Harvard Women's Law Journal, 24*, 255–277.

Miller, N. (2001). Stalking investigation, law, public policy, and criminal prosecution as problem solver. In J. A. Davis (Ed.), *Stalking crimes and victim protection: Prevention, intervention, threat assessment, and case management* (pp. 387–424). Boca Raton, FL: CRC Press.

Mullen, P. E., Pathé, M., & Purcell, R. (2000). *Stalkers and their victims.* Cambridge, UK: Cambridge University Press.

Mullen, P. E., Pathé, M., Purcell, R., & Stuart, G. W. (1999). Study of stalkers. *American Journal of Psychiatry, 156*, 1244–1249.

National Institute of Justice. (1993). Project to develop a model antistalking code for states. Washington, DC. Retrieved July 23, 2003, from *http://www.ojp. usdoj.gov/ocpa/94Guides/DomViol/welcome.html.*

Orion, D. (1998). *I know you really love me.* New York: Dell.

Packard, A. (2000). Does proposed federal cyberstalking legislations meet constitutional requirements? *Community Law and Policy, 5*, 505–519.

Palarea, R., Zona, M. A., Lane, J. C., & Langhinrichsen-Rohling, J. (1999). The dangerous nature of intimate relationship stalking: Threats, violence and associated risk factors. *Behavioral Sciences and the Law, 17*, 269–283.

Pappas, D. (1996). When a stalker's hot pursuit turns coldly calculated chase in Minnesota: How specific need expressions of intent be or do actions speak louder than words ? *Hamline Law Review, 20*, 371–393.

Phillips, L., Quirk, R., Rosenfeld, B., & O'Connor, M. (2004). Is it stalking? Perceptions of stalking among college undergraduates. *Criminal Justice and Behavior, 31*, 73–96.

Purcell, R., Pathé, M., & Mullen, P. E. (2001). A study of women who stalk. *American Journal of Psychiatry, 158*, 2056–2060.

Roberts, K. A. (2002). Stalking following the breakup of romantic relationships: Characteristics of stalking former partners. *Journal of Forensic Sciences, 47*, 1070–1077.

Rosenfeld, B. (2000). Assessment and treatment of obsessional harassment. *Aggression and Violent Behavior, 5*(6), 529–549.

Rosenfeld, B. (2003). Recidivism in stalking and obsessional harassment. *Law and Human Behavior, 27*, 251–265.

Rosenfeld, B. (2004). Violence risk factors in stalking and obsessional harassment: A review and meta-analysis. *Criminal Justice and Behavior, 31*, 9–36.

Rosenfeld, B., & Harmon, R. (2002). Factors associated with violence in stalking and obsessional harassment cases. *Criminal Justice and Behavior, 29*, 671–691.

Schwartz-Watts, D., & Morgan, D. (1998). Violent versus non-violent stalkers. *Journal of the American Academy of Psychiatry and Law, 26,* 241–245.

Schwartz-Watts, D., Morgan, D. W., & Barnes C. J. (1997). Stalkers: The South Carolina experience. *Journal of the American Academy of Psychiatry and Law, 25,* 541–545.

Spitzberg, B. H., & Cupach, W. R. (2003). What mad pursuit ? Obsessive relational intrusion and stalking related phenomena. *Aggression and Violent Behavior, 8,* 345–375.

Tjaden, P., & Theonnes, N. (1998). *Stalking in America: Findings from the National Violence Against Women Survey.* Washington, DC: National Institute of Justice Centers for Disease Control and Prevention.

U.S. Department of Justice. (2001). *Report to Congress on Stalking and Domestic Violence.* Washington, DC: Author.

Wiggens, B. (2000). Stalking humans: Is there a need for federalization of anti-stalking laws in order to prevent recidivism in stalking? *Syracuse Law Review, 50,* 1067–1112.

Zona, M., Sharma, K., & Lane, J. C. (1993). A comparative study of erotomanic and obsessional subjects in a forensic sample. *Journal of Forensic Sciences, 38,* 894–903.

6 Sexual Harassment in the Workplace

A Legal and Psychological Framework

MAUREEN O'CONNOR
BRIGITTE VALLABHAJOSULA

> His conversations were very vivid. He spoke about acts
> he had seen in pornographic films involving such matters
> as women having sex with animals and films showing
> group sex or rape scenes. He talked about pornographic
> materials depicting individuals with large penises or large
> breasts involved in various sex acts. On several
> occasions, [he] told me graphically of his own sexual
> prowess.[1]

The "conversations" described in the epigraph did not occur in the backroom of a bar nor on the set of a pornographic movie.
Rather, they occurred between now-Law Professor Anita Hill and now-
U.S. Supreme Court Justice Clarence Thomas when she worked as his
assistant at the Department of Education, and then at the Equal Employment Opportunity Commission (EEOC), the federal agency charged
with implementing sexual discrimination law, including the law against
sexual harassment. "Sexual harassment" is not a new phenomenon, nor
is it a rare occurrence. But the Hill/Thomas controversy brought it into
public consciousness in an unprecedented manner, sparking a national
debate and generating a sharp increase in EEOC complaints alleging sex-

115

ual harassment.[2] These increases can be quantified in various ways—claims more than doubled between 1991 and 1993 (Beiner, 1999); sexual harassment charges filed with the EEOC and state and local fair employment practice agencies increased by 150% in the 4 years after the Hill/Thomas hearings (Casellas, 1998); the proportion of discrimination claims based on sexual harassment increased from 40% of gender-based claims in 1991 to 64% of gender claims in 1999 (Goodman-Delahunty, 1999). According to Ross (1996), the percentage of companies reporting sexual harassment claims made within their organization increased from a little over half in 1991 to over 70% by 1995. In the years since those explosive hearings, psychologists, lawyers, and employers have focused tremendous energy and attention on sexual harassment. A veritable industry of consultants and experts now offer training and technical assistance to companies desperately trying to comply with changing sexual harassment law (Bisom-Rapp, 2001). But, yet, has consensus emerged about what constitutes sexual harassment? Have the courts articulated a clear path for employers and employees to follow? Have psychologists uncovered the answers to questions about the behavior underlying sexual harassment complaints?

This chapter provides an overview of the development of the legal protection against sexual harassment. More specifically, it will trace the development of the concept of sexual harassment from Catherine MacKinnon's (1979a) groundbreaking book in 1979, through the articulation of the legal cause of action by the EEOC, and finally, through the important U.S. Supreme Court cases that have given shape and form to sexual harassment as unlawful sexual discrimination. This legal overview also includes focused attention on the elements required to prove sexual harassment, as well as recent controversies in sexual harassment law in the workplace.[3] Additionally, this chapter highlights the psycholegal nature of sexual harassment, since virtually every feature of a legal claim of sexual harassment raises psychological questions that have been, or should be, the subject of psychological research and practice. Further, the most important contributions psychologists have made to the development of our understanding of sexual harassment are discussed as they relate to the legal claim of sexual harassment. In summary, this chapter provides the reader with a sound grasp of important legal doctrine and psychological knowledge about sexual harassment.

HOW BIG A PROBLEM IS SEXUAL HARASSMENT?

Sexual harassment is no longer an odd curiosity about which most Americans have only passing interest and less awareness. Allegations of

abusive social sexual conduct in the workplace are common in many settings touching the lives of workers ranging from blue-collar employees
to the powerful public officials . . . sexual harassment allegations are
part of the psychological reality of our culture and our times. (Wiener &
Gutek, 1999, p. 507)

As the quotation suggests, formal complaints filed with the EEOC
and in lawsuits around the country have increased substantially in the
last decade. But tracking formal complaints only tells us about the harassment that becomes public, and as we know from many areas of
crime reporting, unreported experiences outweigh those that are reported formally. In the case of sexual harassment, numerous efforts have
been undertaken to ascertain a reasonable prevalence level for the
behavior. In 1980, 1987, 1988, and 1994, the United States Merit Systems Protection Board (USMSPB) conducted extensive surveys in which
federal employees were asked if they had experienced any of the following unwanted behaviors while on the job: sexual teasing, jokes, remarks
or questions, sexual gestures or looks, leaning over, deliberate touching,
pinching or cornering, letters or telephone calls, pressure for dates or
sexual favors, or actual or attempted assault or rape (United States Merit
Systems Protection Board, 1995). In 1980, 42% of the women and 15%
of the men who responded reported experiencing sexual harassment on
the job. The corresponding percentages from the 1987 survey were 42%
of women and 14% of men, and from the 1994 survey, 44% of women
and 19% of men. The most often reported behaviors were sexual teasing, jokes, questions, or remarks followed by sexual looks or gestures,
deliberate touching, pinching, leaning over, or cornering. In the 1994
survey, 4% of women and 2.5% of men also reported attempted assault
or rape (United States Merit Systems Protection Board, 1995).

Later studies have found a range of prevalence rates across different
work environments. For example, in a survey of second-year residents
who were chosen randomly from an American Medical Association database, 63% of women reported at least one instance of sexual harassment or discrimination during their internship (Daugherty, Baldwin, &
Rowley, 1998). Similarly, O'Hare and O'Donohue (1998), in a survey of
students, staff, and faculty at a large Midwestern university, found that
69% of women reported having experienced at least one incident of gender harassment, 53% reported an experience of unwanted sexual attention, 12% acknowledged having felt it necessary to sexually cooperate
with a coworker in order to be treated adequately at work, and 6% reported having faced reprisals for refusing to cooperate sexually at work.
Almost 11% of this sample reported having been threatened for refusing
sexual cooperation, and 9% reported having been offered bribes for

their cooperation. Further, among a national sample of Canadian women, 51% had experienced at least one type of sexual harassment, while the average subject had experienced four different types of sexual harassment (Gruber, Smith, & Kauppinen-Toropainen, 1996). Also, a review of 18 research studies of public and private employees and university students in the United States and Canada yielded percentages from 28 to 75% of women experiencing some form of sexual harassment (Gruber, 1997). Sexual harassment, particularly the "hands-off" kind, appears to affect approximately 50% of women in the workplace in the industrialized nations that have participated in surveys, making sexual harassment one of the most common ways women are sexually victimized (Sbraga & O'Donohue, 2000).

But it is not only women who experience sexual harassment in the workplace. A survey of nearly 1,000 male workers found that just under 50% of the men had experienced at least one incident involving potential sexual harassment at work, and that other men were the perpetrators in over half of these incidents (Waldo, Berdahl, & Fitzgerald, 1998). Recent data suggest that upwards of 10% of reported claims of sexual harassment come from males. A 1999 survey reported that 81% of complaints involved female targets and male perpetrators, 9% involved male targets with female perpetrators, and 10% involved same-sex harassment (Society for Human Resources Management, 1999, cited in Grossman, 2003). Another study found that 5.4% of all sexual harassment lawsuits between 1986 and 1995 were brought by men (Juliano & Schwab, 2001). The EEOC's recent statistics show that 14.9% of charges filed with that agency are filed by male complainants, up from 9.1% in 1992 (see, generally, Grossman, 2003, note 9).

One of the significant challenges to the gathering of accurate prevalence and impact data is the failure of most measurement instruments to deal with the definition of sexual harassment. If no definition is provided by the researcher, then it is difficult to know by what standard people are responding. If a definition is provided, it may or may not correspond to the legal definitions set forth in the following sections.

DEFINITIONS OF SEXUAL HARASSMENT

Her boss often insulted her because of her gender and often made her the target of unwanted sexual innuendos. . . . in front of others, he suggested that the two of them "go to the Holiday Inn to negotiate [her] raise." He occasionally asked her and other female employees to get coins from his front pants pocket. He made sexual innuendos about her [. . .] clothing. [After a few months], she complained to him about his conduct. He said he was surprised that Harris was offended, claimed he was only joking, and apologized. (*Harris v. Forklift Systems, Inc.*, 510 U.S. 17, 20 (1993))

What is sexual harassment? How you answer that question depends on many things, not the least of which is knowing what definition you are using to decide, and perhaps, whether you are in a court of law or watching a daytime talk show. In any case, defining sexual harassment is not easy. While the behavior that now might be described as sexual harassment has been around for as long as people have worked together, the term itself has only been in use for approximately 30 years (Forell & Matthews, 2000). The term has described behaviors ranging from sexist jokes or untoward glances to rape. What one person perceives as "sexual harassment" another might see as harmless flirtation. The range of behaviors that are grouped together as sexual harassment exacerbates the problem of precision.

The first prominent attempt to define the term as a legal wrong came in 1979, in Catherine MacKinnon's (1979a) groundbreaking book, *Sexual Harassment of Working Women.*[4] In the book, MacKinnon clearly saw sexual harassment as a form of power over and domination of women by men. She defined the term as "the unwanted imposition of sexual requirements in the context of a relationship of unequal power" (p. 1). Since then, the concept has expanded beyond situations involving unequal power. Many would now agree that sexual harassment is manifested when sexual or sexualized behavior occurs that is inappropriate for the context and is unwanted by a participant or observer (Sbraga & O'Donohue, 2000). Yet, except for the most innocuous behaviors and the most serious, little consensus has emerged about what constitutes sexual harassment (see, for example, Epstein, Saute, Oglensky, & Gever, 1995).

Psychological efforts to define sexual harassment have tended to focus on the experience of victimization or level of offensiveness or trauma inherent in the behavior. One prominent sexual harassment scholar defined sexual harassment psychologically as "an unwanted sex-related behavior at work that is appraised by the recipient as offensive, exceeding her resources, or threatening her well-being" (Fitzgerald, Swan, & Magley, 1997, p. 20). Other scholars have focused less on precisely defining the concept and more on trying to categorize the behaviors that might be considered sexual harassment. Various categorizations have been developed. For example, Gruber (1992) categorized sexually harassing behaviors as follows: (1) pressure for dates/relationships, (2) sexual comments, (3) sexual posturing, (4) sexual touching, and (5) sexual assault. Similarly, in a number of investigations, Fitzgerald and her colleagues developed a model of sexual harassment that includes three types of behavior: (1) *gender harassment*, behavior that is insulting, hostile, and degrading, but not for the purpose of sexual cooperation; (2) *unwanted sexual attention*, behavior of a sexual nature that is unwelcome, offensive, and unreciprocated; and (3) *sexual coercion*, extortion of sexual cooperation in return for job-related considerations (see, for example, Fitzgerald, Gelfand, & Drasgow, 1995; Gelfand, Fitzgerald, & Drasgow, 1995; see also, Till, 1980). More recently, Rotundo, Nguyen, and Sackett (2001) also included acts such as obscene phone calls and belittling of the target's competence in their classification scheme of sexually harassing behaviors.

Another way to conceptualize sexual harassment is to think about an underlying theoretical/psychological framework that might explain the behavior. If we had a better grasp on *why* such behaviors occur, we might have a better chance at (1) defining it more precisely and (2) proscribing it more effectively. As early as 1981, Nieva and Gutek identified a number of psychological models that rested on differing assumptions or explanations for why sexual harassment would occur at the workplace (see also Gutek, 1985, pp. 12–18; Sbraga & O'Donohue, 2000). The following models may explain the development and maintenance of sexually harassing behavior:

Sociocultural Model

This model focuses on the larger political and social context in which sexual harassment occurs. Specifically, this model proposes that sexual harassment at work is an extension of male dominance in the society in which the organizations is embedded (MacKinnon, 1979b). It posits that many workers bring their stereotypes and gender roles into their workplace and that women and men are socialized for stereotyped interactions to occur. Men are expected to display aggressive and dominating behaviors, while women remain more passive; consequently, men view their behaviors as justified and natural, and disregard the negative consequences for women (Sbraga & O'Donahue, 2000).

Evolutionary Model

According to this model, sexual harassment is natural behavior that is the normal consequence of the stronger sex drive of men. This higher sex drive, in turn, results in sexually aggressive behavior at work. It is suggested that evolution has produced different reproductive strategies in women and men, which creates a conflict of interest that is played out in many workplaces. More specifically, men seek to maximize their reproductive success and, thus, emit sexually harassing behaviors in order to improve the probability of gaining sexual access to more females (Sbraga & O'Donahue, 2000).

Organizational Model

This model assumes that companies facilitate sexual harassment by creating situations and power hierarchies that set the stage for sexually harassing behavior to occur. As a result, individuals in positions of authority are provided with the opportunity to exploit workers in lower positions. This organizational model asserts that institutional power differentials and policies may create an environment ideally suited for the development and maintenance of sexually harassing behaviors.

Sex-Role-Spillover Model

According to Gutek and Morasch (1982), workers bring gender-based expectations for behavior into the workplace even though these beliefs may be inappropriate to it. Because gender identity is more salient than the worker identity, women and men may fall back on these gender-based expectations in their workplace. Thus, conflicts are more likely to arise in situations in which the work roles of the particular genders are discrepant with the sex-role stereotypes; situations in which gender is made more pronounced and is recognized over the work role. Therefore, women are more likely to experience sexually harassing behavior in non-traditional work situations (Sbraga & O'Donahue, 2000).

Person × Situation Model

According to Pryor and his associates (Pryor, Giedd, & Williams, 1995), men who have a propensity to sexually harass do so when they are in situations that prime a proponent connection between power and sex. Such men admit that under certain circumstances they would commit various types of sexual harassment; they do not, however, commit sexually harassing behavior all the time. Instead, their proclivities to harass become primed by certain situational cues, such as working in an environment where harassing behavior is condoned or at least not actively discouraged.

Despite these efforts to articulate a theoretical framework for understanding this behavior, overall the various models have been inadequately tested, and can be criticized as overly simplistic. To date much of the research has either sought to describe its prevalence among adults (e.g., Gruber, 1998; Welsh & Nierobisz, 1997; Williams, Giuffre, & Dellinger, 1999) or has asked about hypothetical scenarios rather than actual events (e.g., Barr, 1993; Katz, Hannon, & Whitten, 1996). Because of the inchoate state of sexual harassment research, basic questions of measurement and definition have only begun to take shape in the literature. Early measures of sexual harassment often lacked validity due to inconsistent question wording, a lack of exhaustive and mutually exclusive categories, and insufficient contextual information (Gruber, 1989; Welsh, 1999; Welsh & Nierobisz, 1997). Recent advances include behaviorally based survey questions, which reduce errors due to varying respondent interpretations, and measures that distinguish between quid pro quo and hostile work environment harassment[5] (Gruber, 1989; Welsh, 1999; Welsh & Nierobisz, 1997).

Despite these recent advances, there is "no unified theoretical framework" of sexual harassment (Welsh, 1999, p. 186), nor is there a universally accepted measure for it. One study, in fact, concluded that data have far outstripped theory, in both quantity and quality in the area of sexual harassment research (Gelfand et al., 1995). Existing theories that have been applied to sexual harassment tend to focus only on its occurrence, without considering the outcomes of harassment. Further, criminological theories as well as theoretical insights from the sociology of law have been underutilized in studies of sexual harassment (Welsh, 1999). Research also suggests that it is not just the societal norms and values, sex-role ideology, natural human design, and organizational policies that drive sexual harassment, but a complex combination of all of these factors. Indeed, according to O'Hare and O'Donahue (1998), a four-factor model taking into account the convergence of factors predicted sexual harassment better than any one of the other models alone.

These psychological efforts at definition and explanation are important to our nuanced understanding of the behavior we are calling sexual harassment. Nevertheless, ultimately, sexual harassment has become a *legal* wrong. And, because lay conceptualizations of behavior differ from legal definitions (see, for example, Gutek et al., 1999; Sbraga & O'Donohue, 2000), it is critically important to understand the legal framework for a sexual harassment claim.

The remainder of this chapter addresses the evolution of the concept of sexual harassment as a legal wrong under Title VII of the Civil Rights Act of 1964 (as amended). As is true for a number of the topics addressed in this book, behavior that had been tacitly accepted for many years, that can look otherwise innocuous to the outside eye, and which had no distinct nomenclature until fairly recently, is now unlawful under certain circumstances. The challenging, line-drawing task of determining lawful (though perhaps annoying or aggravating) versus unlawful behavior has proven to be particularly challenging for U.S. courts. MacKinnon (1979b) had it right when she recognized early on that "between the clear coercion and the clear mutuality, exists a murky area where power and caring converge. Here arises some of the most profound issues of sexual harassment, and those which the courts are least suited to resolve" (p. 54).

Since the promulgation of the EEOC's guidelines in 1980, the *legal* definition of sexual harassment has slowly taken shape through lower court struggles and several key U.S. Supreme Court decisions, which are discussed in some detail later,[6] though many unanswered questions remain. Yet, through the patchwork of cases and scholarship, we have been given guidance to structure our understanding of sexual harassment. We turn to an overview of the framework for determining sexual harassment under the law.

THE LEGAL FRAMEWORK
FOR SEXUAL HARASSMENT

Sexual inquiries, jokes, remarks, or innuendoes sometimes can raise the specter of coercion, but they more predictably have the effect of reminding a woman that she is viewed as an object of sexual derision rather than a credible coworker. . . . Treatment that sexualizes women workers prevents them from feeling, and prevents others from perceiving them, as equals in the workplace. (Abrams, 1989, pp. 1207–1208)

While sexually harassing behavior is not new, sexual harassment as a legal wrong is much more recent. Sex discrimination more broadly became unlawful under the antidiscrimination provisions of Title VII of the Civil Rights Act of 1964.[7] Title VII itself, however, contains no specific language prohibiting sexual "harassment." Instead, it prohibits "discriminat[ion] against any individual with respect to . . . compensation, terms, conditions, or privileges of employment, *because of such individual's . . . sex*."[8] Title VII was also directed toward challenges based on impermissible sex stereotypes, such as those present in *Price Waterhouse v. Hopkins*, 490 U.S. 228 (1989). In that case, Ms. Hopkins was not granted partnership at Price Waterhouse because of her "rough" edges and her need to attend "charm school," although she had met objective goals for performance and income generation. Social psychologist Dr. Susan Fiske played a crucial role in *Price Waterhouse*, explaining to the court through her expert testimony how these comments were likely the product of sex stereotyping which, the Court held, impermissibly influenced the firm's decision (see Fiske, Bersoff, Borgida, Deaux, & Heilman, 1991).

A narrow reading of Title VII might have restricted it to such equal treatment or stereotype analyses. Instead, however, through a series of important legal decisions beginning in 1976, the courts have interpreted the statute to include sexual harassment, slowly recognizing it as discrimination on the basis of sex within the meaning of Title VII.[9] In the first reported case, *Williams v. Saxbe*, 413 F. Supp. 654 (D.D.C. 1976), the plaintiff alleged that she had had a good working relationship with her supervisor until she refused his sexual advance, and thereafter she suffered unwarranted reprimands and refusals to respond properly to her work, and was treated as not competent. The court struggled even with these facts, because Title VII was not intended to prohibit all boorish behavior (which this clearly was), but rather *discriminatory* behavior. The defendant here argued that anyone, whether male or female, who refused the sexual advances of a supervisor would have received the same treatment as this plaintiff, so it was not *discrimination* "because of . . . sex" as required by Title VII. While this argument held some appeal, the court ultimately concluded that Congress had intended to prohibit behavior that had the effect of creating an "artificial barrier to employment which was placed before one gender and not the other despite the fact that both genders were similarly situated" (p. 658), and here, the plaintiff faced barriers because of her supervisor's behavior.

Four years later, the EEOC issued guidelines for how to deal with sexual harassment under Title VII, guidelines that (as amended) are still in use today. The guidelines defined sexual harassment as follows:

> unwelcome sexual advances, requests for sexual favors, and other verbal or physical conduct of a sexual nature constitute sexual harassment when (1) submission to such conduct is made either explicitly or implicitly a term or condition of an individual's employment, (2) submission to or rejection of such conduct by an individual is used as the basis for employment decisions affecting such individual, or (3) such conduct has the purpose or effect of unreasonably interfering with an individual's work performance or creating an intimidating, hostile, or offensive working environment. (Section 703)

While the courts are not required to follow agency guidelines such as these in deciding particular cases, they have generally deferred to the expertise of the EEOC and have relied upon these guidelines as the starting point for analysis in any case. The crucial feature of this definition is that it essentially delineates two types of sexual harassment: *quid pro quo* and hostile work environment sexual harassment.[10]

Quid Pro Quo Sexual Harassment

Classic *quid pro quo* harassment occurs when a supervisor grants or withholds a job benefit based on a subordinate's (un)willingness to comply with sexual advances (*Burlington Industries, Inc. v. Ellerth*, 524 U.S. 742, 753-754 (1998)). The following facts paint a clear picture of this form of harassment. A woman whom we will call Norma is hired by a hotel restaurant to work the day shift. This necessitates her working closely with the restaurant manager, James. Several weeks after she started, James began to make sexual advances toward her, verbally and in writing. He wrote her notes and letters, pressing them into her hand when she was serving, placing them inside menus that she distributed to patrons of the restaurant, or slipping them into her purse. He telephoned her at home or at work and made sarcastic, leering comments about her personal and sexual life. Norma was frightened and embarrassed by this behavior. She continually rejected James's suggestions and rebuffed his advances by telling him that she was not interested in him personally, and that his suggestions and advances were distressful and unwanted. With no positive response from her, the explicit sexual advances ceased after several months, but then the employment atmosphere and working conditions became difficult and very uncomfortable. She was excluded from meetings of the staff; James lied to the other staff about her, and made it difficult for her to perform her job. The company refused to fire him or even change his shifts, so Norma quit and filed her lawsuit (for a case with similar facts, see, *Rogers v. Loews L'Enfant Plaza Hotel*, 526 F. Supp. 523 (D.C.D.C., 1981)). The courts recognized this form of harassment early on and have had less difficulty dealing with these claims.

Hostile Work Environment Sexual Harassment

In contrast to *quid pro quo* harassment, the courts had more difficulty identifying the discriminatory nature of a hostile work environment. It was not until 1986 that the U.S. Supreme Court stated affirmatively that a hostile work environment could give rise to a Title VII violation, extending a well-established axiom from racial and national origin discrimination cases that "Title VII affords employees the right to work in an environment free from discriminatory intimidation, ridicule, and insult" (*Meritor Savings Bank v. Vinson*, 477 U.S. 57, 65 (1986); see also *Harris v. Forklift Systems, Inc.*, 510 U.S. 17 (1993)).

In *Meritor*, the Court held that hostile work environment harassment occurs when an employee is subjected to *unwelcome sexual con-*

duct that is *sufficiently severe or pervasive* as to *alter the conditions* of the victim's employment and create an *abusive working environment*. A number of recent class action lawsuits exemplify the types of situations that have given rise to successful hostile work environment claims, and demonstrate that, unfortunately, hostile work environments are not a thing of the past. The accusations included the following:

- The workplace was a place where women were propositioned, told their place is in the home, and confronted by pornographic pictures affixed to male workers' toolboxes (Lawsuit filed in 2003 against the U.S. Mint).
- On the factory floor, some men felt free to grope women or to ask them to bare their breasts. Men would display lewd photographs and commonly refer to women in the crudest of terms. (Class action and private lawsuits against Mitsubishi Corporation ended in 1998 with $44 million in settlements).

A number of the elements of any legal claim of sexual harassment (whether *quid pro quo* or hostile work environment) have posed particular challenges to both the legal system and to psychologists trying to study and inform that system. These are discussed here.

CHALLENGING FEATURES
OF SEXUAL HARASSMENT LAW

A legal claim of unlawful workplace sexual harassment is in large part a factual claim at the heart of which is the contest of credibility. (Burns, 1995, p. 194)

People who bring a sexual harassment claim bear the initial burden of establishing a number of key elements in their sexual harassment case. More specifically, the person bringing a sexual harassment law suit, the plaintiff, must establish three basic elements of the claim: (1) that the plaintiff was subjected to "unwelcome conduct," (2) that the conduct was based upon sex, and (3) that it caused harm. Each part of the legal requirement of sexual harassment must be shown by a preponderance of the evidence (which essentially means that it is more likely than not), while the defendant need only disprove one part of the legal test in order to prevail. These requirements apply whether the underlying behavior fits within either *quid pro quo* or hostile work environment sexual harassment. In hostile work environment claims, the legal standard for proof of harm is that the conduct was "sufficiently severe or pervasive" to alter the conditions of the work environment or to be abusive (Burns, 1995). Each of these challenging elements contain significant psychological content as well as having legal parameters set by case law, and are examined in turn.

"Unwelcome" Conduct

> Testimony was adduced to the effect that the plaintiff initiated conversations with co-workers, including [the defendant], as to topics of a sexual nature. Further, [the defendant] and other witnesses testified that many of the crude and explicit comments that plaintiff claimed were made by defendant (and several of which he admitted) followed equally crude and explicit comments by the plaintiff. (*Socks-Brunot v. Hirschvogel, Inc.*, 184 F.R.D. 113 (1999)).

Can a person who engages in the type of sexual banter described in this quotation be a victim of sexual harassment? Was the behavior here "unwelcome"? The concept of "unwelcomeness" of the alleged sexual advances, which has been called the "gravamen of any sexual harassment claim" by the U.S. Supreme Court (*Meritor*, p. 68) was designed to distinguish between consensual relationships in the workplace and unlawful sexual harassment. But, does it do so? In practice, at least, it has had a number of unintended consequences for sexual harassment plaintiffs. First, it has often had the effect of "putting the victim on trial," focusing attention on the victim's behavior before and during the harassment rather than on the accused harasser's conduct (Burns, 1995, p. 196). Second, it has opened the door to inquiry into the plaintiff's prior sexual conduct, abuse, and even mental health history. Third, it has placed a premium on the plaintiff's postharassment behavior, particularly whether the plaintiff formally complained about the offending behavior.

> Given their recent vintage, sexual harassment suits presented unique opportunities to shape the cause of action with a heightened awareness of the traditional sexist doctrines which the feminist efforts to reform rape laws highlighted. The fact that many federal courts jettison such opportunities daily, that the worst of rape litigation stands more as an example followed than one rejected, is the most persuasive and painful evidence of the durability of sexism in the law's judgment of the sexual relations of men and women. (Estrich, 1991, p. 816)

As Burns (1995) thoughtfully explained, so much of a successful sexual harassment claim turns on whether the plaintiff can tell a credible story. In our own research, the credibility of the plaintiff is an important predictor of sexual harassment judgments (see, for example, O'Connor, Gutek, Stockdale, Geer, & Melançon, 2004). While the importance of a coherent story is true in many cases (see Pennington & Hastie, 1991), it is especially true in the he said–she said world of unwanted versus consensual sexual conduct.[11] Whether the plaintiff is deemed to be telling a credible story of harassment may turn less on whether she said "no" or told the harasser that the conduct made her uncomfortable and more on the match between her claim and her behavior before and during the alleged offending behavior.

This issue is highly reminiscent of the battle that has been waged against probing the *victim's* behavior in sexual assault cases. As one prominent legal scholar remarked: "unwelcomeness has emerged as the doctrinal stepchild of the rape standards of consent and resistance, and shares virtually all of their problems" (Estrich, 1991, p. 827). There, "consent" of the victim was a defense to sexual assault charges. Here, although "voluntariness" in the sense of consent is not a defense to a sexual harassment claim (according to *Meritor* p. 825), a complainant's behavior, speech, and dress are relevant as a matter of law in determining whether the conduct was unwelcome (*Meritor*; see also Burns, 1985; Stockdale, O'Connor, Gutek, & Geer, 2002).

Another avenue that defendants pursue for discrediting a plaintiff's claim that the conduct was unwelcome is to investigate the plaintiff's *prior* sexual life or mental status (Stockdale et al., 2002). Focus on a complainant's prior sexual experiences (unwanted or otherwise) or her mental health could, it is argued, be relevant to determining whether a current workplace interaction constitutes consensual social relations or unwanted sexual advances. It could also, however, be used to discredit or discourage a plaintiff from proceeding with the lawsuit (Estrich, 1991, p. 828–829). As a result, Congress revised the federal rape shield laws in 1994. Federal Rule of Evidence 412 now bars the admission of evidence offered to prove that the victim engaged in other sexual behavior or to prove the victim's sexual predisposition, (Fed. R. Evid. 412(a)(1)–(2)), unless the probative value outweighs the danger of harm to the victim and of unfair prejudice to any party (Fed. R. Evid. 412(b)(2)). However, such case-by-case determinations do not provide much solace either to plaintiffs concerned about public exposure of their past or to defendants who are trying to defend against accusations from a plaintiff whom they believe welcomed their advances.

In its policy guidelines, the EEOC has stated that the best way for a woman to prove that the conduct was unwelcome is by *complaining* immediately. Recent U.S. Supreme Court decisions have placed additional emphasis on this requirement, particularly in relation to whether an employer will be held liable for the acts of its employees or agents, which are discussed later ("Employer Liability").

Consider the following exchange during the Clarence Hill confirmation hearings:

> SENATOR SPECTER: . . .understanding of the fact that you're 25 and that it's your—you're shortly out of law school and the pressure that exist in this world. . . . But even considering all of that, given your own expert standing and the fact there you have the chief law enforcement officer of the country on this subject and whole purpose of civil rights law is being perverted right in the office of the Chairman with one of his own female subordinates—what went through your mind, if anything, on whether you ought to come forward at that stage, because if you had you'd stop this man from being head of the EEOC perhaps for another decade. What went through your mind? I know you decided not to make a complaint, but did you give that any consideration, and if so how could you allow this kind of reprehensible conduct to go on right in the headquarters without doing something about it? (Clarence Thomas confirmation: Hearing of the Senate Judiciary Committee, 102d Congress, October 11, 1991).

> MS. HILL: That's a very good question. And I'm sure that I cannot answer that to your satisfaction. That is one of the things that I have tried to do today. I have suggested that I was afraid of retaliation. I was afraid of damage to my professional life. And I believe that you have to understand that response—and that's one of the things that I have come to understand about harassment—this response, this kind of response, is not atypical. And I can't explain. It takes an expert in psychology to explain how that can happen. But it can happen, because it happened to me. (Clarence Thomas confirmation: Hearing of the Senate Judiciary Committee, 102d Congress, October 11, 1991)

Professsor Hill has it at least partially correct—psychologists have demonstrated that it is not necessarily a typical reaction to affirmatively complain about sexual harassment (Brooks & Perot, 1991; DuBois, Knapp, Faley, & Kustis, 1998; Gutek, 1985; Schneider, Swan, & Fitzgerald, 1997; research summarized by Gutek & Koss, 1993), though it is not as clear that we can explain *how* it happens in these various ways (see Fitzgerald, Swan, & Fischer, 1995). Fitzgerald, Swan, and Fischer (1995) explain that no one response strategy is the norm, that both internal versus external responses are common. They describe two types of responses in addition to the active complainer who does go through established channels and makes a formal complaint. Other typical responses include the "silent tolerator," who simply puts up with the behavior until the breaking point and who then leaves the organization and brings a lawsuit; the "instigator-in-kind" who goes along with the behavior and even, perhaps, participates in it to a point, and then reaches a breaking point as well. These responses, though perhaps typical psychologically, pose serious challenges legally because they seriously undermine the target's claim that she did not "welcome" the behavior.

In addition to the many reasons for choosing not to complain, a woman may have difficulty naming the behavior when it occurred (sometimes the conduct involves sexual innuendo and ambiguity) (Kidder, Lafleur, & Wells, 1995).

"Because of . . . Sex"

Title VII is an anti*discrimination* law. It does not prohibit all boorish behavior in the workplace or elsewhere. It specifies "sex" as one of the protected categories within its reach, such that harassment not based on sex (or race, religion, color, or national origin) is not actionable under Title VII. Consequently, a plaintiff who seeks to bring a Title VII claim for harassment must first establish that the harassment was because of his or her membership in the protected class.

The key inquiry in determining whether sexual harassment was "because of . . . sex" is whether members of one sex have been subjected to unwelcome conduct or disadvantageous conditions of employment to which members of the opposite sex were not subjected (see *O'Shea v. Yellow Technical Services*, 185 F.3d 1093 (10th Cir. 1999); *Harris*).

Early on in the development of sexual harassment law, some defendants argued that general sexualized environments, while inappropriate, perhaps, were not sex-based discrimination because they were not aimed at the individual women workers (see, for example, *Robinson v. Jacksonville Shipyards, Inc.*, 760 F. Supp. 1486 (M.D. Fla. 1991)). As Burns (1995) explains, however, this argument was effectively defeated by compelling psychological expert testimony on sex stereotyping. Such evidence included the presence of factors that make it more likely that stereotyping will occur, including the proportion of women in the workforce, priming (or features in the environment that make sex stereotypes more salient), an unprofessional ambience, and the absence of clear company norms that would make such conduct unprofessional (Burns, 1995, p. 199; see generally Deaux, 1995; Gutek, 1985).

More recently, courts have had little difficulty finding that the "because of . . . sex" requirement is satisfied when the victim and the harasser are of the opposite sex, either because it is assumed that the conduct was motivated by sexual desire, or because the manner in which the harasser treated members of the respective sexes, in the absence of

sexual advances, showed that the sexual harassment occurred on the basis of sex (see *Oncale v. Sundowner Offshore Services, Inc.*, 523 U.S. 75
(1998)).

The challenge for the courts based on this requirement, then, has
come in the more recently evolving same-sex harassment cases. The U.S.
Supreme Court first dealt with the issue of whether same-sex harassment
could come within the antidiscrimination framework at all in *Oncale* in
1998. In that case, a man worked as a roustabout on an all-male, eight-
person crew on an offshore oil rig. According to his allegations, he was
forcibly subjected to sex-related, humiliating actions against him by coworkers and supervisors. The issue in the case was whether same-sex harassment qualified under Title VII's proscriptions against hostile environment sexual harassment. The Court said "yes," stating that a
plaintiff in a same-sex case must prove that the conduct "was not merely
tinged with offensive sexual connotations, but actually constituted discrimination *because of sex*," considering the "social context in which
particular behavior occurred and was experienced by its target" (*Oncale*,
p. 81, emphasis added).[12]

How, then, does one show that the discrimination is because of sex
when all parties are of the same sex? Since discrimination based on sexual orientation is *not* prohibited under Title VII, at least one court has
said that the "because of . . . sex" requirement must mean something
different than "because of . . . sexual orientation" (see, for example,
Dandan v. Radisson Hotel Lisle, 2000 WL 336528 (N.D. Ill. March 28,
2000)).[13] No doubt, it will be quite some time before this latter requirement is fully understood and its implications are clear.

Harm Caused by Sexual Harassment

> As a result of Mr. Hardy's behavior, Ms. Harris became extremely anx-
> ious, embarrassed, and would sometimes shake uncontrollably. She in-
> dicated that she did not want to go to work, that she could not sleep, that
> she cried and drank frequently, and that her relationships with her fam-
> ily had become strained. Her physician prescribed tranquilizers and
> sleeping pills for her, noting her high level of anxiety. (Paetzold &
> O'Leary-Kelly, 1996, pp. 97–98, describing the plaintiff in *Harris*)

It is, by now, well accepted that exposure to some forms of sexual
harassment can be harmful to the individual (psychologically, physically,
somatically) as well as to the organization (in terms of lost productivity,
turnover, and litigation).[14] Yet, not every wayward glance, even if "unwelcome" and given "because of" the target's sex will be considered a
sufficiently legal harm to justify liability for sexual harassment in the le-

gal system (Hanisch, 1996). After describing the basics about individual consequences of the behavior, this chapter turns to a discussion of the legal parameters for translating that harm into legal liability and remedy.

Psychological Consequences

Sexual harassment has significant personal and professional consequences (see Gutek & Koss, 1993). Specifically, victims of sexual harassment may develop psychological and somatic symptoms that mirror those of victims of other types of sexual assaults (Kilpatrick, Dansky, & Saunders, 1994). Indeed, victims often report depression, anxiety, irritability anger, uncontrolled crying, fatigue, headaches, weight loss, gastrointestinal and dental problems, confusion, shame, guilt, embarrassment, denial, and isolation (Dansky & Kilpatrick, 1997; Gutek & Koss, 1993; Jorgenson & Wahl, 2000). Research has also shown that the lifetime risk of developing posttraumatic stress disorder (PTSD) or major depression is significantly higher for female victims of sexual harassment than for women who report never having been harassed (Dansky & Kilpatrick, 1997). Further, the effect of sexual harassment on the mental status of victims is long lasting. More specifically, one-tenth of sexual harassment victims in Dansky and Kilpatrick's (1997) study had PTSD, and one in five victims showed depression after an average of 11 years since the harassment incidents. In addition, victims report decreased job performance and job satisfaction, disruption in their careers, and adversely affected earning potentials (Dansky & Kilpatrick, 1997; Gutek & Koss, 1993).

PTSD also provides a viable explanation for the reluctance of many victims of sexual harassment to report that behavior. PTSD is experienced by individuals in situations "following exposure to an extreme traumatic stressor involving direct personal experience of an event that involves actual or threatened death or serious injury, or other threats to one's physical integrity" (American Psychiatric Association, 1994, p. 424). Included in the types of injuries or threats that can lead to PTSD are sexual assaults and physical attacks, both of which are experienced by victims of sexual harassment (see, for example, *Nichols v. American National Insurance Co.*, 154 F.3d 875 (8th Cir. 1998)(attempted rape); *Gretzinger v. University of Hawaii*, 156 F.3d 1236 (1998) (plaintiff sexually assaulted on numerous occasions)). A person suffering from PTSD "commonly makes deliberate efforts to avoid thoughts, feelings, or conversations about the traumatic event, and to avoid activities, situations, or people who arouse recollections of it (American Psychiatric Association, 1994, pp. 424–425).[15]

Even assuming that a target can show that particular conduct was unwelcome and that she was subjected to it because of her sex, she must also demonstrate that some harm resulted from it. Determining "harm" encompasses a number of considerations. What types of behavior will satisfy the harm requirement? *Quid pro quo* harassment is generally assumed to be harmful (Burns, 1995), whereas hostile work environment harms are more complicated to discern. How hostile or abusive does an environment have to be? And, from whose perspective?

Legal Framework

SCOPE OF THE HARM REQUIREMENT

The U.S. Supreme Court addressed the question of legal harm in 1993. In that case, *Harris v. Forklift Systems*, 510 U.S. 17 (1993), the Court held that a plaintiff need not demonstrate a tangible psychological injury in order to prove a sexual harassment claim. The effects described in the quotation opening this section on "Harm Caused by Sexual Harassment" had been described by the district court as no doubt resulting from Ms. Harris's supervisor's annoying behavior, but that court did not believe that harm was significant enough to cause tangible psychological injury, which was the standard in that federal circuit at the time. In rejecting such a strict requirement, the U.S. Supreme Court noted that "Title VII comes into play before the harassing conduct leads to a nervous breakdown" (*Harris*, p. 22). So long as the environment could reasonably be perceived, and is perceived, as abusive or hostile, "there is no need for it also to be psychologically injurious" (*Harris*, p. 22). Though the Court conceded that this is not a particularly precise, mathematical standard, it concluded that it was a fair interpretation of Title VII's intent.

LEVEL OF HARM REQUIRED IN HOSTILE WORK ENVIRONMENT CASES

> Ms. Jones alleged that while she was employed by the state . . . , the governor of that state summoned her to a hotel room, where the alleged harassment took place. . . . [He then] attempted to grope her and then exposed himself while asking her to perform a sex act. (Allred & West, 1998)

The incident described in this quotation took place over the course of 15 minutes. One of the crucial issues in that case was whether a one-time, relatively short encounter could be *sufficiently* severe or pervasive to state a claim of hostile work environment sexual harassment—even if the defendant was the then-Governor of Arkansas and later President of the United States! This challenging component of sexual harassment law raises two issues: First, what behaviors are sufficiently severe or pervasive to be illegal, and second, from whose perspective should that determination be made?

What Is a Sufficiently *Severe or Pervasive Hostile Work Environment?* "Not all offensive workplace behavior violates the law" (*Smith v. Sheahan*, 189 F.3d 529, 534 (7th Cir. 1999)). According to the EEOC, the behavior must alter the conditions of employment and create an abusive working environment to give rise to a claim of sexual harassment. To determine whether that has occurred, courts look at whether the harassment was "sufficiently severe or pervasive to alter the conditions of employment and create an abusive working environment" (*Meritor*, pp. 57, 67).

How does one determine whether the offensive conduct is "*sufficiently* severe or pervasive" to constitute discrimination? What is "sufficient"? Courts have treated this as a question of fact, not as a precisely drawn line, thereby necessitating a review of all of the circumstances in the case (*Williams v. General Motors Corp.*, 187 F.3d 553 (6th Cir. 1999); *Harris* (1993)). In *Harris*, the Court articulated relevant factors for consideration, which include (1) the frequency of the discriminatory conduct, (2) its severity, (3) whether it was physically threatening or humiliating, or a mere offensive utterance, and (4) whether it unreasonably interfered with an employee's work performance. So, for example, one particularly egregious act (such as sexual assault) might be sufficient legally, whereas one minor act (one sexual insult) might not. Alternatively, numerous and repeated minor acts (a daily barrage of relatively minor, yet offensive comments) over a long period of time might be sufficient, whereas sporadic, occasional rude jokes might not.

Nonetheless, translating these commonsense requirements into legal decision making has proven problematic in many cases. In general, the more severe the behavior, the less frequently it needs to occur in order to be found sexually harassing. Whereas one instance of sexual assault may be considered sexual harassment, less egregious behaviors, such as sexual jokes and remarks, would need to occur frequently over a period of time. It is not possible, however, to categorize behaviors as always being severe or pervasive enough to meet the legal test. Instead, the court will examine the personal and professional relationship between the parties, the reactions of the plaintiff and other workers to the behavior, the nature and atmosphere of the workplace, and the male–female ratio.

From Whose Perspective Is Harm Evaluated? In determining severity and pervasiveness, whose perspective is relevant? If it is the plaintiff or target of the behavior, then some might argue that such a standard would not be fair to the defendant if that particular plaintiff is especially sensitive and would find a wayward glance to be sexually harassing (what one court called concerns for the "hypersensitive plaintiff," *Ellison v. Brady*, 924 F.2d 871 (9th Cir. 1991)). Yet, if it required the harasser's intent to harass, no self-respecting harasser would admit to this and short of that, it would be difficult to prove. The courts have attempted to resolve this issue by developing a two-pronged approach to this question. First, the target of the behavior must subjectively perceive the environment to be harassing to her (or him) (*Harris*). Second, that environment must have been sufficiently severe or pervasive from an objective perspective, from the perspective of a reasonable person, to have altered the conditions of the workplace (*Faragher v. City of Boca Raton*, 524 U.S. 775 (1998)). This guards against that hypersensitive plaintiff by providing a legal buffer that juries or judges can use to measure the behavior—would a reasonable person in that same situation have felt sexually harassed?

One of the issues that developed because of this approach is the question of whether male jurors and judges (not to mention employers, workers, and lawyers) would be able to take the perspective of a reasonable person in such a way that they would truly understand a woman's experience in a sexual harassment situation. Having been criticized for using the "reasonable person" standard, which was in effect still very much a "reasonable *man*" standard, some courts have shifted the inquiry to a "reasonable *woman*" standard when the victim is female (see, e.g., *Ellison v. Brady*, 924 F.2d 872 (9th Cir. 1991)). No doubt, what a man might find "harmless and innocent," a reasonable woman may find "highly offensive" (see Gutek, 1985). Indeed, while men and women agree that sexual coercion constitutes sexual harassment, they do not necessarily agree that sex-stereotyped jokes or repeated requests for dates after refusal do constitute it (Gutek & O'Connor, 1995; Rotundo et al., 2001). Thus, a woman may perceive that sexual harassment has occurred after a number of the more harmless types of social-sexual behaviors have taken place, whereas a man may be less inclined to do so (Rotundo et al., 2001). Further, research evidence indicates that men's and women's perceptions of sexual harassment are influenced by the position or role of the harasser relative to the harassee (e.g., supervisor, peer, subordinate) (Rotundo et al., 2001). Less severe or more ambiguous behaviors seem to generate the greatest gender difference and are more common than the more extreme forms (Frazier, Cochran, & Olson, 1995; Gutek & O'Connor, 1995). However, when social-sexual behaviors are so benign that they are not harassment, the gender gap closes (Gutek & O'Connor, 1995).

Courts have taken different approaches to this question, some relying on the reasonable woman standard and others on the reasonable person (Gutek et al., 1999). The U.S. Supreme Court has yet to formally rule on the proper standard, though it has continued to refer to the "reasonable person" (see, e.g., *Harris*, 1993). Meanwhile, psychologists have demonstrated that at least for mock jurors, the reasonable woman standard by itself may have only a small impact on verdicts (see Gutek et al., 1999; Wiener et al., 2002). These perspective issues, paired with evidence that women define a wider range of behaviors as harassing, or with evidence that many men are also sexually harassed, may eventually give rise to the implementation of a refined legal standard that focuses on the point of view of a more-nuanced reasonable victim.

EMPLOYER LIABILITY

Why does sexual harassment persist despite nearly three decades of attempts to eliminate it? While courts have developed a comprehensive set of legal rules governing workplace harassment, the incidence of harassment has not changed. That is true, in part, because the rules of employer liability for harassment are calculated to ensure that employers adopt basic policies and procedures with respect to workplace harassment, not, surprisingly, to ensure that they actually prevent it. (Grossman, 2003, p. 3)

Assume that all three of the elements of a sexual harassment case have been shown (unwelcome conduct, engaged in because of target's sex, causing harm). The question then arises, who should pay for the harm caused by the harassment?[16] Sexual harassment is treated as a civil, rather than a criminal, wrong (Stein, 1999). As such, people who believe they have been sexually harassed may bring lawsuits to receive monetary damages (for lost wages, psychological harm) and orders from the court to be compensated for other harms they have suffered, such as loss of the job.[17] Of course, some sexually harassing behavior might also run afoul of criminal laws (e.g., sexual assault), and in that situation, a perpetrator might also be prosecuted for the crime.[18] But the victim's primary recourse is through a civil lawsuit. And, if anyone is to pay damages, it is almost always the employer, rather than the individual perpetrator.

But when is an employer liable for the sexually harassing acts of its employees? This question has been a vexing one for the courts, which, until recently, had only vague agency principles to guide them (employers would be liable for harms caused by employees acting "within the scope" of their employment). In a series of decisions in the late 1990s, the U.S. Supreme Court dealt directly with the issue of employer liability for the sexually harassing behavior of its supervisors and employees and developed a set of clearer rules (see *Burlington Industries, Inc. v. Ellerth*, 524 U.S. 742 (1998); *Faragher v. City of Boca Raton*, 524 U.S. 775 (1998); see also *Kolstad v. American Dental Association*, 527 U.S. 526 (1999)). Where an employee has suffered some tangible harm in the workplace (demotion, termination, etc.) because of a supervisor's harassing behavior, the employer has no real defense to the lawsuit even if the employer technically was not aware of the harassment by the supervisor. It will be held vicariously liable for the actions of that supervisor, the idea being that an employer is ultimately responsible for hiring, training, and supervising that supervisor, and the supervisor only has the power to grant or withhold job benefits *because of* his supervisory power.[19]

Where a harassed employee has *not* suffered any adverse action on the job, however, the rules are slightly different.[20] The Supreme Court, in *Faragher* and *Burlington* enunciated a two-pronged affirmative defense to liability that is available to the employer in those situations when the targeted employee has suffered no tangible loss (in other words, the employee had to endure the harassment, but was not demoted, fired, or otherwise adversely affected in terms of employment benefits). An employer seeking to assert this defense must demonstrate that (1) it exercised reasonable care in preventing or promptly correcting any sexually harassing behavior; and (2) the employee unreasonably failed to take advantage of the preventive and/or corrective opportunities offered by the employer, or otherwise failed to avoid the harm.

The EEOC has suggested that reasonable care "generally requires an employer to establish, disseminate, and enforce an anti-harassment policy and complaint procedure and to take other reasonable steps to prevent and correct harassment" (Equal Employment Opportunity Commission, Enforcement Guidance on Vicarious Employer Liability for Unlawful Harassment by Supervisors, EEOC Notice No. 915-002, 14 (1999)). The presence or absence of a sexual harassment policy is not a guaranteed defense, but employers are being advised to have one in place. This has led to an increased focus on so-called "zero-tolerance" policies, which are now considered by some to be the "lynchpin" to preventing and defending sexual harassment claims (Powers, Kinder, & Keeney, 1999).[21] However, there is little empirical evidence for the effectiveness of such policies, and they may in fact allow employers to mask existing harassment problems in the workplace (Stockdale, Bisom-Rapp, O'Connor, & Gutek, 2004). They are more likely serving as liability-prevention strategies rather than sexual harassment elimination strategies.

In addition, an employer may still be able to avoid liability if the harassed employee fails to complain of the harassment (*Madray v. Publix Super Mkts., Inc.*, 30 F. Supp. 2d 1371 (S.D. Fla. 1998)). This is important because, at least in part, it places the onus on the affected employee to take "proper" action in response to harassment—to assertively complain. Yet, as was discussed earlier, psychological evidence suggests that targets of sexual harassment respond in varied ways. Failure to complain may itself be reasonable, if the harasser is the plaintiff's direct supervisor or an individual responsible for administering the sexual harassment policy (*Wilson v. Tulsa Junior College*, 164 F.3d 534 (10th Cir. 1998)). Courts, however, may be reluctant to accept a plaintiff's "excuse" for not complaining. As one court explained:

> Every employee who feels harassed by a supervisor will at some level fear the inevitable unpleasantness which will result from complaining to the employer. Confrontation is by its very nature unpleasant. To allow an employee to circumvent the reasonable complaint requirements of *Faragher* and *Burlington*, by making conclusory allegations of feared repercussions, however, would effectively eviscerate an affirmative defense which the Supreme Court clearly went to great effort to craft in order to stem the tide of unwarranted lawsuits. (*Fierro v. Saks Fifth Avenue*, 13 F. Supp. 2d 490 (S.D.N.Y. 1998)).[22]

Social science research tells us that fear of loss of job, of not being believed, and of embarrassment are not fears of mere "unpleasantness," and these fears are not unfounded. Only 32% of victims in the United States Merit System Protection Board (1994) study who filed grievances or complaints with the government found that it made things better; 47% found that it made things worse. Victims are also concerned with the potential effects on their families, their children, and their spouses (Morgan, 1999). The narrative of the plaintiff in *Nichols v. Frank*, 42 F.3d 503 (9th Cir. 1994), provides a chilling example:

> I tried to kill myself because I just didn't know how to tell my husband, you know, what was going on. . . . I was afraid that he would take my children and divorce me. And so I was just stuck. I was stuck between the two [the harasser and her husband] and there was no one I could talk to. I was afraid other people wouldn't believe me, so I was really stuck with both. Say, if I went and told anybody on him, on the supervisor I would lose my job. My husband and I had just recently bought a house and that house depended on my earnings, and I didn't want to lose everything. And that job was so important to the support of my family, so I was just stuck with the two. (p. 507)

Courts may not be sympathetic to employees who claim not to have known about existing policies (especially where they have been posted at least somewhere, or included in handbooks), nor to those who delay reporting beyond the timeline in the policy. Courts are also divided with respect to the reasonableness of a plaintiff complaining outside the employer's "official" policy dictates.

Is the Court's solution to employer liability a sound one? As of 1998, when sexual harassment claims were still climbing, it was difficult if not impossible to find tangible evidence of the effectiveness of sexual harassment training or sexual harassment policies in actually curbing sexually harassing behavior. In one study, 97% of the organizations that had sexual harassment claims filed against them had written policies against sexual harassment, 63% provided training, and 86% reported having established formal processes to investigate complaints (Society for Human Resources Management, 1999, cited in Dranoff, Dobrich, Maatman, & Lamel, 2002). Only time (and better assessment of the effectiveness of policies and training) will provide the answer.

CONCLUSION

This chapter presented a framework for understanding the law of sexual harassment and recognizing its crucial psychological underpinnings. The juxtaposition of law, psychology, and policy is drawn starkly in the domain of sexual harassment. The legal parameters of sexual harassment cases depend on behavioral assumptions and practices, while the psychological reality of sexual harassment today is much determined by how it transpires in the legal and policy arena. Understanding one domain requires some facility with the other.

Through consultation, expert testimony, and *amicus* briefs, psychologists are contributing substantially to the development of sexual harassment law, and this formal interaction needs to continue so that the knowledge and expertise gained from our research and clinical experience with sexual harassment can best inform legal doctrine. In this chapter, we saw how certain elements of sexual harassment law do not mesh with current psychological knowledge about people involved in sexually harassing situations, such as whether and how they might complain, or why they might stay in a workplace setting that they believe is a hostile and abusive environment. These understandings can and should be brought to bear in legal and policy reforms so as to move the law toward greater effectiveness in preventing and managing sexual harassment.

ACKNOWLEDGMENTS

We would like to thank Renée Melançon for her significant contributions to earlier drafts of this chapter.

NOTES

1. Testimony of Professor Anita Hill, United States Senate Confirmation Hearings, September 1991. Audio available at *http://www.historychannel.com/speeches/archive/speech_124.html*.
2. A number of other factors occurred in 1991 that no doubt added to the sharp increase in sexual harassment claims, most notably the passage of the Civil Rights Act of 1991, which allowed plaintiffs to recover compensatory and punitive damages, see 42 U.S.C. § 1981a(c) (1994).
3. Many of the principles and practices from the employment context also apply to another important area, sexual harassment in the schools, though sexual harassment in that context (dealt with under Title IX of the 1972 Education amendments in addition to Title VII) raises unique issues as well that are beyond the scope of this chapter. For helpful overviews of the topic, see McCarthy, 2001; Paludi, 1997.
4. In a 1978 book, Lin Farley described sexual harassment as "unsolicited nonreciprocal male behavior that asserts a woman's sex role over her function as worker" (pp. 14–15).
5. For clarification of these types of sexual harassment, see the section "The Legal Framework for Sexual Harassment."
6. Relevant cases discussed include *Meritor Savings Bank v. Vinson*, 477 U.S. 57 (1986); *Harris v. Forklift Systems, Inc.*, 510 U.S. 17 (1993); *Oncale v. Sundowner Offshore Services, Inc.*, 523 U.S. 75 (1998); and *Burlington Industries, Inc. v. Ellerth*, 524 U.S. 742 (1998).
7. Historians of Title VII point out that "sex" was added to the list of protected classes at the last possible moment as a last-ditch effort by opponents of the legislation to defeat it (on the theory that no one in their right mind would pass antidiscrimination laws that were so broad as to include sex discrimination) (Freeman, 1991), but it was added, the bill was passed, and the rest, as they say, is herstory!
8. Other categories protected under the statute include race, religion, color, or national origin. Neither disability nor sexual orientation are to this day included under Title VII's protected classes, though disability discrimination in various forms is prohibited by a number of other federal laws; see, for example, Title I of the Americans with Disabilities Act (Title I) and Section 504 of the Rehabilitation Act. Many types of discrimination are prohibited by many state antidiscrimination laws (see, for example, New York Executive Law § 296 which prohibits employment discrimination; California Labor Code § 1102.1., which prohibits discrimination based on sexual orientation). With the exception of Alabama and Mississippi, all states and the District of Columbia have enacted antidiscrimination statutes that prohibit sexual harassment as a form of unlawful sex discrimination, and most states now follow Title VII's standards when analyzing sexual harassment claims under the state's antidiscrimination statute. Specifically, state courts now recognize both *quid pro quo* and hostile environment sexual harassment, and frequently follow the federal standards for analyzing both types of claims (see *Steinberg v. Hoshijo*, 960 P.2d 1218 (Haw. 1998)). It should also be noted that claims of sexual harassment can be based on alternative legal theories, on tort or contract law (such as, intentional infliction of emotional distress or

tortious interference with contract), criminal law (in a case involving assault or sexual assault), wrongful discharge or whistleblower laws (in the case of termination or retaliation for complaining), or even prostitution laws (Gray, 2000–2001).

9. More recently, a number of scholars, notably Franke (1997), have questioned whether antidiscrimination law is the best or most effective framework for deciding sexual harassment cases. See also note 12.

10. The U.S. Supreme Court has adopted the EEOC's framework, although in *Burlington Industries* it recently clarified the point that, while the two categories of harassment are a useful analytic tool, there is not necessarily a clear demarcation of the two in terms of legal doctrine, and they may only be relevant in proving the threshold of whether a plaintiff can establish discrimination.

11. Unwanted sexual conduct also occurs, of course, between members of the same sex, where the same issues can arise. Same-sex harassment will be discussed more generally later.

12. For a more complete discussion of the issues raised by same-sex harassment cases, which are beyond the scope of this chapter, see for example, Bobak, 2002. It should be noted that significant legal scholarship has traced the difficulties in developing coherent legal doctrine on this point to the mistaken decision to locate sexual harassment legal challenges within a "sex" discrimination framework that focused on sexual conduct or on male–female relationships, rather than a "sexism" framework (see, for example, *Franke*, 1997), or a "gender subordination" framework (see, for example, *Abrams*, 1998; see also Schultz, 1998). For a thorough review and critique of these reconceptualization efforts and the Court's response, see Schwartz, 2002.

13. The *Oncale* Court did not elaborate on the definition of "because of . . . sex" in the context of same-sex claims. This has led to discrepancies among lower courts' interpretations of *Oncale* (see, for example, *Higgins v. New Balance Athletic Shoe, Inc.*, 194 F.3d 252 (1st Cir. 1999); *Schmedding v. Tnemec Co.*, 187 F.3d 862 (8th Cir. 1999)). Consequently, cases in which a heterosexual harasses another heterosexual, or a homosexual harasses another homosexual are probably actionable. In contrast, cases in which a heterosexual harasses a homosexual are considered antigay harassment because of sexual orientation, and, thus, may fail to satisfy the "because of . . . sex" element (*Rene v. MGM Grand Hotel*, 243 F.3d 1206 (9th Cir. 2001)). Further, sexual harassment inflicted on both female and male victims does not constitute discrimination on the basis of sex since neither sex suffers disparate treatment (*Holman v. Indiana*, 211 F.3d 399 (7th Cir. 2000)).

14. Organizational costs also include absenteeism, requests for transfers, and increased use of employee assistance services (Knapp & Kustis, 1996), as well as losing productive hours investigating claims of sexual harassment. U.S. government estimates put annual costs of sexual harassment at $267.3 million (United States Merit System Protection Board, 1987). It has been estimated that the cost of sexual harassment for each Fortune 500 company, averages $6.7 million per year, excluding legal fees (Sbraga & O'Donahue, 2000).

15. Perpetrators of sexual harassment also face a number of outcomes if allegations against them are investigated and proven, and possibly even if they are not proven. More specifically, perpetrators may experience personal and professional reprisals for their harassing behavior. They may face humiliation and embarrassment. They may also experience strained relationships with coworkers, lowered productivity, and, consequently, demotions, loss of jobs, and potentially becoming less employable due to a record of sexual harassment (Sbraga & O'Donahue, 2000).

16. The question of how much should be paid is not an easy one either. After the Civil Rights Act of 1991, sexual harassment plaintiffs are eligible for monetary damages, both compensatory and punitive (up to certain limits), though plaintiffs can only re-

cover punitive damages when they work for a private sector employer that acted with malice or in reckless disregard of the employee's rights (Conte, 1997). Note that, also under the 1991 Act, plaintiffs were given the right to a jury trial in sexual harassment cases. Psychological damages are particularly challenging to assess.

17. A person who feels he or she has experienced sexual harassment must take several steps before taking the case to court, however. First, many companies have sexual harassment policies and complaint procedures. Although not explicitly required by law, bringing an initial complaint to the employer will often bolster future legal action and stymie an employer's argument that it is not liable because it was not aware of the situation. In addition, a complaint to one's employer may be enough to halt the harassing behavior. In many instances, however, the person to whom a woman must complain—her supervisor or manager—is the very person committing the harassment. In this situation, a target may file a complaint with the harasser's superior or a human resource representative, for example, or may take action outside the company. A claim must also be filed with the EEOC.

18. Note that for those in the military, sexual harassment is dealt with as a crime that can lead to dishonorable discharge or incarceration, and military targets are generally not permitted to bring civil lawsuits (Stein, 1999). For a detailed discussion of sexual harassment in the military, which is beyond the scope of this chapter, see Niebuhr (1997).

19. For a more detailed discussion of the concept of vicarious liability in sexual harassment cases, see White (1999).

20. As previously discussed, in order to establish a hostile environment case, a plaintiff must show that she was subjected to unwelcome sexual conduct that was sufficiently severe or pervasive to alter the conditions of her employment and create an abusive environment (*Harris*; *Meritor*). It is interesting to note that while these two types of sexual harassment appear discrete, and raise separate and distinct issues, the most recent U.S. Supreme Court cases on sexual harassment have downplayed the distinction, particularly in the context of determining employer liability (*Burlington*, 1998).

21. For a spirited critique of the zero-tolerance approach, and current sexual harassment policies more generally, as resulting in a sanitized workplace in which sexuality and intimacy are suppressed, see Schultz, 2003.

22. While the EEOC has explained that an employee is reasonable in not using a policy where (1) the "complaint mechanism entails a risk of retaliation," (2) "there were obstacles to complaints," and (3) "the complaint mechanism was not effective" (Equal Employment Opportunity Commission Compliance Manual, 1999, p. 31), courts have applied a more narrow approach. A plaintiff's refusal to report harassment because of possible repercussions has met with mixed results in providing a plaintiff with an excuse for not reporting sexual harassment or delaying reporting harassment. In fact, in many cases courts have held that such fears would not excuse an employee's failure to report the harassment early on (see, for example, *Fierro v. Saks Fifth Avenue*). Courts in these cases characterized the victim's fears as unsubstantiated, too generalized, or lacking in any objectively reasonable basis.

REFERENCES

Abrams, K. (1989). Gender discrimination and the transformation of workplace norms. *Vanderbilt Law Review, 42*, 1183–1248.

Abrams, K. (1998). The new jurisprudence of sexual harassment. *Cornell Law Review, 83*, 1169–1230.

Allred, G., & West, J. S. (1998, October 28). Sexual harassment. *National Law Journal, 21*, Section: Employment law, B12.

American Psychiatric Association. (1994). *Diagnostic and statistical manual of mental disorders* (4th ed.). Washington, DC: Author.

Barr, P. A. (1993). Perceptions of sexual harassment. *Sociological Inquiry, 63*, 460–470.

Beiner, T. M. (1999). The misuse of summary judgment in hostile environment cases. *Wake Forest Law Review, 34*, 71–134.

Bisom-Rapp, S. (2001). An ounce of prevention is a poor substitute for a pound of cure: Confronting the developing jurisprudence of education and prevention in employment discrimination law. *Berkeley Journal of Employment and Labor Law, 22*, 1–47.

Bobak, D. L. (2002). Hampel v. Food Ingredients Specialties, Inc.: To prove that your same-sex co-worker sexually harassed you, first prove that he was sexually attracted to you. *Capital University Law Review, 30*, 911–946.

Brooks, L., & Perot, A. R. (1991). Reporting sexual harassment: Exploring a predictive model. *Psychology of Women Quarterly, 15*, 31–47.

Burns, S. E. (1995). Issues in workplace sexual harassment law and related social science research. *Journal of Social Issues, 51*, 193–207.

Casellas, G. F. (1998). The Equal Employment Opportunity Commission: Challenges for the twenty-first century. *University of Pennsylvania Journal of Labor and Employment Law, 1*, 1–14.

Conte, A. (1997). Legal theories of sexual harassment. In W. O'Donohue (Ed.), *Sexual harassment: Theory, research and treatment* (pp. 5–28). Boston: Allyn & Bacon.

Dansky, B. S., & Kilpatrick, D. G. (1997). Effects of sexual harassment. In W. O'Donahue (Ed.), *Sexual harassment: Theory, research and treatment* (pp. 151–174). Boston: Allyn & Bacon.

Daugherty, S. R., Baldwin, D. C., Jr., & Rowley, B. D. (1998). Learning, satisfaction, and mistreatment during medical internship: A national survey of working conditions. *Journal of the American Medical Association, 279*, 1194–1199.

Deaux, K. (1995). How basic can you be? The evolution of research on gender stereotypes. *Journal of Social Issues, 51*(1), 11–20.

Dranoff, S., Dobrich, W., Maatman, G. L., & Lamel, L. (2002). *Effective management of risk in the legal profession, hitting the brick wall: Sexual harassment revisited* (676 PLI/Lit. 421) (Litigation and Administrative Practice Course Handbook Series, PLI Order No. H0-00FC). New York, NY: Practicing Law Institute.

DuBois, C. L. Z., Knapp, D. E., Faley, R. H., & Kustis, G. A. (1998). An empirical examination of same- and other-gender sexual harassment in the workplace. *Sex Roles, 39*, 731–749.

Epstein, C. F., Saute, R., Oglensky, B., & Gever, M. (1995). Glass ceilings and open doors: Women's advancement in the legal profession. *Fordham Law Review, 64*, 291–449.

Equal Employment Opportunity Commission. (1999). *Enforcement guidance on vicarious employer liability for unlawful harassment by supervisors* (EEOC Notice No. 915-002). Washington, DC: Author.

Equal Employment Opportunity Commission (2003). *Sexual harassment charges EEOC and FEPAs combined: FY 1992–2002.* Retrieved December 15, 2003 from *http://www.eeoc.gov/stats/harass.html*

Estrich, S. (1991). Sex at work. *Stanford Law Review, 43,* 813–861.

Farley, L. (1978). *Sexual shakedown: The sexual harassment of women on the job.* New York: McGraw-Hill.

Fiske, S. T., Bersoff, D. N., Borgida, E., Deaux, K., & Heilman, M. E. (1991). Social science research on trial: Use of sex stereotyping research in *Price Waterhouse v. Hopkins. American Psychologist, 46,* 1049–1060.

Fitzgerald, L. F., Gelfand, M. J., & Drasgow, F. (1995). Measuring sexual harassment: Theoretical and psychometric advances. *Basic and Applied Social Psychology, 17,* 425–445.

Fitzgerald, L., Swan, S., & Fischer, K. (1995). Why didn't she report him? The psychological and legal implications of women's responses to sexual harassment. *Journal of Social Issues, 51*(1), 117–138.

Fitzgerald, L. F., Swan, S., & Magley, V. J. (1997). But was it really sexual harassment? Legal, behavioral, and psychological definitions of the workplace victimization of women. In W. O'Donohue (Ed.), *Sexual harassment: Theory, research and treatment* (pp. 5–28). Boston: Allyn & Bacon.

Forell, C. A., & Matthews, D. M. (2000). *A law of her own: The reasonable woman as a measure of man.* New York: New York University Press.

Franke, K. M. (1997). What's wrong with sexual harassment? *Stanford University Law Review, 49,* 691–772.

Frazier, P. A., Cochran, C. C., & Olson, A. M. (1995). Social science research on lay definitions of sexual harassment. *Journal of Social Issues, 51,* 21–37.

Freeman, J. (1991). How "sex" got into Title VII: Persistent opportunism as a maker of public policy. *Law and Inequality: A Journal of Theory and Practice, 9*(2), 163–184.

Gelfand, M. J., Fitzgerald, L. F., & Drasgow, F. (1995). The structure of sexual harassment: A confirmatory analysis across cultures and settings. *Journal of Vocational Behavior, 47,* 164–177.

Goodman-Delahunty, J. (1999). Pragmatic support for the reasonable victim standard in hostile workplace sexual harassment cases. *Psychology, Public Policy, and Law, 5*(3), 519–555.

Gray, J. A. (2000–2001). Sexual harassment, prostitution, and the tort of abusive discharge: An analysis and evaluation of recent legal developments. *Buffalo Women's Law Journal, 9,* 169.

Grossman, J. L. (2003). The culture of compliance: The final triumph of form over substance in sexual harassment law. *Harvard Women's Law Journal, 26,* 3–75.

Gruber, J. E. (1989). How women handle sexual harassment: A literature review. *Social Science Research, 74,* 3–7.

Gruber, J. E. (1992). A typology of personal and environmental sexual harassment: Research and policy implications for the 1990's. *Sex Roles, 26,* 447–464.

Gruber, J. E. (1997). An epidemiology of sexual harassment: Evidence from North America and Europe. In W. O'Donohue (Ed.), *Sexual harassment: Theory, research, and treatment* (pp. 84–98). Boston: Allyn & Bacon.

Gruber, J. E. (1998). The impact of male work environments and organizational policies on women's experiences of sexual harassment. *Gender and Society, 12*, 301–320.

Gruber, J. E., Smith, M. D., & Kauppinen-Toropainen, K. (1996). An exploration of sexual harassment experiences and severity: Results from North America and Europe. In M. S. Stockdale (Ed.), *Sexual harassment in the workplace: Perspectives, frontiers, and response strategies* (pp. 151–173). Newbury Park, CA: Sage.

Gutek, B. A. (1985). *Sex and the workplace: The impact of sexual behavior and harassment on women, men, and organization.* San Francisco: Jossey-Bass.

Gutek, B. A., & Koss, M. P. (1993). Changed women and changed organizations: Consequences of and coping with sexual harassment. *Journal of Vocational Behavior, 42*, 28–48.

Gutek, B. A., & Morasch, B. (1982). Sex-ratios, sex-role spillover, and sexual harassment of women at work. *Journal of Social Issues, 38*(4), 55–74.

Gutek, B. A., & O'Connor, M. (1995). The empirical basis for the reasonable woman standard. *Journal of Social Issues, 51*, 151–166.

Gutek, B. A., O'Connor, M., Melançon, R., Geer, T., Done, R., & Stockdale, M. (1999). The utility of the reasonable woman legal standard in hostile environment sexual harassment cases: A multimethod, multistudy examination. *Psychology, Public Policy and Law, 5*, 596–629.

Hanisch, K. A. (1996). An integrated framework for studying the outcomes of sexual harassment: Consequences for individuals and organizations. In M. Stockdale (Ed.), *Sexual harassment in the workplace: Perspectives, frontiers, and response strategies* (pp. 174–198). Newbury Park, CA: Sage.

Jorgenson, L. M., & Wahl, K. M. (2000). Psychiatrists as expert witnesses in sexual harassment cases under Daubert and Kumho. *Psychiatric Annals, 30*(6), 390–396.

Juliano, A., & Schwab, S. J. (2001). The sweep of sexual harassment cases. *Cornell Law Review, 86*, 548–602.

Katz, R. C., Hannon, R., & Whitten, L. (1996). Effects of gender and situation on the perception of sexual harassment. *Sex Roles, 34*, 35–42.

Kidder, L. H., Lafleur, R. A., & Wells, C. V. (1995). Recalling harassment, reconstructing experience. *Journal of Social Issues, 51*, 53–67.

Kilpatrick, D. G., Dansky, B. S., & Saunders, B. E. (1994). *Sexual harassment in the workplace: Results from the National Women's Study* [Monograph]. Charleston, SC: Crime Victims Research and Treatment Center, Department of Psychiatry and Behavioral Sciences, Medical University of South Carolina.

Knapp, D. E., & Kustis, G. A. (1996). The real "disclosure": Sexual harassment and the bottom line. In M. S. Stockdale (Ed.), *Sexual harassment in the workplace: Perspectives, frontiers, and response strategies* (pp. 199–213). Newbury Park, CA: Sage.

MacKinnon, C. A. (1979a). *Sexual harassment of working women.* New Haven, CT: Yale University Press.

MacKinnon, C. A. (1979b). The social causes of sexual harassment. In E. Wall (Ed.), *Sexual harassment: Confrontations and decisions* (pp. 51–79). Buffalo, NY: Prometheus Books.

McCarthy, M. (2001). Students and targets and perpetrators of sexual harassment: Title IX and beyond. *Hastings Women's Law Journal, 12,* 177–214.

Morgan, P. (1999). Risking relationships: Understanding the litigation choices of sexually harassed women. *Law and Society Review, 33*(1), 201–226.

Niebuhr, R. E. (1997). Sexual harassment in the military. In W. O'Donohue (Ed.), *Sexual harassment: Theory, research, and treatment* (pp. 250–262). Boston: Allyn & Bacon.

Nieva, V. F., & Gutek, B. A. (1981). *Women and work: A psychological perspective.* New York: Praeger.

O'Connor, M., Gutek, B. A., Stockdale, M. S., Geer, T., & Melançon, R. (2004). Predictors of sexual harassment judgments: More than sex of the rater. *Law and Human Behavior, 28,* 69–95.

O'Hare, E., & O'Donohue, W. (1998). Sexual harassment: Identifying risk factors. *Archives of Sexual Behavior, 27,* 561–579.

Paetzold, R., & O'Leary-Kelly, A. (1996). The implications of U.S. Supreme Court and circuit court decisions for hostile environment sexual harassment. In M. S. Stockdale (Ed.), *Sexual harassment in the workplace: Perspectives, frontiers, and response strategies* (pp. 85–104). Newbury Park, CA: Sage.

Paludi, M. A. (1997). Sexual harassment in schools. In W. O'Donohue (Ed.), *Sexual harassment: Theory, research, and treatment* (pp. 225–240). Boston: Allyn & Bacon.

Pennington, N., & Hastie, R. (1991). A cognitive theory of juror decision making: The story model. *Cardoza Law Review, 13,* 5001–5039.

Powers, Kinder, & Keeney. (1999). Prevent sexual harassment the right way. *Rhode Island Employment Law Letter, 4*(4), 6–8.

Pryor, J. B., Giedd, J. L., & Williams, K. B. (1995). A social psychological model for predicting sexual harassment. *Journal of Social Issues, 51,* 69–84.

Ross, J. J. (1996). *The employment law year in review* (547 PLI/Lit. 9) Litigation and Administrative Practice Course Handbook Series, PLI Order No. H4-5237). New York: Practicing Law Institute.

Rotundo, M., Nguyen, D., & Sackett, P. R. (2001). A meta-analysis review of gender differences in perceptions of sexual harassment. *Journal of Applied Psychology, 86,* 914–922.

Sbraga, T., & O'Donohue, W. (2000). Sexual harassment. *Annual Review of Sex Research, 11,* 258–286.

Schneider, K. T., Swan, S., & Fitzgerald, L. F. (1997). Job-related and psychological effects of sexual harassment in the workplace: Empirical evidence from two organizations. *Journal of Applied Psychology, 82,* 401–415.

Schultz, V. (1998). Reconceptualizing sexual harassment. *Yale Law Journal, 107,* 1683–1732.

Schultz, V. (2003). The sanitized workplace. *Yale Law Journal, 112,* 2061–2193.

Schwartz, D. S. (2002). When is sex because of sex? The causation problem in sexual harassment law. *University of Pennsylvania Law Review, 150,* 1697–1794.

Stein, L. W. (1999). *Sexual harassment in America: A documentary history.* Westport, CT: Greenwood Press.

Stockdale, M. S., Bisom-Rapp, S., O'Connor, M., & Gutek, B. A. (2004). Coming to terms with zero-tolerance sexual harassment policies. *Journal of Forensic Psychology Practice, 4*(1), 65–78.

Stockdale, M. S., O'Connor, M., Gutek, B. A., & Geer, T. M. (2002). The relationship between prior sexual abuse and reactions to sexual harassment: Literature review and empirical study. *Psychology, Public Policy, and the Law, 8,* 64–95.

Till, F. J. (1980). *Sexual harassment: A report on the sexual harassment of students.* Washington, DC: National Advisory Council on Women's Educational Program.

United States Merit System Protection Board. (1995). *Sexual harassment in the federal workplace: Trends, progress, continuing challenges.* Washington, DC: U.S. Government Printing Office.

Waldo, C. R., Berdahl, J. L., & Fitzgerald, L. F. (1998). Are men sexually harassed? If so, by whom? *Law and Human Behavior, 22,* 59–79.

Welsh, S. (1999). Gender and sexual harassment. *Annual Review of Sociology, 25,* 169–190.

Welsh, S., & Nierobisz, A. (1997). How prevalent is sexual harassment: A research note on measuring sexual harassment in Canada. *Canadian Journal of Sociology, 22,* 505–522.

White, R. H. (1999). There's nothing special about sex: The Supreme Court mainstreams sexual harassment. *William and Mary Bill of Rights Journal, 7,* 725–753.

Wiener, R. L., & Gutek, B. A. (1999). Advances in sexual harassment research, theory, and policy. *Psychology, Public Policy, and Law, 5*(3), 507–518.

Wiener, R. L., Hackney, A., Kadela, K., Rauch, S., Seib, H., Warren, L., & Hurt, L. E. (2002). The fit and implementation of sexual harassment law to workplace evaluations. *Journal of Applied Psychology, 87,* 747–764.

Williams, C., Giuffre, P., & Dellinger, K. (1999). Sexuality in the workplace: Organizational control, sexual harassment, and the pursuit of pleasure. *Annual Review of Sociology, 25,* 73–93.

PART II

Sexualized Violence against Children

While Part I of this volume deals with problems that could be viewed as societally "overconforming" behavior,[1] Part II deals with societal amnesia and psychological repression on a society-wide scale. The problem of child sexual abuse,[2] addressed in this section, is fundamentally different from rape, spousal abuse, stalking, and sexual harassment.

There are few, if any, societies that have considered adult sex with children normal. However, for reasons that are still not well understood, and regardless of the overwhelming evidence that child sexual abuse has been present (even rampant) in many if not most societies, there is a strange denial of its existence, even today. As opposed to rape, which took a long time to be perceived as a wrong, particularly against the female victim, and also spousal abuse, which until quite recently was perceived as a normal part of marriage, child sexual abuse has been perceived largely as wrong—but as absent or very rare. Current research on child sexual abuse continues to deal with the issue that child reporters of sexual abuse are not believed. In fact, there is a current controversy as to whether children can accurately report that something has happened to them. This is true even though much research shows that most children when properly questioned, even at young ages, do know and can tell if something sexual has been done to them. Surprisingly, there is also a counterforce that proclaims that adult sex is good for children, or at least not harmful. This view is held in spite of clear evidence that children are traumatized by adult sexuality foisted upon them, and suffer very clear harm in a variety of different ways for long periods of time, if not permanently. Thus, human society seems to have great difficulty be-

149

lieving that child sexual abuse is occurring, even while it is. This controversy also extends to adults who report that they suffered child sexual abuse, particularly when their recall of the abuse has been delayed (i.e., they do not clearly remember and report it until much later).[3] New research on memory, particularly under conditions of trauma or high emotional excitation, gives some explanations of how amnesia and dissociation can occur for highly charged events. However, there continues to be a popular mistrust of these psychological phenomena when they relate to child sexual abuse, although they are commonly accepted when applied to other traumas, such as the World Trade Center disaster.

Issues of child sexual abuse and delayed recall of child sexual abuse are addressed in the following chapters, which constitute Part II of this volume.

NOTES

1. Overconforming behavior refers to behavior that is generally accepted in milder forms. Thus, it is only a problem because there is *more* of the behavior than is usually acceptable. For example, from this point of view, it is rape when a man presses *too forcefully* for sex, spousal abuse is the result of a man hitting his wife *too hard*, stalking is when a suitor pursues his love object *too much*, and sexual harassment occurs when someone is *too sexually explicit* at work.
2. For details on child sexual abuse and related references, see Chapter 7, this volume.
3. For details on delayed recall of child sexual abuse and related references, see Chapter 8, this volume.

7 Child Sexual Abuse

ERNA OLAFSON

DEFINITIONS

Definitions of what constitutes child sexual abuse vary among studies, and the term encompasses a wide range of criminal behaviors. Contact child sexual abuse includes private parts touching between victim and perpetrator, oral sex, and penetrating rape of the vagina, anus, or mouth. Some perpetrators also show pornography to children, use their child victims to produce pornography, expose their private parts to children, and/or force children to engage in sexual acts with each other. Perpetrators differ in their approaches to children, so that some child sexual abusers engage in extensive grooming before assaulting children sexually, whereas others simply attack their child victims without preliminaries.

Children's symptoms are more severe when sexual abuse is by parent figures, when it is penetrating, when it is accompanied by aggression, when there are multiple abusers, or when it is repeated over months or years (Kendall-Tackett, Williams, & Finkelhor, 1993; Putnam, 2003). Penetrating rape results in very high rates of posttraumatic stress disorder among both child and adult victims, among the highest for any form of interpersonal violence, including combat (Bloom & Reichert, 1998; Kessler, Sonnega, Bromet, Hughes, & Nelson, 1995). However, for all

151

kinds of child sexual abuse, including nonviolent fondling, up to 40% of victims present with few or no symptoms at any one time (Putnam, 2003). Longitudinal studies show that a "sleeper effect" may be operating in many of these children, in which apparently unharmed victims become symptomatic in the year or two following initial assessment (Finkelhor & Berliner, 1995; Putnam, 2003). Indeed, one study showed that sexually abused children who showed fewest initial symptoms evidenced the most marked deterioration over time (Gomez-Schwartz, Horowitz, & Cardarelli, 1990).

"Mild" child sexual abuse is unique among interpersonal crimes in a manner that has contributed to a long history of confusion and denial in Western popular culture, professional opinion, and the law about whether sexual contact between an adult and a child is criminal and wrong. Most criminal acts perpetrated upon children are also crimes if perpetrated upon adults. It is a crime to batter, lock up, starve, isolate, or rape an adult or a child. It is also a crime to engage in the grooming and nonviolent genital fondling of a child who appears to have assented and to be enjoying the sexual touching. By contrast, it is not a crime to court and engage in nonviolent genital fondling or sexual intercourse with a nondependent adult who consents and enjoys the genital touching. Indeed, since the recent United States Supreme Court decision in *Lawrence v. Texas*, 123 S. Ct. 2472 (2003), sexual activity between consenting homosexual adults is now decriminalized throughout the United States. A child's age, dependent status, and inability to consent make nonviolent child sexual abuse both criminal and wrong, even when the child does not appear to be physically or emotionally damaged by the encounter (Finkelhor, 1979).

Feminists have not been alone in identifying men as the primary perpetrators of sexual crimes against children, but feminists were among the first to break centuries of silence about child sexual abuse, linking this silence explicitly to institutionalized patriarchy. As psychiatrist Judith Herman wrote in 1981, "Without a feminist analysis, one is at a loss to explain why the reality of incest was for so long suppressed by supposedly responsible professional investigators, why public discussion of the subject awaited the woman's liberation movement, or why the recent apologists for incest have been popular men's magazines" (Herman, 1981, p. 3). In surviving patriarchal cultures, silence and shame persist. Japan's only expert on classroom sexual abuse of girls, Akido Kamei, reported recently on the persistent Japanese "myth" by which rape victims, not perpetrators, are blamed. Akido added that although child sexual molestation and rape are commonplace in Japan, victims rarely come forward, and when they do, they are blamed and shamed and the perpetrators lightly punished if at all (French, 2003). A recent World Health

Organization study of violence and health finds that in those patriarchal cultures that maintain strong notions of family honor, women are blamed for sexual assaults while men go unpunished (Krug, Dahlberg, Mercy, Zwi, & Lozano, 2002). To alleviate family shame and restore family honor, young rape victims are forced to marry their rapists or they are murdered, often by brothers who are very likely to face no criminal conviction for thus "cleansing" their families (Krug et al., 2002, pp. 160, 163–164). A study of female homicides in Alexandria, Egypt, for example, revealed that in 47% of all murder cases, girls or women were murdered by their own family members after they had been "defiled" by rape (Krug et al., 2002, p. 93).

THE IMPACT OF CHILD SEXUAL ABUSE ON CHILDREN AND ADULT SURVIVORS

What do we know today about the effects of child sexual abuse on children? Current research studies document outcomes in three basic categories—psychiatric disorders, dysfunctional behaviors, and neurobiological dysregulation.

Regarding psychiatric disorders, women with child sexual abuse histories are 3–5 times more likely to have one or more episodes of major depression in their lifetimes than women without such a history. Indeed, when the history of child sexual abuse in women is controlled for, the gender difference in depression rates between males and females disappears (Whiffen & Clark, 1997). Sexually abused boys have more pervasive and severe short- and long-term symptoms than do sexually abused girls, but boys are far less likely than girls to be sexually abused (Putnam, 2003). Other associations between child sexual abuse and psychiatric disorders in clinical and community samples include substance abuse, suicide risk, posttraumatic stress, and dissociative disorders.

Of the many behavioral and conduct disorders that are associated with having been sexually abused as a child, sexualized behaviors have been the most closely linked. Both male and female victims are more likely to engage in high-risk sexual behaviors and thus to be more vulnerable to sexually transmitted diseases such as HIV (Brown, Lourie, Zlotnick, & Cohn, 2000; Cunningham, Stiffman, Dore, & Earls, 1994; Krug et al., 2002; Parillo, Freeman, Collier, & Young, 2001). Sexually abused adolescent girls are more likely than nonabused girls to have early pregnancies (Fiscella, Kitzman, Cole, Sidora, & Olds, 1998; Herrenkohl, Herrenkohl, Egolf, & Russo, 1998; Rainey, Stevens-Siman, & Kaplan, 1995; Romans, Martin, & Morris, 1997; Stevens-Simon & Reichert, 1994). One study has shown far higher rates of attention-deficit/hyperactivity disorder (ADHD) diagnoses in sexually abused girls than in their matched comparison group of nonabused girls. It appears likely that many children with apparent ADHD may be suffering from posttraumatic symptoms that superficially resemble the symptoms of ADHD (Putnam & Trickett, 1997).

The neurobiological research outcomes are the most recent and the most troubling. A longitudinal study by Putnam, Trickett, and their colleagues that compared sexually abused and nonabused girls has shown negative results for the hypothalamic–pituitary–adrenal (HPA) axis, the sympathetic nervous system, and possibly the immune system in the victimized girls (De Bellis, Chrousos, et al., 1994; De Bellis, Lefter, Trickett, & Putnam, 1994; Putnam, 2003). A dysregulated HPA axis compromises stress and anxiety management. A charged-up sympathetic nervous system is associated with increased resting and stressed heart rates, irritability, and sleep disturbances (Perry, Pollard, Blakley, Baker, & Vigilante, 1995). Chronic severe stress appears to be toxic to the developing brain of the infant and preschooler; thus Michael De Bellis and his colleagues found significantly smaller brains and lower IQs in abused children by the time they were 5 or 6 than in matched controls, a neuroanatomical effect that was stronger for boys than for girls (De Bellis et al., 1999).

BRIEF HISTORY

The two great waves of Western European and American feminist activism, one in the late 19th and one in the late 20th century, brought all forms of violence against girls and women, including child sexual abuse, to public awareness. During feminism's first wave but unconnected with it, physicians in Germany, France, and Vienna after 1860 brought attention to the high rates of violence and sexual assault to children, debated issues of memory and suggestibility, and, in three early papers by Sigmund Freud, described the psychological effects of child sexual abuse on boys and girls (Herman, 1981, 1992; Masson, 1984; Olafson, Corwin, & Summit, 1993). After 1896, Freud changed his mind and began to explain patient accounts of incest as autoerotic fantasies. Meanwhile, Pierre Janet in Paris, one of the pioneers in the study of trauma and dissociation, remained focused on abuse and trauma and was virtually forgotten for almost a century. It was Freud, not Janet, who dominated mental health paradigms in the Anglo-American world until late in the 20th century. Janet was rediscovered by Ellenberger at about the same time that the second-wave feminist critique of Freud and the emergence of biological psychiatry began to chip away at Freud's dominance in the late 20th century (Ellenberger, 1970; Olafson et al., 1993; van der Kolk & van der Hart, 1989).

Public Minimization of Child Sexual Abuse

For about 50 years between the two great waves of feminist activism and professional discovery, that is, from roughly the end of World War I until about 1970, public and policy attention to all forms of sexual violence and to child maltreatment in general was minimal. In the Victorian era, there had been strong and effective efforts to protect children from physical abuse, sexual abuse, and neglect, public attention that carried over into the early years of the 20th century and then, mysteriously, waned. As historian George K. Behlmer (1982) has written, "There remains to be explained the curious decline of public interest in child abuse between 1920 and the early 1960's" (p. 225). Child psychiatrist Lenore Terr (1990) wrote about these mid-20th century years in child psychiatry, "Childhood psychic trauma was assumed to be understood while simultaneously being ignored" (p. 10).

Child sexual abuse was never completely forgotten of course, and there continued to be some criminal prosecutions (Myers, 2004; Olafson, 2002; Olafson et al., 1993). For the most part, however, the professionals and the media who focused on child sexual abuse during the middle years of the 20th century minimized both its prevalence and its impact. As late as 1975, Henderson wrote in a standard American psychiatric textbook that incest victims numbered only one in a million in the English-speaking world and that incestuous daughters often initiate and collude in the incest and do not appear to be injured by it (p. 1536). When a patient described a history of incest, mental health professionals and social workers in predominantly Freudian traditions were trained to "think fantasy." As Herman summarized the situation in 1981, "The legacy of Freud's inquiry into the subject of incest was a tenacious prejudice, still shared by professionals and laymen alike, that children lie about sexual abuse. This belief is by now so deeply ingrained in the culture that children who dare to report sexual assaults are more than likely to have their complaints dismissed as fantasy" (p. 11).

Victim Blaming

For most of the 20th century, when child victims were not viewed as liars, they were labeled as sex delinquents. When a man sexually assaulted a child (or a woman), it was the victim, not the offender, who was blamed and held accountable for this crime. The offender became invisible and was not held to account. Freud's student, Karl Abraham

(1907/1927), began the trend in professional writing with a 1907 paper titled, "The Experiencing of Sexual Trauma as a Form of Sexual Activity," in which he wrote that child victims unconsciously desired sexual assaults; the evidence he cited was that the children did not run, resist, or call for help. Janet was writing at the time about traumatic dissociation in studies that garnered little attention, so that it would take two generations before psychiatrist Roland Summit, in his landmark 1983 paper, would eloquently argue that small victims are more likely to freeze like rabbits than they are to fight or flee. Abraham had written in 1907 that a 9-year-old girl in one of his case studies "allowed herself to be seduced" (Abraham, 1907/1927, p. 52). Abraham's use of the language of seduction rather than of criminal assault, coupled with his reflexive victim-blaming, becomes clearer when one applies Abraham's sentence to other crimes. Sentences such as "The child allowed herself to be robbed," "The child allowed herself to be beaten," or "The child allowed herself to be murdered" reveal the absurdity of Abraham's arguments.

A generation after Abraham, outstanding professionals such as psychologist Loretta Bender, creator of a major psychological instrument, the Bender–Gestalt, echoed the victim-blaming theme by describing child sexual abuse victims as "sex delinquents" (Bender & Blau, 1937). Bender and Blau wrote that given the emotional placidity, the charming and attractive personalities, and the apparent lack of psychological symptoms in the children they were studying, "It is not remarkable that frequently we considered the possibility that the child might have been the actual seducer rather than the one innocently seduced" (p. 514). Bender and Blau did not merely summarize their cases but included case vignettes for each child, vignettes that reveal that these were anything but placid and symptom-free children. One case summary refers to the child's "emotional disturbance" that appeared to depress her IQ test scores. Case vignettes for the other children document the children's irritability, sullenness, severe behavioral problems, repetitive sexual acting out, school difficulties, extreme restlessness, and even one child's repeatedly expressed fear that her father (the alleged offender) was going to murder her. However, Bender and Blau's case vignettes also included references to the "charm" and "attractiveness" of some of these children. One such victim, an 11-year-old boy of "average intelligence," was described as having a "frankly hedonistic attitude" toward sex, and this vignette concluded, "There is no doubt that the boy was the seducer of the adult in this case" (Bender & Blau, 1937, pp. 509–510).

Victim accountability and offender invisibility continued in the mainstream literature through the 1950s and 1960s. San Francisco's prestigious Langley Porter Psychiatric Institute, in a study funded by the state of California, described the sexually abused children they studied as "participating victims" or "seductive" girls who were generally un-damaged by child sexual abuse (Weiss, Rogers, Darwin, & Dutton, 1955; see also Olafson, 2002; Olafson et al., 1993; Salter, 1988, 1995, 2003, for detailed historical accounts). In their influential and very widely read studies at mid- century, Alfred Kinsey and his colleagues (Kinsey, Pomeroy, & Martin, 1948; Kinsey, Pomeroy, Martin, & Geb-hard, 1953) went so far as to argue that there was no reason, apart from adult overreactions, for children to be psychologically damaged by hav-ing their genitalia touched by adults, and Kinsey chided the many women in his surveys who had reported being upset as children by sex-ual contacts with adult men (Kinsey et al., 1953).

Thus, in the mental health fields, breaking the silence about child sexual abuse did little to hold perpetrators accountable. Through a cen-tury of Western professional literature about child sexual abuse by main-stream medical professionals as well as by a libertarian fringe, the "se-ductive," "participating," or "consenting" child victim became a fixture by which offenders were overlooked and their offenses against children decriminalized, while their young victims or their mothers were scruti-nized and held responsible for the children's victimization (Herman, 1981, 1992; Olafson, 2002; Olafson et al., 1993).

As late as 1978, while professional awareness of child sexual abuse was finally becoming established, psychiatrist Alayne Yates argued that even prolonged father–daughter incest left the girls she had evaluated "emotionally unscathed" (p. 120). Yates concluded, "There is an impor-tant lesson to be learned from non-coercive father-and-daughter incest. Early erotic pleasure by itself does not damage the child. It can produce sexually competent and notably erotic young women. Childhood is the best time to learn, although parents may not always be the best teach-ers" (p. 121). Yates's case studies include references to girls eroticized by incest who, at ages 9 and 12, behaved "seductively" toward other adult men or who "initiated" and enjoyed sex play with the boys in the neigh-borhood. Yates wrote nothing about the risks these sexualized girls faced of disease, early pregnancy, and future revictimization by sexual assault or rape. She described these sexualized behaviors as signaling erotic competence rather than traumatic sexualization.

Mother Blaming

Meanwhile, the family systems theorists of the late 20th century impli-cated mothers in father–daughter incest, so that incestuous fathers were described as passive puppets acting out maternal homosexual fantasies toward their daughters or as sexually deprived men turning to their daughters because their wives were prudish or frigid (Giaretto, 1982; Lustig, Dresser, Spellman, & Murray, 1966; see also the analyses in

Myers, 1998; Olafson, 2002; Olafson et al., 1993; Salter, 1988, 2003). Giaretto's (1982) nationwide self-help program, Parents United, described all parties in the incestuous family, including the offender, as "unconscious victims of a dysfunctional system." Giaretto's Parents United program taught nonoffending mothers to assume coresponsibility for the father's sexual abuse of their daughters (p. 38). As one adolescent incest victim reportedly commented on his experience with one family systems psychotherapist, "I think that therapist forgets who is the fucker and who is the fuckee" (Salter, 2003, p. 57).

CHILD SEXUAL ABUSE IN THE LAW: THE HISTORY

Psychiatric skepticism about child sexual abuse spilled over into American law. John Henry Wigmore's (1904/1978) famous and enormously influential *Treatise on Evidence* warned that women and girls who accuse men of sexual abuse, especially girls who accuse their fathers, must be examined by medical professionals, because of a female predisposition to bring false accusations of sexual assault against respectable men. In support of this theory, Wigmore cited case reports of two girls, ages 7 and 9, whom he described as pathological liars, even though the original case reports, which Wigmore did not fully include in his *Treatise*, document that the girl of 7 had gonorrhea, and the 9-year-old girl's vagina was so inflamed and swollen that the doctor was unable to examine her (cited in Herman, 1981, p. 11).

Attorney John Myers, the leading expert on child sexual abuse and the law in the United States, writes that during the first half of the 20th century, Wigmore (as cited in Myers, 2004, p. 374) was the most influential legal scholar in the United States regarding evidence in court. His words about girls and women deserve repetition in full.

> Modern psychiatrists have amply studied the behavior of errant young girls and women coming before the courts in all sorts of cases. Their psychic complexes are multifarious, distorted partly by inherent defects, partly by diseased derangements or abnormal instincts, partly by bad social environments, partly by temporary physiological or emotional conditions. One form taken by these complexes is that of contriving false charges of sex offenses by men. The unchaste mentality (let us call it) finds incidental but direct expression in the narration of imaginary sex incidents of which the narrator is the heroine or the victim. On the surface the narration is straight-forward and convincing. The real victim, however, too often in such cases is the innocent man . . . No judge should ever let a sex offense charge go to the jury unless the female complainant's social history and mental makeup have been examined and

testified to by a qualified physician. It is time that the courts awakened
to the sinister possibilities of injustice that lurk in believing such a witness without careful psychiatric scrutiny.

Myers summarizes this remarkable passage by pointing out that
Wigmore is arguing that girls and women are so likely to fantasize or lie
about sex that every single female who brings a sex offense charge
against a man should be examined by a psychiatrist (Myers, 2004). Generations of judges and attorneys were influenced by this passage, which
often formed part of judges' instructions to juries in rape and sexual assault cases through much of the 20th century, until feminist activism and
books like Susan Brownmiller's (1975) *Against Our Will: Men, Women
and Rape* began to change both attitudes and the law.

What about the actual prosecution picture during the years of denial? Myers tells us that "child abuse" did not receive a separate heading
in the *Index to Legal Periodicals and Books*, a major research resource
for attorneys, until 1970, and "child sexual abuse" only in 1990.
Searching the *Index* under the category "Rape," Myers has read every
law review article about child sexual abuse that he could find for the
years from 1888 to 1975, a chore less difficult than it sounds because so
little was written on the topic in those years. Most of what was published about the rape of both women and children in these years cast
doubt on victim veracity.

However, Myers found that when cases came to court, the criminal
prosecution of child sexual abuse did not mirror this skepticism. In the
absence of national statistics about the criminal prosecution of child sexual abuse, Myers estimates that prosecutions increased slowly from
1900 to about 1980, after which prosecutions increased exponentially.
Looking at smaller samples of all rape caseloads state by state before
1975, Myers found that the majority of rape victims were children ages
2–16. Percentages of child victims ranged from 67 to 83% of all cases,
and convictions in these child rape victim cases were frequent. Child sexual abuse prosecution rates were low in these years, and it is likely that
only the very strongest cases, such as those with medical evidence, were
brought to court. In only a small minority of child sexual assaults—perhaps as few as 10% of cases—do children have any physical evidence
upon medical examination.

THE MODERN PERIOD: 1970–1990

The unprecedented and sustained public and professional attention to all
forms of child maltreatment can be dated back into the period of

minimization about child sexual abuse. In 1962, pediatrician Henry Kempe and colleagues published a very influential paper about battered children (Kempe, Silverman, Steele, Droegmueller, & Silver, 1962). Child abuse reporting laws were passed in every state between 1963 and 1967, with physical violence to children as their focus (Pleck, 1987). These laws did not explicitly include child sexual abuse. Fontana's 1964 book, *The Maltreated Child*, did not include child sexual abuse. The 1968 edition of Helfer and Kempe's *The Battered Child* did not include child sexual abuse. There were nevertheless occasional cracks in the professional wall of denial. Thus, DeFrancis in the United States wrote in 1969, as Ferenczi had written in Vienna in 1933, that victims of sex crimes experience trauma, shame, and anxieties, and that the experience is damaging to them (Ferenczi, 1955; first published in German in 1933). DeFrancis's was one of the earliest large-scale studies of child sexual abuse, and he alerted readers that his findings pointed to the probability of an enormous national incidence, greater than that for physical abuse. DeFrancis (1969) bemoaned the fact that society had failed to recognize this substantial problem. This was about to change.

In 1974, Congress passed Walter Mondale's influential Child Abuse Prevention and Treatment Act, which included child sexual abuse in its definitions of maltreatment. By 1976, every state had a law requiring professionals to report child sexual abuse, although these laws still vary in their details from state to state (Myers, 2004). By the late 1970s, there was an outpouring of professional, feminist, and popular literature about child sexual abuse and incest (Olafson, 2002; Olafson et al., 1993). As Myers (2004) writes, by the mid 1980s research and writing on child sexual abuse had "exploded" (p. 388).

Grassroots/Professional Alliances

Unlike those in the first great wave of interest at the end of the 19th century, the late 20th-century activists in child sexual abuse formed alliances between the grassroots and the professions, so that feminist activists and adult survivors teamed up with social workers, psychologists, pediatricians, and even some psychiatrists to advance knowledge and create social policy in this area (Corwin, 2002; Olafson, 2002). The grassroots/professional alliances about child sexual trauma mirrored similar alliances elsewhere during the 1970s. Vietnam veterans teamed with psychiatrists to lobby for the creation and inclusion of a new diagnosis, posttraumatic stress disorder (PTSD) in the 1980 edition of the *Diagnostic and Statistical Manual of Mental Disorders* (DSM-III, American Psychiatric Association, 1980). Battered women and shelter staff teamed with mental health professionals for recognition of the battered woman syndrome (L. E. Walker, 1979). Rape survivors and the professionals who worked with them advocated for recognition of rape trauma syndrome (Burgess & Holstrom, 1974). This extraordinarily creative period of intellectual, political, and social activism is well documented in Herman's *Trauma and Recovery* (1992, 1997). During the 1980s, as professionals from these diverse areas of interpersonal violence studies came to recognize commonalities in the symptom patterns they were seeing, they joined to offer a new diagnosis for disorders associated with prolonged and severe trauma. They gave this proposed diagnosis various names, from "violence disorders" (with the unfortunate acronym VD), to "disorders of interpersonal violence," to "complex posttraumatic stress disorder" (Herman, 1992), to the category submitted to—and rejected by—the American Psychiatric Association's (1994) DSM-IV Committee, the awkward DESNOS, or "disorders of extreme stress not otherwise specified" (Corwin, 1992; Pelcovitz et al., 1997).

Formation of Professional Societies

The modern period has also been fertile in the creation of new professional societies that focus on interpersonal trauma and child abuse. Kempe and his colleagues founded the International Society for Prevention and Treatment of Child Abuse and Neglect (*ISPCAN.org*) in 1977; the society publishes *Child Abuse and Neglect* and sponsors international and regional conferences. In 1985, psychiatrist David L. Corwin and his colleagues summoned a National Summit to develop a diagnostic category for the sexually abused child, and although participants did not agree on a diagnosis, they did agree to found a new society, the American Professional Society on the Abuse of Children (APSAC). APSAC publishes *Child Maltreatment* and the *APSAC Advisor*; has many strong state chapters; sponsors conferences; issues guidelines, study guides, and child maltreatment handbooks; and conducts investigative interview and trauma treatment training programs (*APSAC.org*). Also founded in the 1980s was the International Society for Traumatic Stress Studies (*ISTSS.org*), which publishes the *Journal of Traumatic Stress* and sponsors conferences about traumatic stress in adults and children.

The year 1985 saw the birth of the child advocacy center movement for child sexual abuse investigations. The National Children's Advocacy Center (NCAC) was established in Huntsville, Alabama, in 1985. By 2003, there were 460 full or associate children's advocacy centers in 49 states. The goals of these innovative programs are to "improve child abuse investigations and reduce stress on children and families. CACs aim to eliminate repetitive interviews for child victims, provide a child-friendly environment for the investigation, use well-trained interviewers, and coordinate forensic investigations by multiple agencies" (Walsh, Jones, & Cross, 2003, p. 3). Child advocacy centers use multidisciplinary teams made up of law enforcement, child protective service, prosecutors, and mental health and medical professionals. Protection and prosecution investigations theoretically co-occur in a child-friendly environment designed to reduce the risks of secondary trauma for alleged child victims. Although remarkably successful, the national CAC movement has experienced inevitable growing pains, including turf or boundary issues with other institutions devoted to child welfare. In addition, the sometimes divergent goals of the criminal justice and social services systems can challenge multidisciplinary team cooperation within advocacy centers (Walsh et al., 2003). Originally designed for child sexual abuse cases alone, most CACs have now expanded to investigate other alleged crimes involving children, such as serious physical abuse and the witnessing of violence to others (Walsh et al., 2003, p. 3).

Mass Day Care Cases

If the 1970s and 1980s were fertile in the creation of new institutions, new definitions, and strong alliances between the professions and the the grassroots, the 1980s and 1990s also saw the emergence of a formidable backlash against these new developments in child protection (Myers, 1994). While many professionals were arguing that children should be believed in child sexual abuse cases, and "Believe the Children" took root as a new organization complete with bumper stickers and lapel buttons, videotaped interviews from a number of mass day care cases revealed suggestive and even coercive questioning by some investigators and cast doubt on children's witness capacity (Bruck, Ceci, & Rosenthal, 1995; Myers, 2004).

Kelly Michaels, who had tended children at the Wee Care Nursery Center in New Jersey, was convicted in 1988 on 115 counts of child sexual abuse involving 115 children ages 3–5. An appellate court overturned the conviction in 1994 and all charges were dropped, *State of New Jersey v. Michaels*, 136 N.J. 299 (N.J. 1994). An *amicus* brief by a Committee of Concerned Social Scientists prepared by psychologists Maggie Bruck and Stephen Ceci documented the flawed interview techniques in this investigation (Ceci & Bruck, 1995). Statements by interviewers to Wee Care children included naming other children who had disclosed abuse and pressuring children by saying that the interviewer would hate to have to tell the child's friends that the child had not wanted to help them. The videotaped interviews are sealed, and investigators wishing copies of the tens of thousands of pages of court transcripts from the Wee Care case must pay to have all names expunged.

The McMartin case, which began in 1983, eventually involved allegations by over 400 children of sexual abuse at three Manhattan Beach, California, preschools. McMartin culminated in what were up to that time the longest and costliest trials in American history, trials that ended in acquittals and hung juries (Ceci & Bruck, 1995; Stanton, 1997). Unlike in the Wee Care case, copies of the McMartin interview tapes still circulate in certain academic and legal circles with warnings that this is the sort of thing that happens when true believers get hold of little children. Segments of the McMartin case videotapes continue to be shown in college classrooms, although there is no evidence that the alleged child victims, who are now adults, have signed releases for the videotaped dissemination of their childhood statements to investigators. A made-for-television drama about the notorious McMartin case has been aired on HBO.

Satanic Ritual Abuse Cases

The backlash against the new developments in child protection was also fed by the satanic ritual abuse phenomenon of the 1980s. Large numbers of adults and children claimed to have been victimized in organized satanic or ritual sexual abuse cult activities that included alleged murders of babies and children by costumed perpetrators, grotesque sexual assaults, consumption of excrement, cannibalism, animal sacrifice, and the breeding of babies for use by the cult (Bottoms, Shaver, & Goodman, 1996). Some responsible and well-trained physicians and psychologists and much of the media, including *MS* magazine, publicized the dangers and consequences of satanic ritual abuse (Rose, 1993). After initially believing that organized satanic ritual abuse rings might possibly exist, FBI investigator Ken Lanning pointed out that investigators in thousands of alleged cases had found no corroborating evidence for child murders or organized ritual criminal cults, although he did not deny that groups of isolated sadistic individuals have always come up with imaginatively horrible ways to torture and sexually assault child victims (Corwin, Olafson, Parker, Derstine, & Bottoms, 1996; Lanning, 1991; Putnam, 1991). In a random sampling of over 3,000 psychologists with a 46% response rate, 13% of respondents reported having encountered adult survivor cases of ritual abuse, and 11% had encountered child cases. Most psychologists described having dealt with only one or two such cases. A small minority who stated they had treated scores of cases accounted for most of the over 700 ritual abuse cases described for this study (Bottoms et al., 1996).

The satanic ritual abuse phenomenon had tragic consequences that included professional excesses and actual malpractice, such as the involuntary psychiatric hospitalization and forced medication of alleged cult members' children. The consequences included ruptured families, interrupted lives, subsequent lawsuits, federal prosecutions, and loss of licensure for some mental health professionals involved. The unfortunate results have included widespread public and media skepticism toward children and adult survivors in less spectacular child sexual abuse cases, a skepticism that survives until the present (Ceci & Bruck, 1995; Putnam, 1997).

CURRENT RESEARCH ON CHILDREN'S MEMORY AND SUGGESTIBILITY

The mass day care center cases such as McMartin and the Kelly Michaels case of the 1980s were at least partially responsible for several subsequent developments. Other day care cases with dozens of alleged victims, such as the San Francisco Presidio nursery school case in the late 1980s, were never brought to trial. Little has been published about the Presidio Nursery School Case, with which I am familiar only because I was an intern at Letterman Army Medical Center from 1986 to 1988 when over 100 children and their families were interviewed and more than half of these cases clinically substantiated (Ehrensaft, 1992). One of the alleged perpetrators in that case has since died of AIDS.

Partly in response to the interviewing shortcomings and flaws during the day care cases that were prosecuted, memory and suggestibility research on children has proliferated. One school, continuing the 1980s research by Goodman, Saywitz, and their associates, conducts analogue studies to show children's strengths as witnesses and works to develop techniques to improve children's witness capacity (see Lyon, 1999, for references and a summary of this research). A new wave of researchers that emerged in the 1990s and is led by psychologists Steven Ceci and Maggie Bruck, answers with analogue studies designed to demonstrate children's memory deficiencies and their vulnerability to suggestion (Lyon, 1999). Bruck and Ceci wrote the *amicus* brief in *New Jersey v. Michaels* that contributed to the reversal of Michaels' conviction (Bruck et al., 1995). Also during the 1990s, international, national, and regional institutions created training programs for law enforcement, social work, medical, and child advocacy center interviewers and investigators to improve and standardize child forensic interviewing approaches and build teamwork among those in various disciplines who interview children and investigate cases. Investigators have taken the lessons learned in research funded because of the child sexual abuse wars and are now applying it to their work with child witnesses to other alleged crimes such as physical abuse and the witnessing of violence to others (Walsh et al., 2003).

On the issues of children's memory and suggestibility, there are emerging areas of agreement and ongoing controversies. Both waves of memory researchers agree that even young children, if properly questioned, can recall and report large amounts of forensically relevant material about personally experienced, salient events (Ceci & Bruck, 1995; Ceci & Huffman, 1997; Saywitz, Goodman & Lyon, 2002; Saywitz & Lyon, 2002). Because of the egocentricity of young children, that is to say, their focus on themselves and close family members to which they are attached, emotional significance for children may not be what adults imagine it to be. Nevertheless, it is now clear that it is very difficult to persuade even the youngest children that negative or painful things happened to their bodies when these experiences did not take place (Ceci, Loftus, Leichtman, & Bruck, 1994). Even when such erroneous memories appear to be implanted, they do not in most cases persist over time (Huffman, Crossman, & Ceci, 1997). It appears to be easier to convince children that they took part in fictional positive experiences, such as, for example, stories about taking a ride in a hot air balloon or helping someone find a lost monkey (Gilstrap & Ceci, 2001). Implanting false memories about implausible events is also more difficult than about plausible events, but here we encounter definitional problems; what does "implausible" mean to a generation reared on the Internet, Harry Potter, and Saturday morning television? (Pezdek & Hinz, 2002).

Although researchers agree that on average children's memories improve and suggestibility decreases as children mature, there are individual and situational differences. It appears that some individuals are more suggestible than others, for reasons linked both to intelligence and personality (Eisen, Winograd, & Qin, 2002). If suggestibility is about memory alone, then developmentally average children from ages 10–12 are nearly as resistant to suggestion as adults are; however, if children's dependent status and possible compliance with the demands of adult authority are included, even adolescents can remain vulnerable (Westcott, Davies, & Bull, 2002). Dependent adults such as battered women or prisoners are, of course, also suggestible in this way, because this dependence-linked "suggestibility" is about false statements, not about false memories. Stressful situations such as appearing in court also impede children's recall and increase their suggestibility (Saywitz & Nathanson, 1993).

The greatest effort, much of the available research funding, and the greatest honors and prizes in the memory wars, especially for those academic researchers who are not also active in child protection, continue to be devoted to guarding against false allegations by children and protecting adults from being falsely accused. At the Summer 2003 Convention of the American Psychological Association, for example, Stephen J. Ceci was awarded the Distinguished Scientific Contribution for the Application of Psychology Award for his research showing the circumstances in which children are susceptible to suggestion, and Elizabeth Loftus was honored for nearly 30 years of research on false memories (Bailey & Dittman, 2003). Loftus was also honored in 2003 in an APA published book honoring 16 psychologists (only two of whom are women) for having "battled the establishment and won" (Zigler, 2003, title page). There has been far less interest in and federal funding devoted to finding ways to help what many professionals believe to be the far greater number of actually sexually abused children who either cannot remember or will not tell when they are questioned about genital touching and child sexual abuse (Freyd, 1996; Lyon, 1995, 2002; Saywitz, Goodman, Nicholas, & Moan, 1991; Sjoberg & Lindblad, 2002; *Stogner v. California*, 123 S. Ct. 2446 (2003)).

RECENT DEVELOPMENTS: 1990–2004

After a generation of media attention, political advocacy, and legal reform, what is the current situation with respect to child sexual abuse in the United States?

Training Programs and Protocols

Child forensic interview manuals and training programs began to be established in the late 1980s and have proliferated since then (Poole & Lamb, 1998). Major national trainers meet in think tanks sponsored by APSAC (American Professional Society on the Abuse of Children, 2003). The National Advocacy Center in Huntsville, Alabama, trains child advocacy center investigators and multidisciplinary teams (Steele, 2003). The American Prosecutor's Research Institute (APRI) has incorporated Minnesota's Cornerhouse semistructured protocol to train multidisciplinary teams throughout the United States (Holmes & Vieth, 2003). San Diego's Children Hospital (Davies et al., 1996), and Bourg, Broderick, and their colleagues in Oregon (Bourg et al., 1999) established strong regional programs during the 1990s and have trained thousands of investigators among them. APSAC founded 5-day interviewing clinics in 1996 and revived them in 2002, and they have since trained investigators in Kentucky, Michigan, Florida, and Massachusetts (American Professional Society on the Abuse of Children, 2003). All these programs teach flexible interviewing approaches that include the use of interview aids such as anatomical drawings and dolls when necessary.

The state of Michigan has mandated a semistructured protocol for use throughout the state that recommends against (but does not prohibit) the use of interview aids such as dolls and drawings (State of Michigan Governor's Task Force on Children's Justice, 1998). In neighboring Wisconsin, Canadian psychologist John Yuille's Stepwise Protocol, one of the very earliest child interview protocols to be developed and disseminated, is widely taught to child abuse investigators. The Stepwise Protocol recommends against the use of anatomical dolls (Yuille, 1996).

Researchers have also developed structured protocols that resemble scripts and that have received a mixed reception among those who interview children (Faller, 2003). Michael Lamb, federally funded by the National Institute of Child Health and Human Development (NICHD), has employed a structured protocol written by the late Kathy Sternberg and colleagues to study hundreds of alleged child sexual abuse cases in Israel, Sweden, England, and the United States, a protocol that offers investigative teams the precise language to use in order to avoid questions that are too specific or leading (Orbach et al., 2000; Sternberg, Lamb, Orbach, Esplin, & Mitchell, 2001). Ongoing peer review and supervision is essential for adherence to the protocol over time. Psychology professor and attorney Thomas D. Lyon has recently modified Sternberg's NICHD script, is field testing it in the Los Angeles area, and finds it most effective with children ages 6 and older who are in at least partial disclosure (Lyon, 2003). Neither version of these structured protocols includes the use of interview aids such as dolls and drawings.

The Childhood Trust Forensic Training Institute in Cincinnati (of which I am the director), established in 1997, teaches both a structured protocol and flexible guidelines. We recognize the advantages of a well-researched, structured protocol for those children who are able and ready to describe their experiences fully. We train investigators in Lyon's adaptation of the NICHD protocol for children ages 6 and older who are in active disclosure. We also recognize the disadvantages of structured protocols for the very large numbers of young, developmentally delayed, reluctant, or traumatized children who cannot or will not talk readily to investigators. For these children, we train investigators to use flexible guidelines that include dolls and drawings. We provide trainees with guidelines for selecting the type of approach each case requires. Structured and supervised small group practice in peer review throughout the training enables investigators to return to their agencies with the skills necessary to maintain and refine their new interviewing skills through ongoing practice, teamwork, and peer review. We offer 1-day advanced trainings to update past trainees in new developments (*http:// www.childhoodtrust.org*). For very reluctant children, the Childhood Trust training also recommends the extended interview protocol developed in Huntsville and piloted in several American advocacy centers (Carnes, Nelson-Gardell, Wilson, & Orgassa, 2001; Carnes, Wilson, & Nelson-Gardell, 1999).

Most of the major investigative interview training programs include updated sections about children's memory and suggestibility, and they all incorporate the indispensable work by forensic linguist Ann Graffam Walker about how to question children using language and sentence structure that is developmentally optimal (A. G. Walker, 1999). Walker writes, "Even very young children can tell us what they know if we ask them the right questions in the right way," and she cites cases demonstrating that children as young as 3 have testified competently and credibly in court (p. 2). Walker shows that young children use words for time, distance, kinship, size, and other matters long before they understand their meaning (p. 3); they have difficulty with pronouns and prepositions, and they become confused when questions are complex. Walker explains that asking preschoolers "when" something happened or "how many times" it happened can produce errors in their answers, because young children will try to answer even those questions they do not understand. They will translate unfamiliar words such as "allegation" into familiar words such as "alligator," or "jury" into "jewelry" (Saywitz & Camparo, 1998; Saywitz & Goodman, 1996; Saywitz et al., 2002). Psychologist Sandra Hewitt, an expert on preschoolers, argues that children can be competent witnesses if they can answer "who," "where," "what," and "what happened" questions (Hewitt, 1999). Hewitt and Walker offer guidelines for the optimal language and sentence structures to use with the very young, as well as linguistic pitfalls to avoid. Every prosecutor and interviewer in the United States should own, learn, and apply the A. G. Walker (1999) manual, which is published by the American Bar Association Center on Children and the Law in Washington, DC.

Applying a very effective team approach, Florida psychologist Dennison Reed and detective Rick Cage train law enforcement/interviewer teams to move quickly on child sexual abuse cases, using rapid police intervention and surprise interviews with alleged perpetrators to increase their confession rates and thus improve conviction rates (Reed & Cage, 2003). Cage and Reed agree with the American Prosecutor's Research Institute's Victor Vieth that the child interview cannot always carry the weight of an entire case, and that good police work, corroborative evidence from the crime scene, and confessions greatly strengthen efforts to protect children and prosecute their offenders (Vieth, 1999).

Prevalence of Abuse and Prosecution Rates

Reporting, substantiation, and prosecution of child sexual abuse cases skyrocketed in the 1980s and into the 1990s. Because it appears that most cases are still not reported to the authorities, the true prevalence of child sexual abuse and incest remains unknown (brief of *amici curiae* by the American Psychological Association, National Association of Counsel for Children, American Professional Society on the Abuse of Children, and California Professional Society on the Abuse of Children in *Stogner v. California*, 123 S. Ct. 2446 (2003); Myers, 1998). Substantiations of child sexual abuse declined significantly during the 1990s. Experts disagree about whether these numbers indicate a decline in actual child sexual abuse prevalence or can be explained otherwise. Sociologist David Finkelhor is among those who argue that there has been a real decline in child sexual abuse in the 1990s, and he offers several possible reasons. These include the general prosperity of the period, increased incarceration rates for offenders, sexual offender and community notification laws nationwide, continued media attention and personal safety education programs for schoolchildren (Finkelhor, 2003).

Those who question the reality of a true decline note that substantiation rates provide only a partial picture of the prevalence of this crime. Lyon recently summarized current research that indicates that most child sexual abuse is still not reported to the authorities because large percentages of both male and female victims never tell anyone about the abuse (brief of *amici curiae* by the American Psychological Association et al., for *Stogner v. California*, 123 S. Ct. 2446 (2003); see also Putnam, 2003, about similar rates of nonreporting in other countries). Even when children do tell adults, one study shows that in 75% of United States cases, adults do not then report these alleged offenses to the authorities (Hanson, 2002; Hanson, Resnick, Saunders, Kilpatrick & Best, 1999). Assaults and rapes by strangers are far more likely to be reported and prosecuted than are similar offenses by family members or friends (Smith & Elstein, 1993).

The United States has no national statistics on the criminal prosecution of child sexual abuse. It is known that with the rediscovery of child sexual abuse after 1980, child sexual abuse prosecutions increased dramatically in the United States (Myers, 2004), but many cases are still not prosecuted, especially when there is no corroborating evidence or when victims are very young. The average age of child witnesses in child sexual abuse cases appears to be about 10 (Lyon, 1995). Even when prosecutors are familiar with the research studies showing that younger children can be competent and nonsuggestible witnesses, these prosecutors are also aware that the general public who make up the jury pool from which fact finders (judges and juries) are drawn is highly skeptical of child witnesses (Brigham, 1998; Vieth, 1999).

The age of consent in the Netherlands, where the propedophile journal *Paidika* is published, has been lowered to 12, but age of consent in the United States continues to be debated. If child sexual abuse is criminal and wrong because children cannot consent, at what age can developmentally average children legally consent? State laws vary from age 14 to one day before age 18. Myers (2004) found that there exist no national data about prosecution rates for substantiated child sexual abuse, but regional studies indicate that prosecutors are less likely to pursue cases when victims have reached puberty and might be viewed as partially "responsible" for the sexual contacts (Gray, 1993, p. 108). Prosecutors are also reluctant to bring cases when victims are very young (Gray, 1993, p. 109; Lyon, 1995). For children and young adults who have developmental disabilities, the issue of consent is complex and difficult, and it is well established in numerous research studies that these children are more likely to experience all forms of abuse and neglect, including sexual assault (Davies, 2003).

When offenders are convicted, sentences for child sexual abuse offenses, including penetrating rape, often amount to little more than a slap on the wrist (Salter, 2003). Many states still release convicted child sexual offenders from prison after only a few years. Although the sexual offender and community notification laws passed throughout the United States in the 1990s are designed to protect children from subsequent offending by these released felons, the effectiveness of these laws has not yet been documented (Hanson, 2002). It has long been established that, in contrast to most violent criminals, child molesters do not "age out" of this criminal behavior (Dickey, Nussbaum, Chevolleau, & Davidson, 2002; Hanson, 2002). Rates of sexual offending for these men continue virtually unchanged until they reach at least 50 years of age, and all too frequently impotent old men continue to sexually assault children. In a recent Midwestern case, for example, a multidisciplinary team interviewed an elderly man in his home. This grandfather had been released years before after serving time for the molestation and rape of his daughter, and he was now accused by two prepubescent granddaughters of fondling them. Impotent because of age and illness, sustained by the oxygen tank at his feet, he still had his persuasive powers, his fingers, and his urge to sexually assault children.

Proponents of Normalizing Adult–Child Sexual Relations

Occasional professional works purporting to show that adult–child sexual contact is normal or does not damage children continue to be published even now. Judith Levine (2002) recommends lowering the age of consent in the United States to 12 and argues that because most normal men are attracted to adolescents, this attraction should not be diagnosed as deviant. In 1998, Bruce Rind and his colleagues published in the American Psychological Association's *Psychological Bulletin* a meta-analysis of studies using college population samples about the impact of child sexual abuse. They concluded that child sexual abuse does not damage children, and they recommended that the word "abuse" be dropped and "adult–child" or "adult–adolescent" sex be substituted instead (Rind, Tromovitch, & Bauserman, 1998). This proposed change in terminology takes us back to an earlier time; Bender and Blau in 1937 did not describe what happened sexually between adults and children as "sexual abuse," but used the words "seduction," "sexual relations," and "promiscuous relations with men" to describe the children's victimization.

The 1998 study by Rind et al. was so methodologically unsound that the first set of peer reviewers rejected it outright and recommended against resubmission to *Psychological Bulletin*. After a change of editors at this journal, the Rind study somehow reached publication, although psychologist Anna Salter reports that at least one reviewer again rejected the paper and the other reviewers (if any) have not come forward (Salter, 2003). When the United States Congress, alerted to the Rind study in a major American Psychological Association journal by radio personality Dr. Laura, passed a resolution condemning it, some professionals defended its publication on the grounds of academic freedom (Salter, 2003). Although academics in subsequent issues of *Psychological Bulletin* and elsewhere criticized the study on methodological grounds (Dallam, 2001, 2002; Ondersma et al., 2001), Rind and his colleagues then attacked their critics as biased by moral and religious zealotry and defended their own work as scientific. Salter reminds us that Rind and his colleagues do not acknowledge their own biases and that they have a history of publications in the propedophile Dutch journal, *Paidika, The Journal of Pedophilia*, where they have written positively about sex between adult men and boys. (See Salter, 2003, pp. 62–66 for a more detailed account of the Rind et al. study and its context.)

Rind (2001) has also written positively about sex between men and adolescent boys in a paper based on his analysis of a study of gay college students at an Ivy League school, 26 of whom reported having engaged in sex with adult men when they were ages 12–17. Most of these college students, Rind states, recalled and described the experiences positively and were as well adjusted in terms of self-esteem as the controls. Rind's paper ends with 26 brief vignettes describing the sexual experiences these 26 subjects had with adult men, including quotations from the subjects. Ivy League college student samples select from only the highest functioning of child sexual abuse survivors, and even among these, the sampling was not random. These are anecdotes, not research findings.

INCEST AND ITS OUTCOMES
IN INTACT AND SEPARATED FAMILIES

It remains true today, as it was in the past, that for those children who are identified and rescued from incest by a father-figure, a number of negative consequences follow. Family income declines precipitously. Mothers are left to cope with their own postdisclosure anger, anxiety, depression, and guilt and so may not be fully available to child victims. In addition, these mother-headed households generally have to move to more modest housing when incestuous father or stepfather income is lost. Maternal support has been robustly shown to be the most crucial factor in children's recovery from child sexual abuse (Cohen & Mannarino, 1996; Elliott & Carnes, 2001). But postdisclosure emotional, financial, legal, and personal pressures upon nonoffending mothers make it challenging to provide this necessary support consistently. In addition, for reasons that are not clear, child abuse victims often blame their mothers for the abuse, and the mother–child relationship suffers significant damage (Jacobs, 1994).

Research also shows that children's posttraumatic symptoms are most effectively alleviated through cognitive-behavioral therapy, but it is only when nonoffending mothers or caretakers participate in therapy that children's depression, sexualized behaviors, and aggression are alleviated (Cohen & Mannarino, 1993; Deblinger & Heflin, 1996). Indeed, one study showed that these symptoms in children reduced even when the mother alone was treated, with no direct psychological interventions for the sexually abused children (Deblinger, Lippman, & Steer, 1996). In a federally funded study, the cognitive-behavioral therapies (CBT) developed by Judith Cohen, by Esther Deblinger, by Anthony Mannarino, and by their respective colleagues was given the highest ranking as a well-supported and efficacious treatment for childhood trauma and maltreatment among the 22 approaches evaluated (Saunders, Berliner, & Hanson, 2003). Trauma-focused CBT is now being adapted in new manuals and widely disseminated throughout the federally funded National

Child Traumatic Stress Network (NCTSN; Saunders, Berliner, & Hanson, 2003).

As for other therapies, the relationship enhancement component of parent–child interaction therapy (PCIT) shows promise in restoring disturbed attachment relationships between nonoffending parents and children in homes where there has been maltreatment (Friedrich, personal communication, 2003; Funderburk, personal communication, 2003). PCIT, which has a strong research base as an intervention for children with behavioral disturbances and their caretakers, is now being adapted for maltreating families, with promising initial results (Friedrich, 1998; Hembree-Kigin & McNeil, 1995; Urquiza & McNeil, 1996).

When incest occurs in the context of separated parents, the situation is bleaker. Although the most recent nationwide study is now more than 10 years old (Thoennes, Pearson, & Tjaden, 1988; Thoennes & Tjaden, 1990), there are many case studies and at least one good regional study documenting the difficulty faced by nonoffending parents— most always mothers—when they try to protect their children from ongoing child sexual abuse in the context of family court proceedings (Faller & Devoe, 1995; Myers, 1997). Most divorcing parents with minor children settle custody issues without going to court, so that custody disputes by divorcing families who have minor children constitute only about 10–15% of cases. Regional studies suggest that when parents are willing to fight for custody, it is often because something is wrong with the other parent. There is some evidence suggesting that in a great many of these cases, one parent is expressing genuine concern about the safety of the children in the other household, whether because of violence, substance abuse, neglect, or child sexual abuse (Pearson & Anhalt, 1994; Statewide Office of Family Court Services, 1992).

Domestic Relations Courts

Given the research findings about the potential dangers of child sexual abuse to children in the context of separated parents, what are family and domestic courts doing? Faller's regional study of several hundred alleged sexual abuse cases in custody disputes shows that in almost 40% of child sexual abuse cases substantiated in her excellent university-based program, judges failed to protect minor children from ongoing unsupervised contact with the alleged offending parent, generally a father, who continued to get sole or joint custody or unsupervised visitation. In one case, the judge not only repeatedly refused to look at the evaluation report but threw it to the floor, and in another case, medical evidence supportive of the sexual abuse allegation was not considered by the court despite 3 years of effort by one mother (Faller & Devoe, 1995).

Why does this happen? Judge Leonard Edwards argued over 15 years ago that domestic relations courts are not structured to investigate alleged crimes. Physical and sexual assaults are crimes, whether perpetrated in the home or on the street (Edwards, 1987). Family court is structured to get parents to agree, to mediate, to conciliate, and so to move cases along. Some states, such as California, have required mediation in all cases where custody is disputed, even when there has been spousal battering (Pearson & Anhalt, 1992). Judge Edwards argued that when crimes against children are alleged in the context of separated parents, cases should be transferred to juvenile court, which is constituted to investigate, and that the juvenile court's decisions should take priority over domestic relations court decisions.

Instead of implementing proposals such as Judge Edwards's, what has happened nationwide is that mothers who allege sexual abuse in the context of custody proceedings are too often vilified as brainwashers, delusional, schizophrenic, alienating parents, or vindictive women who are using the children to bargain for property (St. Charles & Crook, 2000). In many cases these protective parents lose custody and even all contact with their children (St. Charles & Crook, 2000). A cottage industry of privately printed and non-peer-reviewed publications, lectures, and court cases by the late Richard Gardner, MD, has fed this regressive trend, the ultimate effect of which has been to make it difficult to protect children from criminal assault when custody is at stake (Bruch, 2001a, 2001b; Dallam, 2002; Faller, 1998; Faller, Corwin, & Olafson, 1993; Wood, 1994).

In one of the oddities of 1980s literature on the topic, mothers in intact families continued to be described as collusive to or partially responsible for ongoing incest (Giaretto, 1982), while at the same time a new backlash literature emerged claiming that divorcing mothers brainwashed their children into false allegations against their ex-spouses. This rapidly changing professional vision of mothers, from incest collaborators in intact families to vindictive brainwashers in separated ones, had in common the urge to blame mothers and excuse fathers (Olafson et al., 1993). These mutually contradictory mother-blaming myths coexisted through much of the 1980s, serving to protect incestuous fathers from being seen and sanctioned and their children from being adequately protected (Caplan & Hall-McCorquodale, 1985). In the context of separated parents, the pervasive myth of the vindictive, brainwashing mother can have tragic consequences. One child is known to have committed suicide after psychiatrist Richard Gardner recommended and the court ordered that he return to live with his father, and there have been uncounted numbers of other tragedies (Carpenter & Kopas, 1998; Pennington, 2000).

There are also a growing number of anecdotal accounts about the misuse of factitious disorder by proxy ("Munchhausen by proxy") diagnoses against mothers who seek to protect children from sexual abuse by estranged husbands (Mart, 2000); I have personally been involved in one such case. Unfortunately, there is little national interest and absolutely no federal money to investigate the current status of child sexual abuse allegations in the context of separated parents, but anecdotal accounts and regional studies such as Faller's suggest that it may be harder to protect children from abuse when custody is disputed than in other circumstances (Faller, 1998). Wigmore's ancient myth of the unstable, lying, vindictive female continues to live on in many domestic relations courts (Czapanskiy, 1993).

Batterers and Custody

It is also well established that battering fathers are far more likely than are nonbatterers to sue for custody, and that when they sue, they are as likely to be awarded joint or sole custody as are nonbatterers (Bancroft & Silverman, 2002; Jaffe, Lemon, & Poisson, 2002). Courts continue to order joint or sole custody to batterers in the face of years of statistics documenting that batterers are far more likely than are nonbatterers to physically and sexually abuse their children (Bancroft & Silverman, 2002; Edleson, 1999; Jaffe et al., 2002). A recent British study indicates that the chronic witnessing of domestic violence has the effect of actually lowering children's IQs on average more deeply than does children's chronic exposure to lead (Koenen, Moffitt, Caspi, Taylor, & Purcell, 2003; Putnam, 2003).

As the witnessing of violence becomes identified as a damaging form of child maltreatment, courts are moving to protect children by holding battered mothers (rather than their batterers) accountable. The threat or the actuality of finding mothers unfit because they fail to protect children from witnessing their own beatings, as has happened in New York City and has become law in the state of Indiana, perpetuates a long history of misguided efforts to hold women accountable for male violence. Organized resistance has already begun. In a 2003 case, *Nicholson v. Scoppetta*, five women sued the Commissioner of the Administration for Children's Services in New York City because they were charged with neglect and had their children removed from their care for allowing their children to witness domestic violence (Otis, 2003). The New York State Court of Appeals and the United States Court of Appeals, Second Circuit, found for the mothers in this class action lawsuit. Advocates for women and children believe that where these new laws and practices are taking hold, women are failing to call the police for protection from batterers because they fear authorities will take away their children (Otis, 2003).

New Approaches

Battering, child abuse, and animal cruelty often coexist in families, a toxic triad that has recently garnered attention in legal and mental health circles (Ascione & Arkow, 1999). Mandating animal control officers to become child abuse reporters, changing state laws so that animal cruelty is a felony rather than a misdemeanor, boarding pets for women and children who seek shelter, and moving quickly to intervene for children who severely abuse pets, are all promising interventions that may help interrupt the intergenerational transmission of physical and sexual violence in families. As part of the Childhood Trust's Forensic Training Institute, psychologist Barbara W. Boat teaches law enforcement, child advocacy center investigators, and social work trainees to team with animal control officers and to include questions about pets as part of the flexible protocol taught in Cincinnati. Given the nationwide backlash against believing children who disclose sexual abuse, one child protection strategy to consider is to convict and imprison "toxic triad" offenders for felony animal abuse and/or domestic violence, even when courts refuse to adjudicate child sexual abuse allegations (Boat, 1995, 1999).

Although there has been no recent federal money to study child abuse allegations in the context of separated parents, federal funding for larger child trauma and maltreatment issues has contributed to the creation of a new institutional structure with enormous potential. Many of the pioneers in the psychobiology of interpersonal victimization are now regional directors in a newly established National Child Traumatic Stress Network (NCTSN), federally funded under the jurisdiction of Health and Human Services, Substance Abuse and Mental Health Services Administration (SAMHSA). This Network has expanded in 2003 to 54 sites nationwide; I am Training Director for Cincinnati's already established Level II site.

A major multisite committee within the NCTSN is revisiting issues of posttraumatic stress disorder (PTSD) and complex PTSD in children, attempting to integrate developmental issues and attachment research into their diagnostic formulations. PTSD was first identified in Vietnam veterans, that is, in adult males. Shoehorning childhood posttraumatic reactions into this structure has always been problematic (American Academy of Child and Adolescent Psychiatry, 1997).

Another multisite NCTSN committee is working to create evidence-based treatments for adolescent rape victims, combining excellent approaches developed and researched by Deblinger (Deblinger & Heflin,

1996), Cohen and Mannarino (1993) for younger children, and Resick and Schnicke (1996) for adult rape victims. Trauma treatment specialists Cohen and Mannarino have traveled to NCTSN sites throughout the country to train providers in their evidence-based treatments for children ages 2–14 who have suffered sexual abuse trauma and other forms of interpersonal violence. Other NCTSN sites are adapting parent–child interaction therapies for nonoffending parents and children to enhance their relationships and repair troubled attachments following child sexual abuse and other traumas.

CONCLUSION

Much remains to be done. Mainstream training programs in counseling, psychology, medicine, psychiatry, and even social work too often still treat child maltreatment in general and child sexual abuse in particular as specialties rather than as central to the etiology of a host of adolescent and adult disorders, health problems, and criminal behaviors. Child abuse histories have now been robustly shown to be associated with subsequent substance abuse, nicotine addiction, depression, anxiety, school failure, adolescent pregnancy, criminal behavior, high-risk sexual behavior and its consequences, suicide, compromised physical health, and even premature death (Anda et al., 1999; Dube, Anda, Felitti, Edwards, & Croft, 2002; Fellitti, 2002; Hillis, Anda, Felitti, & Marchbanks, 2001; Putnam, 2003). It is time, and well past time, to integrate child abuse and trauma studies into mainstream university curricula and professional training programs. The issues are central, not peripheral.

By the early 21st century, the issue of child sexual abuse has become a legitimate focus of professional attention while increasingly separated from second-wave feminism, which has generally moved on to other issues. As child sexual abuse becomes absorbed into the larger field of interpersonal trauma studies, child sexual abuse studies and intervention strategies have become degendered and largely unaware of their political origins in modern feminism and other vibrant political movements of the 1970s. One may hope that unlike in the past, this rediscovery of child sexual abuse that began in the 1970s will not again be followed by collective amnesia. The institutionalization of child maltreatment interventions in federally funded centers, national and international societies, and a host of research studies (in which the United States continues to lead the world), offers grounds for cautious optimism. Nevertheless, as psychiatrist Judith Herman (1992) argues cogently, "The systematic study of psychological trauma . . . depends on the support of a political movement" (p. 9). In the United States, a strong political movement with a focus on interpersonal trauma and child sexual abuse does not now exist. To the extent that the second wave of feminism, at least in academic settings, has become fragmented, preoccupied with identity politics and theory, and marginalized, there exists a danger that public policy attention to child sexual abuse prevention, evaluation, and treatment may correspondingly fragment and weaken in the early 21st century.

ACKNOWLEDGMENTS

I am grateful to John E. B. Myers for access to unpublished material from his forthcoming book, *A History of Child Protection in America*.

REFERENCES

Abraham, K. (1927). The experiencing of sexual trauma as a form of sexual activity. In K. Abraham (Ed.), *Selected papers* (pp. 47–62). London: Hogarth. (Original work published 1907)

American Academy of Child and Adolescent Psychiatry. (1997). Practice parameters for the forensic evaluation of children and adolescents who may have been physically or sexually abused. *Journal of the American Academy of Child Adolescent Psychiatry, 36*(10S), 37S–56S.

American Professional Society on the Abuse of Children (APSAC). (2003). News of the organization. *APSAC Advisor, 15*(3), 15.

American Psychiatric Association. (1980). *Diagnostic and statistical manual of mental disorders* (3rd ed.). Washington, DC: Author.

American Psychiatric Association. (1994). *Diagnostic and statistical manual of mental disorders* (4th ed.). Washington, DC: Author.

Anda, R. F., Croft, J. B., Felitti, V. J., Nordenberg, D., Giles, W. H., Williamson, D., & Giovino, G. A. (1999). Adverse childhood experiences and smoking during adolescence and adulthood. *Journal of the American Medical Association, 3*(282), 1652–1658.

Ascione, F. R., & Arkow, P. (1999). *Child abuse, domestic violence, and animal abuse: Linking the circles of compassion for prevention and intervention.* West Lafayette, IN: Purdue University Press.

Bailey, D. S., & Dittman, M. (2003). Ceci and Loftus honored for memory work. *Monitor on Psychology, 34*(9), 29.

Bancroft, L., & Silverman, J. G. (2002). *The batterer as parent: Addressing the impact of domestic violence on family dynamics.* Thousand Oaks, CA: Sage.

Behlmer, G. K. (1982). *Child abuse and moral reform in England, 1870–1908.* Stanford, CA: Stanford University Press.

Bender, L., & Blau, A. (1937). The reaction of children to sexual relations with adults. *American Journal of Orthopsychiatry, 7*, 500–518.

Bloom, S. L., & Reichert, M. (1998). *Bearing witness: Violence and collective responsibility.* New York: Haworth Maltreatment and Trauma Press.

Boat, B. W. (1995). The relationship between violence to children and violence to animals: An ignored link? *Journal of Interpersonal Violence, 10*(4), 229–235.

Boat, B. (1999). Abuse of children and abuse of animals: Using the links to inform child assessments and protection. In P. Arkow & F. Ascione (Eds.), *Child abuse, domestic violence and animal abuse: Linking the circles of compassion for prevention and intervention* (pp. 83–100). West Lafayette, IN: Purdue University Press.

Bottoms, B. L, Shaver, P. R., & Goodman, G.S. (1996). An analysis of ritualistic and religion-related child abuse allegations. *Law and Human Behavior, 20*(1), 1–34.

Bourg, W., Broderick, R., Flagor, R., Kelly, D. M., Ervin, D. L., & Butler, J. (1999). *A child interviewer's guidebook*. Thousand Oaks, CA: Sage.

Brigham, J. C. (1998). Adults' evaluations of characteristics of children's memory. *Journal of Applied Developmental Psychology, 19*(1), 15–39.

Brown, L., Lourie, K., Zlotnick, C., & Cohn, J. (2000). Impact of sexual abuse on the HIV-risk-related behavior of adolescents in intensive psychiatric treatment. *American Journal of Psychiatry, 157*, 1413–1415.

Brownmiller, S. (1975). *Against our will: Men, women and rape*. New York: Bantam Books.

Bruch, C. S. (2001a). Parental alienation syndrome: Junk science in child custody determinations. *European Journal of Law Reform, 3*(3), 383–404.

Bruch, C. S. (2001b). Parental alienation syndrome and parental alienation: Getting it wrong in child custody cases. *Family Law Quarterly, 35*, 527–552.

Bruck, M., Ceci, S. J., & Rosenthal, R. (1995). Amicus brief for the State of New Jersey v. Michaels. *Psychology, Public Policy, and the Law, 1*, 272–322.

Burgess, A. W., & Holstrom, L. L. (1974). Rape trauma syndrome. *American Journal of Psychiatry, 131*, 981–986.

Caplan, P. J., & Hall-McCorquodale, I. (1985). Mother-blaming in major clinical journals. *American Journal of Orthopsychiatry, 55*, 345–353.

Carnes, C. N., Nelson-Gardell, D., Wilson, C., & Orgassa, U. C. (2001). Extended forensic evaluation when sexual abuse is suspected. *Child Maltreatment, 6*, 230–242.

Carnes, C. N., Wilson, C., & Nelson-Gardell, D. (1999). Extended forensic evaluation when sexual abuse is suspected: A model and preliminary data. *Child Maltreatment, 4*(3), 242–254.

Carpenter, M., & Kopas, G. (1998, May 31). Casualties of a custody war. *Pittsburgh Post-Gazette*, p. A1. Retrieved August 19, 2002, from *http://www.post-gazette.com*.

Ceci, S. J., & Bruck, M. (1995). *Jeopardy in the courtroom: A scientific analysis of children's testimony*. Washington, DC: American Psychological Association.

Ceci, S. J., & Huffman, M. L. C. (1997). How suggestible are preschool children? Cognitive and social factors. *Journal of the American Academy of Child and Adolescent Psychiatry, 36*, 948–957.

Ceci, S. J., Loftus, E. F., Leichtman, M. D., & Bruck, M. (1994). The possible role of misattributions in the creation of false beliefs among preschoolers. *International Journal of Clinical and Experimental Hypnosis, 42*(4), 304–320.

Cohen, J. A., & Mannarino, A. P. (1993). A treatment model for sexually abused preschoolers. *Journal of Interpersonal Violence, 8*, 115–131.

Cohen, J. A., & Mannarino, A. P. (1996). A treatment outcome study for sexually abused preschool children: Initial findings. *Journal of the American Academy of Child and Adolescent Psychiatry, 35*, 42–50.

Corwin, D. L. (1992). Sexually abused children's symptoms and disorders of extreme stress not otherwise specified: Does this proposed psychiatric diagnosis fit? In A. W. Burgess (Ed.), *Child trauma I: Issues and research* (pp. 87–116). New York: Garland.

Corwin, D. L. (2002). An interview with Roland Summit. In J. R. Conte (Ed.), *Critical issues in child sexual abuse* (pp. 1–27). Thousand Oaks, CA: Sage.

Corwin, D. L., Olafson, E., Parker, K. A., Derstine, R. B., & Bottoms, B. (1996, June). *A ritual sexual abuse allegation with evidence of unintentional indoctrination: Clinical, legal and scientific perspectives.* Fifth National Colloquium of the American Professional Society on the Abuse of Children, Chicago, IL.

Cunningham, R., Stiffman, A., Dore, P., & Earls, F. (1994). The association of physical and sexual abuse with HIV risk behaviors in adolescence and young adulthood: Implications for public health. *Child Abuse and Neglect, 18*, 233–245.

Czapanskiy, K. (1993). Domestic violence, the family, and the lawyering process: Lessons from studies on gender bias in the courts. *Family Law Quarterly, 27*, 247–277.

Dallam, S. J. (2001). The effects of child sexual abuse: Comment on Rind, Tromovitch, and Bauserman (1998). *Psychological Bulletin, 127*(6), 715–733.

Dallam, S. J. (2002). Science or propaganda? An examination of Rind, Tromovitch and Bauserman (1998). *Journal of Child Sexual Abuse, 9*(3–4), 109–134.

Davies, D. (2003, June 22–26). American Professional Society on the Abuse of Children (APSAC) Forensic Interview Clinics Curriculum, Cape Cod, MA.

Davies, D., Cole, J., Albertella, G., McCulloch, L., Allen, K., & Kekevian, H. (1996). A model for conducting forensic interviews with child victims of abuse. *Child Maltreatment, 1*(3), 189–199.

De Bellis, M. D., Chrousos, G. P., Dorn, L. D., Burke, L., Helmers, K., Kling, M. A., Trickett, P. K., & Putnam, F. W. (1994). Hypothalamic–pituitary–adrenal axis dysregulation in sexually abused girls. *Journal of Clinical Endocrinology and Metablism, 78*, 249–255.

De Bellis, M., Keshavan, M., Clark, D., Casey, B. J., Giedd, J. N., Boring, A. M., Frustaci, K., & Ryan, N. D. (1999). Developmental traumatology, part II: Brain development. *Biological Psychiatry, 45*, 1259–1284.

De Bellis, M. D., Lefter, L., Trickett, P. K., & Putnam, F. W. (1994). Urinary catecholamine excretion in sexually abused girls. *Journal of the American Academy of Child and Adolescent Psychiatry, 33*, 320–327.

Deblinger, E., & Heflin, A. H. (1996). *Cognitive behavioral interventions for treating sexually abused children.* Thousand Oaks, CA: Sage.

Deblinger, E., Lippman, J., & Steer, R. (1996). Sexually abused children suffering posttraumatic stress symptoms: Initial treatment outcome findings. *Child Maltreatment, 1,* 310–321.

DeFrancis, V. (1969). *Protecting the child victim of sex crimes committed by adults.* Denver, CO: Children's Division, American Humane Society.

Dickey, R., Nussbaum, D., Chevolleau, K., & Davidson, H. (2002). Age as a differential characteristic of rapists, pedophiles, and sexual sadists. *Journal of Sex and Marital Therapy, 28,* 211–213.

Dube, S. R., Anda, R. F., Felitti, V. J., Edwards, V. J., & Croft, J. B. (2002). Adverse childhood experiences and personal alcohol abuse as an adult. *Addictive Behaviors, 27*(5), 713–725.

Edleson, J. L. (Ed.). (1999). Interventions and issues in the co-occurrence of child abuse and domestic violence [Special issue]. *Child Maltreatment, 4*(2).

Edwards, L. (1987). The relationship of juvenile and family courts in child abuse cases. *Santa Clara University Law Review, 27*(2), 201–278.

Ehrensaft, D. (1992). Preschool child sex abuse: The aftermath of the Presidio case. *American Journal of Orthopsychiatry, 62*(2), 234–244.

Eisen, M. L., Winograd, E., & Qin, J. (2002). Individual differences in adults' suggestibility and memory performance. In M. L. Eisen, G. S. Goodman, & J. A. Quas (Eds.), *Memory and suggestibility in the forensic interview* (pp. 205–234). Hillsdale, NJ: Erlbaum.

Ellenberger, H. E. (1970). *The discovery of the unconscious: The history and evolution of dynamic psychiatry.* New York: Basic Books.

Elliott, A. N., & Carnes, C.N. (2001). Reactions of nonoffending parents. *Child Maltreatment, 6*(4), 314–331.

Faller, K. C. (1998). The parental alienation syndrome: What is it and what data support it? *Child Maltreatment, 3*(2), 100–115.

Faller, K. C. (2003). *Understanding child sexual maltreatment.* Thousand Oaks, CA: Sage.

Faller, K. C., Corwin, D. L., & Olafson, E. (1993). Research on false allegations of sexual abuse in divorce. *APSAC Advisor, 6*(3), 6–10.

Faller, K. C., & DeVoe, E. (1995). Allegations of sexual abuse in divorce. *Journal of Child Sexual Abuse, 4*(4), 1–25.

Felitti, V. J. (2002). The relation between adverse childhood experiences and adult health: Turning gold into lead. *Permanente Journal, 6*(1), 44–47.

Ferenczi, S. (1955). Confusion of tongues between adults and the child: The language of tenderness and passion. In M. Balilant (Ed.), *Final contributions to the problems and methods of psycho-analysis* (pp. 156–167). London: Hogarth Press. (Original work published 1933)

Finkelhor, D. (1979). What's wrong with sex between adults and children? Ethics and the problem of sexual abuse. *American Journal of Orthopsychiatry, 49*(4), 692–697.

Finkelhor, D. (2003, February 5). *Sham or champagne: The controversial decline in sexual abuse cases.* Paper presented at the 17th annual San Diego Conference on Child and Family Maltreatment, San Diego, CA.

Finkelhor, D., & Berliner, L. (1995). Research on the treatment of sexually abused children: A review and recommendations. *Journal of the American Academy of Child and Adolescent Psychiatry, 34*(11), 1408–1423.

Fiscella, K., Kitzman, H., Cole, R., Sidora, K., & Olds, D. (1998). Does child abuse predict adolescent pregnancy? *Pediatrics, 101*, 620–624.

Fontana, V. (1964). *The maltreated child: The maltreatment syndrome in children.* Springfield, IL: Charles C. Thomas.

French, H. W. (2003, June 29). Victims say Japan ignores sex crimes committed by teachers. *New York Times*, p. A4.

Freyd, J. J. (1996). *The logic of forgetting childhood abuse: Betrayal trauma.* Cambridge, MA: Harvard University Press.

Friedrich, W. N. (1998). *Treating sexual behavior problems in children: A treatment manual.* Available from the author at the Mayo Clinic, Department of Psychiatry and Psychology, Rochester, MN 55905.

Giaretto, H. (1982). *Integrated treatment of child sexual abuse: A treatment and training manual.* Palo Alto, CA: Science and Behavior Books.

Gilstrap, L., & Ceci, S. J. (2001). The difficulties inherent in integrating clinical wisdom and empirical research regarding forensic interviews. *Contemporary Psychology APA Review of Books, 46*(2), 159–162.

Gomez-Schwartz, B., Horowitz, J. M., & Cardarelli, A. P. (1990). *Child sexual abuse: The initial effects.* Newbury Park, CA: Sage.

Gray, E. (1993). *Unequal justice: The prosecution of child sexual abuse.* New York: Free Press.

Hanson, R. F., Resnick, H. S., Saunders, B. E., Kilpatrick, D. G., & Best, C. (1999). Factors related to the reporting of childhood sexual assault. *Child Abuse and Neglect, 23*, 559–569.

Hanson, R. K. (2002). Recidivism and age: Follow-up data from 4,673 sexual offenders. *Journal of Interpersonal Violence, 17*, 1046–1054.

Helfer, R. E., & Kempe, C. H. (Eds.). (1968). *The battered child.* Chicago: University of Chicago Press.

Hembree-Kigin, T. L., & McNeil, C. B. (1995). *Parent–child interaction therapy.* New York: Plenum Press.

Henderson, D. J. (1975). Incest. In A. M. Freedman, H. I. Kaplan, & B. J. Sadock (Eds.), *Comprehensive textbook of psychiatry* (2nd ed.). Baltimore, MD: Williams & Wilkins.

Herman, J. L. (1981). *Father–daughter incest.* Cambridge, MA: Harvard University Press.

Herman, J. L. (1992). *Trauma and recovery.* New York: Basic Books.

Herman, J. L. (1997). *Trauma and recovery* (Rev. ed.). New York: Basic Books.

Herrenkohl, E., Herrenkohl, R., Egolf, B., & Russo, M. (1998). The relationship between early maltreatment and teenage parenthood. *Journal of Adolescence, 21*, 291–303.

Hewitt, S. K. (1999). *Assessing allegations of sexual abuse in preschool children: Understanding small voices.* Thousand Oaks, CA: Sage.

Hillis, S. D., Anda, R. F., Felitti, V. J., & Marchbanks, P. A. (2001). Adverse childhood experiences and sexual risk behaviors in women: A retrospective cohort study. *Family Planning Perspectives, 33*(5), 206–211.

Holmes, L. S., & Vieth, V. I. (2003). Finding Words/Half a Nation: The forensic interview training program of CornerHouse and APRI's National Center for Prosecution of Child Abuse. *APSAC Advisor, 15*(1), 4–8.

Huffman, M. L., Crossman, A. M., & Ceci, S. J. (1997). "Are false memories permanent?": An investigation of the long-term effects of source misattributions. *Consciousness and Cognition, 6,* 482–490.

Jacobs, J. L. (1994). *Victimized daughters: Incest and the development of the female self.* New York: Routledge.

Jaffe, P. G., Lemon, N. K. D., & Poisson, S. E. (2002). *Child custody and domestic violence: A call for safety and accountability.* Thousand Oaks, CA: Sage.

Kempe, C. H., Silverman, F. N., Steele, B. F., Droegmueller, W., & Silver, H. K. (1962). The battered child syndrome. *Journal of the American Medical Association, 181,* 17–24.

Kendall-Tackett, K. A., Williams, L. M., & Finkelhor, D. (1993). Impact of sexual abuse on children: A review and synthesis of recent empirical studies. *Psychological Bulletin, 113,* 164–180.

Kessler, R. C., Sonnega, A., Bromet, E., Hughes, M., & Nelson, C. B. (1995). Posttraumatic stress disorder in the national comorbidity survey. *Archives of General Psychiatry, 52,* 1048–1060.

Kinsey, A. C., Pomeroy, W. P., & Martin, C. E. (1948). *Sexual behavior in the human male.* Philadelphia: Saunders.

Kinsey, A. C., Pomeroy, W. F., Martin, C. E., & Gebhard, P. H. (1953). *Sexual behavior in the human female.* Philadelphia: Saunders.

Koenen, K. C., Moffitt, T. E., Caspi, A., Taylor, A., & Purcell, S. (2003). Domestic violence is associated with environmental suppression of IQ in young children. *Development and Psychopathology, 15,* 297–311.

Krug, E. G., Dahlberg, L. L., Mercy, J. A., Zwi, A. B., & Lozano, R. (Eds.). (2002). *World report on violence and health.* Geneva: World Health Organization.

Lanning, K. V. (1991). Ritual abuse: A law enforcement view or perspective. *Child Abuse and Neglect, 15,* 171–173.

Levine, J. (2002). *Harmful to minors: The perils of protecting children from sex.* Minneapolis: University of Minnesota Press.

Lustig, N., Dresser, J., Spellman, S., & Murray, T. (1966). Incest: A family group survival pattern. *Archives of General Psychiatry, 14,* 31–40.

Lyon, T. (1995). False allegations and false denials in child sexual abuse. *Psychology, Public Policy, and Law, 1*(2), 429–437.

Lyon, T. D. (1999). The new wave in children's suggestibility research: A critique. *Cornell Law Review, 84,* 1004–1087.

Lyon, T. D. (2002). Scientific support for expert testimony on child sexual abuse accommodation. In J. R. Conte (Ed.), *Critical issues in child sexual abuse: Historical, legal, and psychological perspectives* (pp. 107–138). Thousand Oaks, CA: Sage.

Lyon, T. D. (2003). Speaking with children: Advice from investigative interviewers. In F. Talley & A. Urquiza (Eds.), *Handbook for the treatment of abused and neglected children.* Needham Heights, MA: Allyn & Bacon.

Mart, E. G. (2000). Factitious disorder by proxy in forensic settings. In E. T. St. Charles & L. Crook (Eds.), *Exposé: The failure of family courts to protect children from abuse in custody disputes—A resource book for lawmakers, judges, attorneys and mental health professionals* (pp. 95–104). Las Gatos, CA: Our Children Our Charitable Future Foundation.

Masson, J. M. (1984). *The assault on truth: Freud's suppression of the seduction theory.* New York: Farrar, Strauss, & Giroux.

Myers, J. E. B. (1994). *The backlash: Child protection under fire.* Thousand Oaks, CA: Sage.

Myers, J. E. B. (1997). *A mother's nightmare—incest: A practical legal guide for parents and professionals.* Thousand Oaks, CA: Sage.

Myers, J. E. B. (1998). *Legal issues in child abuse and neglect* (2nd ed.). Thousand Oaks, CA: Sage.

Myers, J. E. B. (2004). *A history of child protection in America.* Philadelphia: Xlibris.

Olafson, E. (2002). When paradigms collide: Roland Summit and the rediscovery of child sexual abuse. In J. Conte (Ed.), *Critical issues in child sexual abuse* (pp. 71–106). Thousand Oaks, CA: Sage.

Olafson, E., Corwin, D. L., & Summit, R. C. (1993). Modern history of child sexual abuse awareness: Cycles of discovery and suppression. *Child Abuse & Neglect, 17*(1), 7–24.

Ondersma, S. J., Chaffin, M., Berliner, L., Cordon, I., Goodman, G. S., & Barnett, D. (2001). Sex with children is abuse: Comment on Rind, Tromovitch, and Bauserman (1998). *Psychological Bulletin, 127*(6), 707–714.

Orbach, Y., Hershkowitz, I., Lamb, M. E., Sternberg, K. J., Esplin, P. W., & Horowitz, D. (2000). Assessing the value of structured protocols for forensic interviews of alleged child abuse victims. *Child Abuse and Neglect, 24*(6), 733–752.

Otis, G. A. (2003, October). *Court may rule on battered women losing custody.* Available online at: *http://www.womensenews.org/article.cfm/dyn/aid/1553/context/archive*

Parillo, K., Freeman, R., Collier, K., & Young, P. (2001). Association between early sexual abuse and adult HIV-risky sexual behaviors among community-recruited women. *Child Abuse and Neglect, 25*, 335–346.

Pearson, J., & Anhalt, J. (1992). *The visitation enforcement program: Impact on child access and child support* (Final report. Grant No. 89M-E-021). Denver, CO: Center for Policy Research. Available from the Center for Policy Research, 1720 Emerson St., Denver, CO 80218.

Pelcovitz, D., van der Kolk, B., Roth, S., Mandel, F., Kaplan, S., & Resick, P. (1997). Development of a criteria set and a structured interview for disorders of extreme stress (SIDES). *Journal of Traumatic Stress, 10*(1), 3–16.

Pennington, H. J. (2000). Testimony before the U.S. House of Representative's judicial committee. In E. T. St. Charles & L. Crook (Eds.), *Exposé: The failure of family courts to protect children from abuse in custody disputes—A resource book for lawmakers, judges, attorneys and mental health professionals* (pp. 181–185). Las Gatos, CA: Our Children Our Charitable Future Foundation.

Perry, B. D., Pollard, R. A., Blakley, T. L., Baker, W. L., & Vigilante, D. (1996). Childhood trauma, the neurobiology of adaptation, and "use-dependent" development of the brain: How "states" become "traits." *Infant Mental Health Journal, 16*, 271–291.

Pezdek, K., & Hinz, T. (2002). The construction of false events in memory. In H. L.

Westcott, G. M. Davies, & R. H. C. Bull (Eds.), *Children's testimony: A handbook of psychological research and forensic practice* (pp. 99–116). West Sussex, UK: Wiley.

Pleck, E. (1987). *Domestic tyranny: The making of American social policy against family violence from colonial times to the present*. New York: Oxford University Press.

Poole, D. A., & Lamb, M. E. (1998). *Investigative interviews of children: A guide for helping professionals*. Washington, DC: American Psychological Association.

Putnam, F. W. (1991). The satanic ritual abuse controversy. *Child Abuse and Neglect, 15*, 175–179.

Putnam, F. W. (1997). *Dissociation in children and adolescents: A developmental perspective*. New York: Guilford Press.

Putnam, F. W. (2003). Ten-year research review update: Child sexual abuse. *Journal of the American Academy of Child and Adolescent Psychiatry, 42*(3), 269–278.

Putnam, F., & Trickett, P. (1997). The psychological effects of sexual abuse: A longitudinal study. *Annals of New York Academy of Science, 821*, 150–159.

Rainey, D., Stevens-Siman, C., & Kaplan, D. (1995). Are adolescents who report prior sexual abuse at higher risk for pregnancy? *Child Abuse and Neglect, 19*, 1283–1288.

Reed, D., & Cage, R. (2003, July). *Investigating child sexual abuse cases with nondisclosing children: Part I*. Eleventh Annual APSAC Colloquium, Orlando, FL.

Resick, P. A., & Schnicke, M. K. (1996). *Cognitive processing therapy for rape victims: A treatment manual*. Thousand Oaks, CA: Sage.

Rind, B. (2001). Gay and bisexual adolescent boys' sexual experiences with men: An empirical examination of psychological correlates in a nonclinical sample. *Archives of Sexual Behavior, 30*(4), 345–368.

Rind, B., Tromovitch, P., & Bauserman, R. (1998). A meta-analytic examination of assumed properties of child sexual abuse using college samples. *Psychological Bulletin, 124*, 22–53.

Romans, S., Martin, J., & Morris, E. (1997). Risk factors for adolescent pregnancy: How important is child sexual abuse? Otago Women's Health Study. *New Zealand Medical Journal, 110*, 30–33.

Rose, E. S. (1993, January/February). Surviving the unbelievable: A first-person account of cult ritual abuse. *Ms.*, 40–45.

Salter, A. (1988). *Treating child sex offenders and victims: A practical guide*. Newbury Park, CA: Sage.

Salter, A. C. (1995). *Transforming trauma: A guide to understanding and treating adult survivors of child sexual abuse*. Thousand Oaks, CA: Sage.

Salter, A. C. (2003). *Pedophiles, rapists, and other sex offenders: Who they are, how they operate, and how we can protect ourselves and our children*. New York: Basic Books.

Saunders, B. E., Berliner, L., & Hanson, R. F. (Eds.). (2003). *Child physical and sexual abuse: Guidelines for treatment* (Final report: January 15, 2003). Charleston, SC: National Crime Victims Treatment and Research Center.

Saywitz, K. J., & Camparo, L. (1998). Interviewing child witnesses: A developmental perspective. *Child Abuse and Neglect, 22*(8), 825–843.

Saywitz, K. J., & Goodman, G. S. (1996). Interviewing children in and out of court: Current research and practice implications. *The APSAC Handbook on Child Maltreatment.* Thousand Oaks, CA: Sage.

Saywitz, K., Goodman, G., & Lyon, T. (2002). Interviewing children in and out of court. In J. Myers, L. Berliner, J. Briere, C. Hendrix, C. Jenny, & T. Reid (Eds.), *The APSAC handbook on child maltreatment* (2nd ed., pp. 349–377). Thousand Oaks, CA: Sage.

Saywitz, K., Goodman, G., Nicolas, G., & Moan, S. (1991). Children's memories of a genital examination involving genital touch: Implications for child sexual abuse. *Journal of Consulting and Clinical Psychology, 59*, 682–691.

Saywitz, K. J., & Lyon, T. D. (2002). Coming to grips with children's suggestibility. In M. L. Eisen, G. S. Goodman, & J. A. Quas (Eds.), *Memory and suggestibility in the forensic interview* (pp. 85–113). Hillsdale, NJ: Erlbaum.

Saywitz, K., & Nathanson, R. (1993). Children's testimony and their perceptions of stress in and out of the courtroom. *Child Abuse and Neglect, 17*(5), 613–622.

Sjoberg, R., & Lindblad, F. (2002). Limited disclosure of sexual abuse in children whose experiences were documented by videotape. *American Journal of Psychiatry, 159*(2), 312–314.

Smith, B., & Elstein, S. G. (1993). *The prosecution of child sexual and physical abuse cases: Final report.* Chicago: American Bar Association Fund for Justice and Education.

Stanton, M. (1997, July/August). U-turn on memory lane. *Columbia Journalism Review,* 44–49.

State of Michigan Governor's Task Force on Children's Justice and Family Independence Agency. (1998). *Forensic Interviewing Protocol* [FIA-PUB-779 (8–98)].

St. Charles, E. T., & Crook, L. (Eds.). (2000). *Exposé: The failure of family courts to protect children from abuse in custody disputes—A resource book for lawmakers, judges, attorneys and mental health professionals.* Las Gatos, CA: Our Children Our Charitable Future Foundation.

Steele, L. C. (2003). Child forensic interview structure: National Children's Advocacy Center. *APSAC Advisor, 15*(4), 2–5.

Sternberg, K. J., Lamb, M.E., Orbach, Y., Esplin, P., & Mitchell, S. (2001). Use of a structured investigative protocol enhances young children's responses to free-recall prompts in the course of forensic interviews. *Journal of Applied Psychology, 86*(5), 997–1005.

Stevens-Simon, C., & Reichert, S. (1994). Sexual abuse, adolescent pregnancy, and child abuse. *Archives of Pediatric Adolescent Medicine, 148*, 23–27.

Summit, R. C. (1983). The child sexual abuse accommodation syndrome. *Child Abuse and Neglect, 7*, 177–192.

Terr, L. (1990). *Too scared to cry: Psychic trauma in childhood.* New York: Harper & Row.

Thoennes, N., Pearson, J., & Tjaden, P. (1988). *Allegations of sexual abuse in custody and visitation cases.* Denver: Association of the Family and Conciliation Courts.

Thoennes, N., & Tjaden, P. (1990). The extent, nature, and validity of sexual abuse allegations in custody/visitation disputes. *Child Abuse and Neglect, 14*, 151–163.

Urquiza, A. J., & McNeil, C. B. (1996). Parent–child interaction therapy: An intensive dyadic intervention for physically abusive families. *Child Maltreatment, 1*, 134–144.

van der Kolk, B. A., & van der Hart, O. (1989). Pierre Janet and the breakdown of adaptation in psychological trauma. *American Journal of Psychiatry, 146*, 1530–1540.

Vieth, V. I. (1999). When a child stands alone: The search for corroborating evidence. *Update, 12*(6), 1–2.

Walker, A. G. (1999). *Handbook on questioning children: A linguistic perspective.* Washington, DC: American Bar Association Center on Children and the Law.

Walker, L. E. (1979). *The battered woman.* New York: Harper & Row.

Walsh, W., Jones, L., & Cross, T. (2003). Children's Advocacy Centers: One philosophy, many models. *APSAC Advisor, 15*(3), 3–6.

Weiss, J., Rogers, E., Darwin, M. R., & Dutton, C. E. (1955). A study of girl sex victims. *Psychiatric Quarterly Supplement, 29*(1), 1–27.

Westcott, H. L., Davies, G. M., & Bull, R. H. C. (2002). *Children's testimony: A handbook of psychological research and forensic practice.* New York: Wiley.

Whiffen, V., & Clark, S. (1997). Does victimization account for sex differences in depressive symptoms? *British Journal of Clinical Psychology, 36*, 185–193.

Wigmore, J. H. (1978, Chadbourn revision). *Evidence in trials at common law.* Boston, MA: Little, Brown. (Original work published 1904)

Wood, C. L. (1994). The parental alienation syndrome: A dangerous area of reliability. *Loyola of Los Angeles Law Review, 29*, 1367–1415.

Yates, A. (1978). *Sex without shame.* New York: William & Morrow.

Yuille, J. (1996). *Investigating allegations of child abuse: An interview protocol.* Training workshop at the 12th Annual Midwest Conference on Child Sexual Abuse and Incest, Madison, WI.

Zigler, E. (2003). *Psychologists defying the crowd: Stories of those who battled the establishment and won.* Washington, DC: American Psychological Association.

8 Memories of Childhood Abuse

Recovered, Discovered, and Otherwise

LAURA S. BROWN

The sexual abuse of a child constitutes one of the most common of human interpersonal traumata. Depending upon the research methodology used to obtain the information, various studies have found that anywhere between one-quarter and one-third of adults in the United States and similar developed, industrialized nations report sexual abuse in their childhood (Briere, 1996). Contrary to the claims of some authors who see the issue of childhood sexual abuse as an invention of late 20th-century feminism (Ofshe & Watters, 1994), sexual abuse of children is not a recent phenomenon. It is described and proscribed in the book of Leviticus in the Old Testament. Charcot, Janet, and Freud all report it occurring to patients, despite Freud's later rejection of these reports as neurotic fantasy (Courtois, 2000). Children have been sexualized in Western and other cultures for millennia—used as prostitutes, victimized by incest, and raped in war.

For as long as the sexual abuse of children has been the subject of study by Western mental health professionals, the phenomenon of memory disturbances in the wake of such abuse has also been described and reported by those same observers (Brown, 2000). Memories of childhood sexual abuse are frequently either overly available, appearing in the form of intrusive thoughts, images, and flashbacks, or they are characterized by partial or full amnesia, difficult or temporarily impossible to retrieve to conscious awareness (Alpert, Brown, & Courtois, 1996). It should surprise no one that sexual abuse of a child may affect the capacity to store, retain, and/or retrieve the details of what happened. Sexual abuse of children is at the very least confusing, may be sexually arousing, and is often frightening and painful (Briere, 1996; Courtois, 2000). All of these forms of autonomic arousal can affect to some degree the functions of memory, interfering with any or all of encoding, storage, retention, and retrieval (Alpert et al., 1996; Pope & Brown, 1996). At every step of the way, the process of remembering and knowing can be affected by the intertwined physiological and emotional dynamics of sexual abuse.

In the early 1990s, the phenomenon of delayed recall of childhood sexual abuse (also referred to as "repressed memory" or "recovered memory") became a topic of fierce debate within scientific and professional circles in North America, Great Britain, and the Netherlands. The controversy focused on two questions. First, was it scientifically possible for a person to remember the trauma of sexual abuse after many years of not knowing of their own experience? Second, was it possible for persons to develop false beliefs about their prior life experiences, specifically false beliefs about having been sexually abused in childhood, in response to suggestions from therapists, books, and other sources?

To quote the findings of the American Psychological Association's (1994) Working Group on Recovered Memories:

> Most people who were sexually abused as children remember all or part of what happened to them. However, it is possible for memories of abuse that have been forgotten for a long time to be remembered. The mechanism(s) by which such delayed recall occur(s) is/are not currently well-understood. It is also possible to construct convincing pseudomemories for events that never occurred. The mechanism(s) by which these pseudomemories is/are constructed are not currently well understood.

This chapter begins at the point where the Working Group (of which the author was a member) ended. In 1994, we could agree that delayed recall occurred; we could not agree about how. We could agree that suggestions could be transformed into false beliefs about one's autobiographical experiences. We could not agree on how easily that could be done. Ten years later, while there is no absolute clarity as to the question of mechanisms for delayed recall, the understanding of the various ways by which it might occur has grown tremendously. There is also greater clarity as to how likely it is that suggestions might lead to false beliefs masquerading as memories.

SEXUAL ABUSE AS AN
INTERPERSONALLY COMPLEX TRAUMA

Unlike many other traumata, sexual abuse carries a complex socio-emotional weight that lends meanings to this experience that are absent for other traumata, even many other interpersonal traumata. These meanings can themselves influence the manner in which a person is able to remember and know of her or his own experience, or, once knowing or remembering, tie that experience to distress or dysfunction in life. Sexual abuse of a child is not an earthquake, easily observed and undeniable, blamed only on geographical forces or divine will. It is most commonly a lengthy, complex process in which the sexually abusive component of the relationship between child and perpetrator is embedded within the dynamics of other relationships, frequently those of care, trust, and dependence. While there are children whose sexual abuse consists of single-episode attacks by strangers, these victims are in the minority. Most commonly, given the nature of this crime, sexual abuse is perpetrated by those who know a child well, and who have regular and easy access to that child; in other words, family members, caregivers, teachers, clergy, coaches, and others with legitimate access to private time with a child.

Sexual abuse of children usually occurs in secret, with the child in isolation from other sources of input about what is happening to her or him as they are touched and invaded. The perpetrator of the abuse is normally known to the child, and there is often a preabuse experience of trust, fear, or both between child and perpetrator. There is no continuum of acceptability in sexual abuse, such as exists for physical or emotional abuse or neglect, where certain early-stage components of the maltreatment fall within the range of what can be called simply bad parenting, rather than abuse. Thus, the experience of being used sexually stands in cognitive and emotional isolation for the child. While many sexual abuse perpetrators engage in behaviors that are retrospectively appraised by others as "grooming" of the child to accept the sexual contact, those grooming behaviors are, in the absence of sexual abuse, no different in form from many types of positive attachments between adults and children. Thus, the confusion for some victims between what constitutes loving, positive connection with an adult, and what the sexual abuse, is also a usual component of the cognitive and emotional matrix into which the memory of sexual abuse must fit.

A sexually abused child may also be forced into social roles, particularly in the case of incest, for which she or he is also unprepared emotionally. For example, a parent may groom a child into incest by first placing that child into a spouse or partnerlike relationship. A nonparental adult may take the child as a confidant, violating emotional boundaries by "gifting" the child with confidences that she or he cannot contain. Finally, perpetrators will frequently impose secrecy on their child victims. At times this may be accompanied by direct threats of violence ("If you tell, I will kill your mother/your dog/you") or loss ("If you tell, they'll make you go away and live in a foster home"). At other times, perpetrators will utilize less overtly violent, more seductive coercion ("You're special; this is our little secret; people wouldn't understand and might be mad at us"). Whatever the means, the child victim learns that she or he is to not know of the events of the sexual abuse outside of the moments of their occurrence, if then.

Additionally, complicated family dynamics are likely to obtain. Family dysfunction other than sexual abuse is common in the lives of sexually abused children (Beitchman, Zucker, Hood, daCosta, & Ackman, 1991; Briere, 1996; Courtois, 2000). Physical violence against the non-sexually offending parent, physical violence by the non-sexually offending parent against the child, emotional abuse, and neglect are all frequently observed. A child who is not told not to tell may nonetheless refrain from coming forward to report sexual abuse due to what she or he observes or intuits may occur to the messenger bearing bad news about a particular family member. A child who is sexually victimized by a non-family member, such as a coach, teacher, or health care provider, may be picked as a target by a predatory perpetrator who can see that this child's welfare is poorly, if at all, attended to by her or his caregivers.

All of these psychosocial factors introduce elements into the equation that further complicate the child's, and later the adult's, capacity to know and make conscious that which has occurred. The inner conflicts evoked for children by sexual abuse are often profound, and damaging by and of themselves. Consequently, memory for the trauma of the abuse will be impacted in some manner for most people who are the victims of this crime.

WHAT IS MEMORY?

The nature of memory has been debated in the field of psychology for most of the past century. At this juncture, the constructivist model first proposed by Bartlett (1932) and later reintroduced by Neisser (1982) holds sway. This model posits that memory is a multistage process in which various factors can affect the capacity to recall; additionally, this model argues that memory is constantly in a process of being reconstructed, so that each time the same event is remembered, it is recalled differently and stored in that new, modified form.

The strong implication of this model is that memory is not an exact representation of events. Rather, it is subject to distortion at each stage of the process of its creation and re-creation. Factors that can in general affect memory include the following:

1. *The person's state of arousal at the time when the memory is formed.* Very high or very low levels of autonomic arousal, such as caused by fear or anger (for high) or peritraumatic (occurring around the time of the trauma) dissociation (for low) can impair the formation of the memory.

2. *Familiarity of the material being stored for recall.* Memories are stored in complex neural networks, in which connections are made between familiar experiences. Extremely unfamiliar experiences may not be well remembered.

3. *Attention.* The remembering person's capacity for attention to the information being stored in memory may be affected by events occurring at the time of memory formation. Studies of the memories of eyewitnesses to criminal assaults have described the "weapon focus" phenomenon, in which the crime victim is so attentive to the gun in the perpetrator's hand that they fail to attend to his or her facial features (Loftus, 1979).

4. *Opportunity for repetition.* The more frequently an event is experienced, the more likely it is that a memory for the repeated event will be stored. However, the specific details of each instance of the event may become confused and blended. For instance, studies of children's recollections for visits to their primary care providers suggested that children developed a "going to the doctor" script, in which elements of various visits were blended into one generic recall of health care visits (Goodman, Bottoms, Schwartz-Kenney, & Rudy, 1991).

Each or all of these factors can be a component of difficulties, distortions, or inaccuracies in an adult's recollection of any childhood experience. When we factor in these complex dynamics, we can begin to see how sexual abuse can affect memory without any special pleading for mechanisms that are unique to the experience of abuse.

There are also general considerations regarding how trauma is remembered that affect the capacity to recall sexual abuse. It is important to note that not all sexual abuse of children falls within the parameters of traumatic stress; frequently, it may be confusing, inappropriately arousing, or disturbing, but will not become traumatic until the adult remembering the experience appraises it as abusive and comes to perceive her or himself as having been at risk.

However, some sexual abuse is clearly traumatic to children. Contact involving penetration, contact involving other forms or threats of violence or harm, and contact involving forms or threats of loss may all rise to the experience of a trauma. Courtois (2000), using a model developed by Wilson (1989), notes that in childhood sexual abuse, there are a number of traumagenic (trauma-inducing) elements, including a "stressor of human design, repeated exposure and physical proximity to the stressor that often increases in severity and physical intrusion over time and over the course of childhood, when the individual is physically and emotionally dependent on caretakers and with whom there is a conflicted relationship and ambivalent attachment" (Courtois, 2000, p. 76). Consequently, it is useful to consider how trauma itself affects the remembering process.

In trauma, somatosensory modalities of processing information are likely to take over from cognitive means. van der Kolk (1996) has noted a range of psychophysiological, neurohormonal, neuroanatomical, and immunological effects of exposure to traumatic stress. These include changes in levels of stress hormones, particularly cortisol; changes in the catecholemine, serotonin, and endogenous opioid systems of the brain; and, with repeated trauma exposure, diminishment of the volume of the hippocampus. van der Kolk's research, using active imaging technology, found that during the recollection of trauma, brains of traumatized individuals were highly activated in the limbic system, particularly the amygdala, and in sensory areas, particularly the visual cortex. However, in these same brains, Broca's area, from which verbal language and speech are derived, was deactivated, as was the prefrontal cortex. These findings strongly suggest that memory for trauma is, in general, stored as sensory and raw affective data that is not yet integrated into the cognitive, verbal form taken by memories for everyday events.

Other research on memory for trauma has found that such memories are different in quality than memory for ordinary events, although the mechanisms by which the information is stored and recalled appear similar. Christianson and Engelberg (1997) note that memories for trauma tend to be quite accurate as to the central details of the event. However, there is usually less than average accuracy of recall for the peripheral details of the trauma. These memories also appeared difficult to access. Duvenage and Dalenberg (1993) noted that memories of childhood trauma were accessible only in response to specific, often unusual, and infrequent cues that contained a wealth of, and unique combination of, somatosensory data not normally present in the remembering person's environment.

These findings suggest that the common human attempt to forget or not think about painful experiences can be seen in the difficulties inherent in remembering trauma, even if the neurobiology of trauma did not also complicate the process of remembering. Trauma creates artificially high or low states of arousal. Trauma is frequently an unfamiliar event, or, if it is familiar through repetition, it constitutes an ongoing violation of the norms of life, something to which a person cannot habituate morally or cognitively. Trauma scatters the attention, so that not all details of an experience will be stored. Thus, the psychobiological phenomenology of trauma interacts with the usual mechanisms of memory storage and retrieval.

HISTORICAL FACTORS:
THE DEBATE OVER DELAYED RECALL

In the middle 1970s, psychotherapy clients, most of them women, began to report in increasing numbers to their therapists that they were remembering having been sexually abused as children after having not remembered or known. A series of books appeared at the end of that decade and the beginning of the next (Armstrong, 1978; Bass & Thornton, 1983; Brady, 1979; Butler, 1978; Herman, 1981; McNaron & Morgan, 1982; Rush, 1980), in which first-person accounts of forgetting and remembering childhood sexual abuse were made available to the general population of mental health providers. Sexual abuse, which had until then been treated as an infrequent occurrence, began to be seen as an almost *uber*-explanatory fiction by some authors (Blume, 1990; Fredrickson, 1992), with every possible symptom or form of distress tracked back to sexual abuse. If a client could not remember sexual abuse, her or his therapist was now taught that she or he had simply not *yet* recalled it. Strategies for assisting clients with remembering (Blume, 1990; Fredrickson, 1992) were published. An "incest survivor" movement grew up, with its own newsletters and conferences.

This movement had a number of notable successes in the arenas of training of mental health professionals, law, and public policy. While sexual abuse had once been a neglected topic in the training of therapists, it now became a frequent focus of postgraduate continuing education and began to be included in the curriculum of a number of training programs. Research on sexual abuse and its effects began to be conducted on both children and adult survivors. This was a necessary corrective against decades in which mental health professionals had helped sexual abuse to become what Rush (1980) dubbed the "best kept secret" about the lives of children.

In the legal realm, adults who remembered sexual abuse began to bring civil lawsuits against their alleged perpetrators. When the Washington State Supreme Court found, in the matter of *Tyson v. Tyson*, 727 P.2d 226 (Wash. 1986)), that the law as then written did not allow the survivor with no memories to bring a civil action after the recovery of knowledge, the Washington State legislature changed the law. Within 2 years of the *Tyson* decision, the statute of limitations for suing began to run at the moment of memory, not from the time of the alleged offense of sexual abuse (for more information about statutes of limitation, see the section "Legal Implications"). More than 20 states followed suit within the next few years to allow such "repressed memory" litigation to take place (Pope & Brown, 1996).

As the discussion of recovered memories of childhood sexual abuse made its move from the confines of the therapy office into the court-room, and affected the pocketbooks and pensions of alleged perpetrators, the nature of the discourse became radically transformed. The decade of the 1990s saw, in response to this transformation, the waxing and (possible) waning of a debate over the delay of recall for childhood sexual abuse. In 1992, with the founding of the False Memory Syndrome Foundation by a man accused of sexual abuse, his wife, their former psychiatrist, and a psychologist who frequently testified as an expert on behalf of accused pedophiles, a controversy arose as to whether it was possible for people to completely forget (e.g., have unavailable to conscious, cognitive recollection) experiences of sexual abuse in childhood, only to have those memories become suddenly available to conscious, cognitive recall during adult life.

The false memory movement, buttressed by its relationship with many leading researchers in the field of declarative memory, argued cogently and persistently that this was impossible, and that reports of "repressed memories" (as they were then referred to in both the popular and scholarly literatures) were a fraud perpetrated on vulnerable clients and a credulous public by ill-trained psychotherapists with a political agenda against families (Loftus & Ketcham, 1994; Ofshe & Watters, 1994). This movement held conferences, pushed (unsuccessfully) for legislative changes (Hinnefeld & Newman, 1997), and inspired ad hominem attacks on therapists and writers who had become identified with the incest survivors movement (Calof, 1998), including myself. I was picketed at my home by false memory activists with signs describing me as a "Voodoo Queen" (Brown, 1998). The message of the false memory movement was that it was relatively easy to create false memories in gullible, suggestible psychotherapy clients. Several persons came forward to retract their claims of childhood sexual abuse, and detailed how therapists had used hypnosis, guided imagery, and other suggestive psychotherapeutic strategies to create false beliefs about their parents and their pasts (Goldstein & Farmer, 1994).

The rise of the false memory movement also spurred many persons within the field of sexual abuse treatment to examine our knowledge and understanding of how delayed recall for childhood sexual abuse might occur. In the intervening decade, those scholars have analyzed what was being done right and what was misguided in earlier attempts to work with people reporting delayed recall of childhood trauma. Out of those analyses has developed a more solid scientific foundation for conceptualizing the various processes that might lead to delayed capacity to recall childhood sexual abuse. Additionally, models of treatment have been revised to integrate both old knowledge and newer, more recent findings on trauma and memory, particularly related to the neurobiology of trauma.

The remainder of this chapter reviews the current state of the science regarding delay of recall for childhood trauma, and describes how both mental health and legal practices have been affected by the findings that have emerged in the past decade. Additionally, the question of whether a "false memory syndrome" can be said to exist is explored in light of the available scientific data.

IS THERE SUPPORT FOR DELAYED RECALL OF CHILDHOOD ABUSE?

To this question, the unequivocal answer of the research literature is "yes." Brown, Scheflin, and Hammond (1998) reviewed all available studies, involving a variety of methodologies, that raised the question of whether persons with a history of childhood sexual abuse reported periods of full or partial amnesia for the abuse. Courtois (2000) revisited and added to their data. The findings from these reviews can be summarized as follows:

1. In nine studies of clinical populations, where the participants were women in various types of mental health treatment, all groups reported high rates of full or partial amnesia for sexual abuse.

2. In eight studies of nonclinical populations, moderate numbers of participants reported full or partial amnesia for experiences of childhood sexual abuse. One study, which surveyed individuals whose recollections had been stimulated by press coverage of sexual abuse accusations against a former priest, reported moderately high rates of both full and partial amnesia for the abuse.

3. In nine random-sample studies, moderate rates of full or partial amnesia were reported. Three of these were studies of psychotherapists and/or practicing psychologists, who reported rates of full or partial amnesia for childhood sexual abuse consistent with the general population.

4. In five prospective studies, individuals who were known,

from legal and/or medical records, to have experienced documented childhood sexual abuse, were queried in late adolescence and/or early young adulthood. Of those queried, between 14 and 38% had full amnesia for the documented abuse that could not be accounted for by developmental factors, or shame or discomfort.

Some of the most interesting data were contained in six case studies reviewed by Brown et al. (1998) and Courtois (2000). In one such study, an individual can be viewed on videotape around the time of the sexual abuse in her childhood, at which time she was able to report and describe the abuse. At the start of the second video, taken when she was a young adult, she is unable to remember the abuse. On the video, her process of beginning to remember can be observed (Corwin & Olafson, 1997). In another study, Schooler and his colleagues (Schooler, Ambadar, & Bendiksen, 1997) describe several cases in which individuals go through several periods of gaining, then losing access to, then regaining, memories of trauma, including adult-onset traumatic events.

Cheit (1998) has developed the Recovered Memory Archive, which can be found on-line at *http://www.brown.edu/Departments/Taubman_Center/Recovmem/Archive.html*. This archive contains detailed information about well-corroborated cases of delayed recall. The majority of the cases posted are those involving allegations of childhood sexual abuse. Cheit requires, for corroboration, such materials as co-victim witness statements, confessions by perpetrators, criminal convictions of perpetrators, medical records, and other similarly solid materials. Anyone wishing to challenge the posting of a given case is invited to do so, and all cases on the site have survived challenge.

The overwhelming weight of the data argues for the reality of delayed recall in the lives of many adults who were sexually abused as children. Delayed recall of trauma appears to occur in almost every type of traumatic stressor (Elliott & Briere, 1995). However, traumata that occur at a younger age, at the hands of caregivers, appear to be the types of trauma most likely to lead to full or partial impairments in memory.

MEMORY, TRAUMA, AND ABUSE: THE TANGLED WEB

As described at the beginning of this chapter, the experience of childhood sexual abuse is a complex, multidimensional phenomenon. It is rarely a single-blow experience, as is true in the case of sexual assault in adulthood. The perpetrator of childhood sexual abuse is rarely unknown to the victim, and frequently has an ongoing relationship with the child encompassing many other dimensions of his or her life. Because of all of these factors, there are multiple hypotheses and multiple possible mechanisms by which memory of childhood sexual abuse, or comprehension and recognition of the events as abusive may be delayed. Each of these possible mechanisms for delay or impairment of recall is discussed in the following sections.

Developmental Issues as Causes for Delayed Recall

Sexual abuse in childhood also does not occur at the same developmental points for each of its victims. This extreme variability in the developmental stages of sexual abuse victims accounts, to some degree, for the variability in the capacity to recall experienced sexual abuse. Most children have little or no verbal, cognitive memory for events that occur prior to approximately age 3, which is generally accepted to be the point at which autobiographical verbal memory may commence. Thus, children sexually abused prior to that age may never have a memory for the event, although Terr (1990) describes cases in which children sexually victimized in child pornography prior to age 3 have been observed to reenact the sexualized behaviors that are memorialized in photos and videos made by the pornographers, suggesting some sort of nonverbal recollection of the experiences.

Similarly, persons sexually victimized at relatively young ages may have incomplete or distorted memories of the experience when they attempt to recall it as adults simply because of the developmental immaturity of their neurological and cognitive mechanisms. Several researchers have documented that young children under the age of 5 are more likely to encode, store, and consequently be able to accurately retrieve memories for neutral or positive events (e.g., going to the zoo) when afforded the opportunity to discuss it with an adult (Fivush, 1996; Tessler & Nelson, 1994). This is apparently even more likely to be true when the memory is of a stressful situation, as researchers studying children's stressful medical experiences have found (Goodman, Quas, Batterman-Faunce, Riddlesberger, & Kuhn, 1996).

Extrapolating from these findings, it is reasonable to posit that children sexually abused at very young ages after the onset of autobiographical memory may develop weak memories for the event because of the absence of what Courtois (2000) refers to as the "social-interactive" effect of sharing the experience in conversation with an adult. The perpetrator of sexual abuse is unlikely, several weeks or months after having forced a child into sexual activity, to sit down with the child and encourage recollection of the experience. Forced silence is more likely; a number of adults who have never entirely forgotten sexual abuse can recall being told, "This never happened," "Forget this," "You dreamed this," and other similar statements aimed at discouraging rather than encouraging memory. Generally, those memories that are weakly retained are extremely difficult to retrieve. The memory may fade entirely, to the point where there is nothing left to retrieve, as is true for our memories of the majority of life events. Or it may require very specific, focused cues to elicit its retrieval because of the extreme weakness of the memory as it was originally encoded, cues of the sort described in research on memory for trauma.

Very young children are also significantly more suggestible than are older children or adults (Zaragoza, 1991). Suggestions by a perpetrator such as described earlier may themselves lead to distortion or weakening of the memory in those sexually abused at young ages. If what is recalled is not coded as abuse, and the memory is not easily available for inspection by the individual, then appraisal of the experience as sexually abusive may never occur, or may only occur after many countersuggestions are made later in life by sources who are as plausible as was the perpetrator. Clinical examples of this are common. For instance, the client who tells a therapist that her uncle "used to love me up all the time" will describe penetrative sexual abuse perpetrated on her when she was age 7. The memory lacks salience as to sexual abuse because of the manner in which it was encoded. Only with reappraisal in adulthood are the emotions of horror, shock, or fear associated with the experience. This late appraisal of a continuous recollection may also be narrated, by those undergoing this narrative transformation, as a sort of recovered or delayed recall, even though the specifics of the events in question have always been available to conscious recollection.

In summary, one possible mechanism for apparent delays or disruptions in the capacity to recall sexual abuse may be simple developmental factors. Memories of childhood sexual abuse are not the only memories of early childhood that return, unbidden and insistent, in adulthood. Many memories that return in this fashion are pleasant ones, triggered by events such as the early birthdays of one's own children, their first days at school, or other emotionally laden childhood experiences that have slipped out of consciousness. Memories of childhood sexual abuse, similarly, may have been "forgotten" simply because nothing in the present called them to mind; when called, they emerge.

Betrayal Trauma and Delayed Recall: Relational Factors

Freyd (1994, 1996), a cognitive psychologist, has posited an elegant sociocognitive model to explicate the forgetting and later recall of childhood sexual abuse. The betrayal trauma (BT) model argues the following:

- Children are dependent upon their caregivers. Children have an evolutionary mandate to create and maintain attachment to their caregivers at all cost, since human children require attachment to adults in order to survive.
- Children also have an evolutionary mandate to detect cheating and betrayal (Cosmides & Tooby, 1992). It is important for humans to know when they have been betrayed, so as to cease connection with the sources of their betrayal.
- When a child is betrayed, in the form of sexual abuse, by a caregiver, the need for attachment trumps the need to know betrayal.
- When a betrayal trauma, in the form of sexual abuse, has taken place, the child develops cognitive mechanisms for sealing off access to the information about the betrayal, in order to maintain the attachment.
- When and if the child no longer requires the attachment for survival (e.g, has become adult and emancipated from the abusive parent), or when the survival of others to whom the person owes a bond of protection (e.g., their own offspring) is threatened, then and only then will it become possible for the person to know of her or his betrayal.

Freyd's model predicts that the closer the relationship between an alleged perpetrator and the victim of childhood sexual abuse, the more likely it is that the victim will have experienced partial or complete inability to recall some or all of the experience of abuse. The need to maintain attachment becomes the factor that interferes with the capacity to know of the abuse. In support of her theory she initially reviewed studies of memory and childhood sexual abuse that were available in the literature by the middle 1990s, the time at which she first published her theory. She found that the studies available to date strongly supported this theory, and that other factors that had been proposed to predict postabuse memory problems, such a severity and intensity of the abuse, did not predict memory problems as well (Freyd, 1996).

Freyd and her colleagues have conducted a series of studies to test her hypotheses empirically, and continue to collect data. In their initial published study, Freyd, DePrince, and Zurbriggen (2001) presented preliminary results from the Betrayal Trauma Inventory (BTI), testing predictions from the BT model about the relationship between forgetting abuse and betrayal by a caregiver. The findings of this study supported their prediction that abuse perpetrated by a caregiver was related to less persistent memories of abuse. This relationship is significant for sexual and physical abuse. Neither age at the time of abuse, nor duration of the abuse, could account for these findings. More recently Freyd (personal communication, 2002) has found further evidence of the relationship between betrayal traumas and impairments in memory.

Dissociation and Memory for Sexual Abuse

Yates and Nasby (1993) have suggested that dissociation, rather than repression, provides the best possible explanation for temporary loss of access to memory for traumatic events. They argue that dissociation—an empirically demonstrable phenomenon with physiological correlates, which has been empirically linked to the trauma response—is the mechanism most likely to account for posttraumatic amnesia. Drawing upon Bower's (1981) model for the influence of affect on memory, they propose a mental mechanism by which memories for trauma may be neurologically and cognitively inhibited from conscious access until the person is exposed to specific disinhibiting retrieval cues. Their suggestions are supported by the work of Bremner, who has performed numerous radiological studies of the brains of traumatized individuals. He and his colleagues (Bremner, Krystal, Charney, & Southwick, 1996) argue that

> what is known about the neurobiology of memory support the idea that special mechanisms may be operative in recall of traumatic events, such as childhood abuse. . . . Changes in brain regions involved in memory may underlie many symptoms . . . including symptoms of amnesia. (p. 72)

Clinically, the return of long-unavailable memories of abuse frequently is observed to have a dissociative quality (Briere, 1996; Courtois, 2000; Pope & Brown, 1996). Intrusive memories of previously un-recalled abuse are experienced as flashbacks, in which the memory is relived and the person regresses, often losing orientation to time, place, and person during the process of remembering.

Inhibitory Memory Processes

Active inhibition is a well-documented memory phenomenon that leads to forgetting of information due to the development of inherent impediments to the retrieval component of remembering. Memories are formed and stored, but their retrieval becomes inhibited. Anderson (1998) suggested how active inhibition might serve as the mechanism for some examples of delayed recall of childhood sexual abuse. In general models of memory, the concept of inhibition is used to refer to forgetting that is motivated. Anderson argues that children may be motivated to forget sexual abuse when the perpetrator is positively construed in the family system. He suggests that active inhibition is particularly likely to occur when the child has other, public relationships with the perpetrator, and explains this via the phenomenon of active inhibition.

Active inhibition expands upon the mental mechanism of inhibition to describe how having multiple associations to one cue may lead to inhibition of one set of associations. This model posits that attention to one thing that is paired with a stimulus cue will actively inhibit retrieval of other things paired with that stimulus cue. Rehearsal of the first pair will inhibit other pairs. Translated into relational terms, this suggests that when a perpetrator is more frequently coded in ways other than sexually abusive, the memory for the sexual abuse will be actively inhibited, pushed aside in the memory system by the more frequent, and frequently rehearsed, construction of the person. For example, if the cue "grandfather" is paired frequently with the construct "good and loving," this pairing will actively inhibit all other pairs. Even if "grandfather" is also paired occasionally with "sexual abuse," the latter pairing, because it is both less frequent and less rehearsed and socially constructed, will be inhibited and less available to recollection. While this memory will be stored, its retrieval will become difficult, and it will be experienced as forgotten.

Summary

Several testable, science-based models exist to explain how some memories of childhood sexual abuse may become unavailable to conscious recollection for lengthy periods following the abuse experience. It appears that no one mechanism accounts for all delays in recall, and that several mechanisms may work together to lead to a particular individual's experience of recovering a memory. As research continues on all of these and other models of memory for trauma, further paradigms for delayed recall may emerge. But the assertions made in the early 1990s by individuals in the false memory movement that it is impossible for reasonably accurate memories to be experienced in this delayed fashion have been well-refuted by the data.

SUGGESTIBILITY AND FALSE BELIEFS

The most powerful talking point for the false memory movement was its assertion that therapists were creating false memories of childhood sexual abuse in vulnerable psychotherapy clients. A number of studies were proffered, indicating that it was possible to create false beliefs about one's life experiences solely in response to suggestion (Hyman, Husband, & Billings, 1995; Hyman & Loftus, 1997; Loftus, 1993: Loftus & Coan, 1994; Loftus & Pickrell, 1995). These studies were used to support the assertion that false beliefs about sexual abuse could be created through simple suggestion. These studies had the following elements in common:

- The events being suggested were unpleasant, but not traumatic. They included being temporarily lost in a shopping mall while a small child; when a small child, pulling down a punchbowl at a wedding; when a small child, going for emergent care of an ear infection.
- None of the events being suggested led to major reevaluation of relationships with important caregivers.
- The persons making the suggestions were either older family members themselves, or represented that they were giving the reports of older family members.
- At most a quarter of research participants integrated the suggestions into their autobiographical narratives as memory.

As noted by Pezdek and her colleagues (Pezdek, 1994, 1998; Pezdek & Banks, 1996; Pezdek & Roe, 1994) the elements of the suggestions in these false memory studies referenced all contained factors that are likely to enhance the power and credibility of a suggestion. That is, the suggestions were plausible, came from authoritative sources, and did not threaten identity or relational schemata.

Pezdek (1994, 1998) reported that when she attempted to replicate these suggestibility studies by varying the plausibility of the events being suggested, her findings were different. Her confederates suggested to their younger siblings that the latter had been the subject of forced enemas. Pezdek described these suggestions as being rejected universally, in some cases with strong affect. She argued that when a suggestion is not plausible, it will not be accepted no matter the authoritative status of the person suggesting it (e.g., an older sibling alleging to have witnessed the event being suggested, the paradigm for the Loftus studies).

The data thus suggest that it may be difficult, but not impossible, to create false beliefs about an individual's life, if what is being suggested is sufficiently plausible. The anecdotal case reports of so-called false memories (Goldstein & Farmer, 1994) describe a process in which therapists increased the credibility of the suggestions, took highly authoritative stances in the therapy, and then made suggestions repeatedly. It appears that, under those conditions, it is possible for a client to develop an autobiographical narrative that is distorted by inaccurate beliefs about childhood sexual abuse.

Several authors (Brown et al., 1998; Courtois, 2000; Pope & Brown, 1996) note that in addition to the factors which may enhance the credibility of a suggestion by a therapist, individual differences in suggestibility are also factors in whether clients, or anyone, might develop inaccurate beliefs about their own lives. These authors suggest that therapists assess the suggestibility levels of their clients, using standardized measures such as the Gudjonsson Scale of Interrogative Suggestibility (Gudjonsson, 1984). These authors also strongly urge therapists to avoid making direct suggestions to clients about what might have happened to them, and to meet client's requests for a firm etiological hypothesis with the willingness to maintain ambiguity.

Pope (1996) carefully reviewed the assertions of the false memory movement regarding the existence of a false memory syndrome. He found that there were no empirical, experimentally derived data to support the existence of such a syndrome, and that many alleged cases of FMS were being so defined by individuals who were accused of being sexual abuse perpetrators, thus biasing their appraisal of the accusatory accounts. A review of subsequent literature has failed to find empirical refutation of Pope's review. Consequently, while it appears to be possible for a small number of persons to develop false beliefs about childhood sexual abuse, there is no evidence to support a diagnosis of a false memory syndrome.

LEGAL IMPLICATIONS

The false memory movement has had a number of effects on the larger cultural context. One of the areas in which this has been most evident has been in the arena of civil litigation. In the late 1980s and early 1990s, 26 states followed the lead of Washington state in amending their civil codes to allow the tolling (or delaying) of the statute of limitations for commencement of a civil action against an alleged perpetrator of childhood sexual abuse (Pope & Brown, 1996). A statute of limitations is the term describing the time period after the alleged act during which it is legally possible to bring actions, either civil or criminal, against an alleged perpetrator. Civil actions, or lawsuits, allow one private party to sue another for monetary damages, while criminal actions are brought by the state or federal government against someone alleged to have violated criminal law. Usually, the statute of limitations begins to run when the alleged act occurs, and is up (i.e., the time to sue is up) after a specified period of years (which will be different in each state, different for civil and criminal matter, and different in state court and federal courts). However, if the statute of limitations is tolled, it may begin to run from the point at which delayed recall first occurs.

These laws for delayed discovery variously allowed civil litigation based on either or both of the conditions of delayed recall, or delayed understanding (e.g., the recall of the abuse was continuous, but the person did not understand that it had harmed them until so informed in adulthood by an authoritative source such as a therapist or instructor). Additionally, a number of other states accepted litigation based on delayed recall on a case-by-case basis. Both black letter law (laws passed by legislatures or Congress) and case law (law based on cases decided at state or federal supreme or appellate court levels) have arisen in response to this issue. Again, as there is enormous variability by jurisdiction, those interested in this matter should consult with an attorney who practices in their area for specific information.

This civil litigation against alleged sexual abuse perpetrators peaked in the early 1990s, and by the end of the decade had almost entirely ceased. The cessation in recovered memory civil suits was due in large part to the efforts of the false memory movement in weakening the bases on which testimony had been offered by experts for plaintiffs in such matters. Additionally, because much of the expert testimony had been based on clinical observation and knowledge, questions were raised as to the admissibility of this testimony under the *Daubert* doctrine.

ADMISSIBILITY OF EXPERT TESTIMONY: *FRYE, DAUBERT, KUMHO*

Experts, such as therapists or forensic evaluators, are allowed to testify in court under several different rules of admissibility of testimony. These rules are defined in what is known as "case law." Case law is law based upon cases decided by high courts, either state or federal supreme courts or courts of appeal. Admission of expert testimony is also affected by the Federal Rules of Evidence, promulgated by the U.S. Congress. For most of the 20th century, a U.S. Supreme Court decision known as *Frye v. U.S.*, 293 F. 1013 (D.C. Cir. 1923), governed whether experts could testify in a court case. The *Frye* doctrine stated that the information being testified to had to be "generally accepted" in the field of scholarship.

In 1993, the Supreme Court came forth with another decision, known as *Daubert* (*Daubert v. Merrell, Dow Pharmaceuticals, Inc.*, 509 U.S. 579, 113 S. Ct. 2786, 125 L. Ed. 2d 469 (1993)). The *Daubert* decision, which is now the standard for admitting expert testimony in all federal cases and which has also been adopted as the standard by some states (although many states still work under a *Frye* standard), sets different hurdles to the admission of expert testimony. *Daubert* makes the trial court judge into the arbiter of whether testimony meets a list of standards for science proposed by the U.S. Supreme Court, including that the information being testified to by the expert has been published in peer-reviewed journals and that there is a known error rate for the phenomenon.

In 1999 the U.S. Supreme Court issued a decision known as *Kumho* (*Kumho Tire Co., Ltd., et al. v. Carmichael et al.*, 526 U.S. 137, 119 S. Ct. 1167, 143 L. Ed. 2d (1999)). The *Kumho* case differentiates "scientific" testimony, which remains governed by *Daubert*, from "technical" testimony, which now comes under the *Kumho* ruling. Most testimony offered by mental health experts appears to fall within the parameters of *Kumho*—for example, one client's results on a psychological test, or the diagnosis of a particular individual.

Mental health professionals who are called to testify must acquaint themselves with the standards for expert testimony that hold sway in the courtroom in which they will appear. If the testifying professional is not a forensic expert, consultation with a forensic practitioner, as well as with one's own attorney, will be helpful in assisting to frame testimony in such a way that it will be admissible, that is, fall within the standards of what an expert is allowed to say in the courtroom.

LAWSUITS AGAINST THERAPISTS

A different type of civil litigation began under the aegis of the false memory movement. It too reached a peak in the early 1990s and then went into decline. This body of litigation consisted of civil lawsuits brought by alleged sexual abuse perpetrators against therapists treating alleged victims. The highly publicized case of *Ramona v. Isabella*, No. 61898 (Cal. Super. Ct. May 13 1994), in which an accused father was awarded civil damages due to negligence by his daughter's therapist, defined the terms of such cases. The trial court judge ruled that Mr. Ramona, by being brought into the therapy session, had been made into a *de facto* client of Ms. Isabella, the therapist, and that she consequently owed him a duty of care. Several other attempts at third-party litigation were dismissed by trial court judges because no evidence existed in those matters that the therapist had created any duty of care to an alleged sexual abuse perpetrator (Brown et al., 1998).

A small but continuing number of cases are being brought against therapists by their own former clients, with the latter alleging creation of false memories through the use of inappropriate suggestive techniques. The feared onslaught of such cases discussed among therapists and proposed at false memory movement conferences (False Memory Syndrome Foundation, 1992) in the middle 1990s has not materialized, however.

The position of testimony based on recovered memory remains ambiguous. In those states where such testimony is admissible by statute because the law itself defines the possibility that memories can be long lost and then recovered, it continues to be offered occasionally. In other states, trial judges have ruled both to admit and to exclude such testimony, again on a case-by-case basis. Judicial rulings in these matters appear to reflect a combination of the judge's level of understanding of the scientific data regarding delayed recall, her or his analysis of how these data comport with *Daubert* or *Frye* standards, and the quality of testimony being offered by experts on either side of the discourse (Brown et al., 1998). Therapists who are not themselves forensically sophisticated are well advised to seek specific forensic training if interested in working as an expert in these matters. Therapists should seek consultation from a forensically experienced colleague if anticipating being called to testify about their own client.

MEMORY FOR CHILDHOOD SEXUAL ABUSE: A LIFTING FOG

One matter that has become clearer with continuing and more sophisticated research is that few people who are subjected to repeated sexual abuse as children remember it all, or remember it well, even when they have never forgotten that abuse occurred, or who perpetrated it. Fragmentary memory is the norm, even for continuous memory (Courtois, 2000). The client who enters therapy remembering that she or he was sexually abused is likely, during the course of treatment, to uncover aspects of the abuse that had not been available to conscious recollection when therapy began. This is because, if therapy is effective, and focuses on the enhancement of functioning (Courtois, 2000; Gold, 2001; Gold & Brown, 1997), the client will develop the emotional capacity to contain more challenging and painful information, and will be able to know more of what is stored in memory.

When the issue of delayed recall is placed into that normative context, its existence becomes more explicable and seems less remarkable. Instead, the delay of recall has become, as it should, a marker of the nature of the abuse. Delayed recall of childhood sexual abuse is most likely to occur when the knowledge of the abuse is itself most challenging to the individual's attachments to family and former caregivers. The person who was repeatedly sexually abused by an otherwise loving parent will have more difficulty knowing of the abuse than a person sexually abused once by a stranger.

Consequently, the presence of delayed recall of childhood sexual abuse should alert therapists to the difficulty of the therapeutic task that lies ahead. The remembering client will not simply be dealing with intrusive knowledge of horrifying experience. Rather, she or he will also be confronting enormous existential challenges, and must encompass the task of reconfiguring attachment relationships (Courtois, 2000; Gold, 2001; Harvey, 1996; Pope & Brown, 1996). Therapists working with these clients are well advised to become knowledgeable as to the most recent standards of practice (Courtois, 2000), so that care can be taken to neither discourage exploration of intrusive recollections, nor make such exploration the sole focus of therapy.

The experience of being sexually abused transforms a child in body, mind, and spirit. To remember and know of this experience is painful, and requires courage and immense inner and social resources. Understanding the dynamics of delayed recall, and the mechanisms by which it occurs, allows therapists to assist their clients in the successful completion of this difficult passage.

REFERENCES

Alpert, J. L., Brown, L. S., & Courtois, C.A. (1996). Symptomatic clients and memories of childhood abuse: What the trauma and child sexual abuse literature tells us. In J. Alpert, L. S. Brown, S. J. Ceci, C. A. Courtois, E. F. Loftus, & P. A. Ornstein, *Final Report of the Working Group on Investigation of Memories of Childhood Abuse* (pp. 1–32). Washington, DC: American Psychological Association.

American Psychological Association. (1994). *Interim report of the Working Group on Investigation of Memories of Childhood Abuse.* Washington, DC: Author.

Anderson, M. (1998, July). *Active forgetting: Evidence for functional inhibition as a source of memory failure.* Presented at the conference on Trauma and Cognitive Science, University of Oregon, Eugene, OR.

Armstrong, L. (1978). *Kiss Daddy goodnight: A speakout on incest.* New York: Pocket Books.

Bartlett, F. (1932). *Remembering: A study in experimental and social psychology.* New York: Macmillan.

Bass, E., & Thornton, L. (Eds.). (1983). *I never told anyone: Writings by women survivors of child sexual abuse.* New York: Harper.

Beitchman, J., Zucker, K., Hood, J., daCosta, G., & Ackman, D. (1991). A review of the short-term effects of childhood sexual abuse. *Child Abuse and Neglect, 16,* 101–118.

Blume, E. S. (1990). *Secret survivors: Uncovering incest and its aftereffects in women*. New York: Wiley.

Bower, G. H. (1981). Mood and memory. *American Psychologist, 36,* 129–148.

Brady, K. (1979). *Father's days*. New York: Seaview.

Bremner, J. D., Krystal, J. H., Charney, D. S., & Southwick, S. M. (1996). Neural mechanisms in dissociative amnesia for childhood abuse: Relevance to the current controversy surrounding the "false memory syndrome." *American Journal of Psychiatry, 153,* 71–82.

Briere, J. (1996). *Therapy for adults molested as children: Beyond survival* (2nd ed., rev. & expanded). New York: Springer.

Brown, D., Scheflin, A. W., & Hammond, D.C. (1998). *Memory, trauma, treatment and the law*. New York: Norton.

Brown, L. S. (1998). The prices of resisting silence. *Ethics and Behavior, 8,* 189–192.

Brown, L. S. (2000). The controversy over delayed recall for trauma: Historical, scientific and political issues. In A. Shalev, R. Yehuda, & A. C. McFarlane (Eds.), *International handbook of human response to trauma* (pp. 195–210). New York: Plenum Press.

Butler, S. (1978). *Conspiracy of silence: The trauma of incest*. San Francisco: New Glide.

Calof, D. (1998). Notes from a practice under siege: Harassment, defamation and intimidation in the name of science. *Ethics and Behavior, 8,* 161–188.

Cheit, R. E. (1998). Consider this, skeptics of recovered memory. *Ethics and Behavior, 8,* 141–160.

Christianson, S. A., & Engelberg, E. (1997). Remembering and forgetting traumatic experiences: A matter of survival. In M. Conway (Ed.), *False and recovered memories* (pp. 230–250). Oxford, UK: Oxford University Press.

Corwin, D. D., & Olafson, E. (1997). Videotapes discovery of a reportedly unrecallable memory of child sexual abuse: Comparison with a childhood interview video-taped 11 years before. *Child Maltreatment, 29,* 91–112.

Cosmides, L., & Tooby, J. (1992). *The adapted mind: Evolutionary psychology and the generation of culture*. New York: Oxford University Press.

Courtois, C. (2000). *Recollections of sexual abuse*. New York: Norton.

Duvenage, C., & Dalenberg, C. (1993, January). *Dissociation, child abuse history and amnesiac barrier strength in a non-clinical population*. Presented at the conference on Responding to Child Maltreatment, San Diego, CA.

Elliot, D. M., & Briere, J. (1995). Posttraumatic stress associated with delayed recall of sexual abuse: A general population study. *Journal of Traumatic Stress, 8,* 629–647.

False Memory Syndrome Foundation. (1992). *Legal aspects of false memory syndrome*. Philadelphia, PA: Author.

Fivush, R. (1996). Young children's event recall: Are memories constructed through discourse? In K. Pezdek & W. Banks (Eds.), *The recovered memory/false memory debate* (pp. 151–168). New York: Academic Press.

Fredrickson, R. (1992). *Repressed memories: A journey to recovery from sexual abuse*. New York: Simon & Schuster.

Freyd, J. (1994) Betrayal-trauma; Traumatic amnesia as an adaptive response to childhood abuse. *Ethics and Behavior, 4*, 307–329.

Freyd, J. J. (1996). *Betrayal trauma: The logic of forgetting abuse.* Cambridge, MA: Harvard University Press.

Freyd, J. J., DePrince, A. P., & Zurbriggen, E. L. (2001). Self-reported memory for abuse depends upon victim-perpetrator relationship. *Journal of Trauma and Dissociation, 2*, 5–17.

Gold, S. N. (2001). *Not trauma alone.* Thousand Oaks, CA: Sage.

Gold, S. N., & Brown, L. S. (1997). Therapeutic responses to delayed recall: Beyond recovered memory. *Psychotherapy: Theory, Research, Practice, Training.*

Goldstein, E., & Farmer, K. (Eds.) (1994). *Confabulations: Creating false memories, destroying families.* Boca Raton, FL: SIRS Books.

Goodman, G. S., Bottoms, B. L., Schwartz-Kenney, B., & Rudy, L. A. (1991). Children's memory for a stressful event: Improving children's report. *Journal of Narrative and Life History, 1*, 69–99.

Goodman, G. S., Quas, J. A., Batterman-Faunce, J. M., Riddlesberger, M. M., & Kuhn, J. (1994). Predictors of accurate and inaccurate memories of traumatic events experienced in childhood. *Consciousness and Cognition, 3*, 269–294.

Gudjonsson, G. H. (1984). A new scale of interrogative suggestibility. *Personality and Individual Differences, 5*, 303–314.

Harvey, M. R. (1996). An ecological view of psychological trauma and trauma recovery. *Journal of Traumatic Stress, 9*, 3–23.

Herman, J. L (1981). *Father–daughter incest.* Cambridge, MA: Harvard University Press.

Hinnefeld, B., & Newman, R. (1997). Analysis of the Truth and Responsibility in Mental Health Practice Act and similar proposals. *Professional Psychology: Research and Practice, 28*, 537–543.

Hyman, I. E., Jr., Husband, T. H., & Billings, F. J. (1995). False memories of childhood experiences. *Applied Cognitive Psychology, 9*, 181–197.

Hyman, I. E., & Loftus, E. F. (1997). Some people recover memories of childhood trauma that never really happened. In P. S. Appbelbaum, L. A. Uyehara, & M. R. Elin (Eds.), *Trauma and memory: Clinical and legal controversies* (pp. 3–24). New York: Oxford University Press.

Legal aspects of false memory syndrome. (1992, June). *False Memory Syndrome Foundation Newsletter,* 1–3.

Loftus, E. F. (1979). *Eyewitness testimony.* Cambridge, MA: Harvard University Press.

Loftus, E. F. (1993). The reality of repressed memories. *American Psychologist, 48*, 518–537.

Loftus, E. F., & Coan, D. (1994). The construction of childhood memories. In D. Peters (Ed.) *The child witness in context: Cognitive, social and legal perspectives.* New York: Kluwer.

Loftus, E. F., & Ketcham, K. (1994). *The myth of repressed memory: False memories and allegations of abuse.* New York : St. Martin's.

Loftus, E. F., & Pickrell, J.E. (1995). The formation of false memories. *Psychiatric Annals, 25*, 720–725.

McNaron, T., & Morgan, Y. (Eds.). (1982). *Voices in the night: Women speaking out about incest*. Minneapolis: Cleis.

Neisser, U. (Ed.). (1982). *Memory observed: Remembering in natural contexts*. San Francisco: Freeman.

Ofshe, R., & Watters, E. (1994). *Making monsters: False memories, psychotherapy, and sexual hysteria*. New York: Scribners.

Pezdek, K. A. (1994). The illusion of illusory memory. *Applied Cognitive Psychology, 8*, 339–350.

Pezdek, K. A. (1998, July). *The recovered memory/false memory debate*. Presented at the conference on Trauma and Cognitive Science, University of Oregon, Eugene, OR.

Pezdek, K. A., & Banks, W. (1996). *The recovered memory/false memory controversy*. New York: Academic Press.

Pezdek, K. A., & Roe, C. (1994). Memory for childhood events: How suggestible is it? *Consciousness and Cognition, 3*, 374–387.

Pope, K. S. (1996). Memory, abuse and science: Questioning claims about the false memory syndrome epidemic. *American Psychologist, 51*, 957–974.

Pope, K. S., & Brown, L. S. (1996). *Recovered memories of abuse: Assessment, therapy, forensics*. Washington, DC: American Psychological Association.

Rush, F. (1980). *The best-kept secret: Sexual abuse of children*. New York: McGraw-Hill.

Schooler, J. W., Ambadar, Z., & Bendiksen, M. (1997). A cognitive corroborative case study approach for investigating discovered memories of sexual abuse. In J. D. Read & D. A. Lindsay (Eds.), *Recollections of trauma: Scientific evidence and clinical practice* (pp. 379–387). New York: Plenum Press.

Terr, L. (1990). *Too scared to cry: Psychic trauma in childhood*. New York: Harper & Row.

Tessler, M., & Nelson, K. (1994). Making memories: The influence of joint encoding on later recall by young children. *Consciousness and Cognition, 3*, 307–326.

van der Kolk, B. A. (1996). The body keeps the score: Approaches to the psychobiology of posttraumatic stress disorder. In B. A. van der Kolk, A. C. McFarlane, & L. Weissath (Eds.), *Traumatic stress: The effects of overwhelming experience on mind, body and society* (pp. 214–241). New York: Guilford Press.

Wilson, J. P. (1989). *Trauma transformation and healing: An integrative approach to theory, research and post-traumatic therapy*. New York: Brunner/Mazel.

Yates, J. L., & Nasby, W. (1993). Dissociation, affect and network models of memory: An integrative proposal. *Journal of Traumatic Stress, 6*, 305–326.

Zaragoza, M. S. (1991). Preschool children's susceptibility to memory impairment. In J. Doris (Ed.), *The suggestibility of children's recollections: Implications for eyewitness testimony* (pp. 27–39). Washington, DC: American Psychological Association.

PART III

Perpetrators of Sexualized Violence and Other Harms against Women and Children

As the discussion in Part II makes clear, there is a significant amount of sexual abuse of children. The question is what to do about the perpetrators. Obviously it is best to eliminate the behavior, but even revising the laws against it or prosecuting the extant laws more vigorously does not accomplish that end. Because sexual molestation and the possible violence associated with it are driven by compulsive psychological needs, it is unlikely that prohibition alone will significantly reduce the behavior. It is not rational decision making that drives pedophiles to molest children, but rather strong sexual urges that are directed toward children. And as anyone knows who has worked with a sexually deviant population, it is extremely difficult to change sexual drives and their objects. Whether it is genetic or socially transmitted, sexuality is encoded early and is very resistant to change. This is true even when the person with perverse behaviors is strongly motivated to change. And, needless to say, arrested pedophiles and rapists rarely seek psychotherapy for their problems. Thus the treatment of sex offenders is important, although difficult.[1] Treatments have been developed, but few claim high success rates. Even treatment that appears to be somewhat successful—in particular, cognitive-behavioral therapy—may not be effective over time because perpetrators, once released, do not voluntarily continue treatment.

213

Failed attempts to treat convicted sex offenders successfully, along with other social factors, have led to two new legal developments. New laws have recently been enacted that attempt to protect citizens, especially children, from sex offenders by either (1) continuing to hold convicted sex offenders after they have served their prison terms (sexual predator laws) or (2) by requiring sex offenders to register with the authorities and to notify the people in their communities upon their release from prison (Megan's laws).[2] Most likely out of the frustration of trying to deal with these problems and a deep fear of the harm that sex offenders do, these laws have recently proliferated—Megan's laws from the early 1990s and sexual predator laws from the late 1990s. Both types of laws have been challenged, first as to the likelihood of their success in reducing the number or severity of sex offenses, and second, legally, as to their constitutionality. Usually, in our justice system, we punish crimes that have already been committed. We do not hold people prospectively, because we think they will commit crimes in the future. And criminals who have already served their time are not required to identify themselves as convicts in their daily lives. In spite of these constitutional problems, sexual predator laws and Megan's laws have withstood strong, repeated constitutional challenges and have been upheld by the U.S. Supreme Court, the ultimate authority on constitutional matters. This may be due to the fact that our society is currently very concerned with law and order and less concerned with the rights and civil liberties of convicted felons. Interestingly, these stringent laws do not seem to be a product of the new wave of feminism. In fact, the political base in support of these laws comes from the right, even the religious right, and is more conservative than progressive. However, the resulting laws benefit the women and children who are the victims of sexual crimes.[3]

Lastly, although this book focuses on wrongs to women and children, there are some notable instances where women commit harms against children—particularly when mothers kill their own children.[4] The media have focused on this recently, but certainly folk tales and folk songs of mothers killing their unwanted children date very far back. Perhaps these crimes are more striking and less understandable now that abortion is widely available. However, there are certain ways in which the treatment of women interacts with their ability to function as mothers or to protect their children. In addition to young girls who cannot psychologically accept their pregnancies, and behave before and after the birth as if they did not have a baby, there are also mothers who, perhaps due to rampant hormonal changes after giving birth, develop or are pushed further into psychotic states. There are also women who are objects of spousal abuse and who either participate with, or fail to stop, their husbands who kill their babies. And then there are women, often the recipients of child abuse and neglect themselves, who are unable to care for or discipline their children appropriately and ultimately lethally harm them.

These issues are addressed in the following chapters, which constitute Part III of this volume.

NOTES

1. For details on the treatment of sex offenders, see Chapter 9, this volume.
2. For details on sexual predator laws and Megan's law, and related references, see Chapter 10, this volume.
3. Although beyond the scope of this book, the political right and new wave feminism have been strange bedfellows on other recent, sex-related issues as well, such as the control of pornography.
4. For details on women who kill their children, and related references, see Chapter 11, this volume.

9 Management and Treatment of the Adult Sexual Offender

WILLIAM D. MURPHY

Sexual violence is highly prevalent in our society, with significant negative consequences for victims. Early studies with adult women on the West coast found rates of sexual abuse prior to the age of 16 of 38% (Russell, 1984) and 45% (Wyatt, 1985). In a national probability sample, Finkelhor, Hotaling, Lewis, and Smith (1990) found abuse rates of 27% in women and 16% in males. In another national probability sample of 4,008 cases, Resnick, Kilpatrick, Dansky, Saunders, and Best (1993) found that 12.6% of their sample reported a completed rape and 14.3% reported other sexual assaults. The National Crime Victim Survey indicated a total of 248,000 rapes and sexual assaults against persons age 12 and above in 2001 (Rennison, 2002). Jones and Finklehor (2001), using data from the National Child Abuse and Neglect Data System found that there were 315,400 reported cases of child sexual abuse in 1998, with 103,600 of these cases substantiated. On the positive side, there has been a decline of 56% in rates of rape/sexual assault from 1993 to 2000, and for substantiated cases of child sexual abuse, a 31% decline from 1992 to 1998 (Jones & Finklehor, 2001; Rennison, 2002).

The impact of sexual victimization on emotional functioning and interpersonal relationships has been well described (Berliner & Elliott, 1996; Burman et al., 1988; Resnick et al., 1993). Sexual abuse has also been linked to women's perceptions of their health status (Koss, Woodruff, & Koss, 1990), and actual health status (Read, Stern, Wolfe, & Ouimette, 1997). Histories of childhood sexual abuse also can be related to future delinquent and criminal behavior; however, this effect is no larger than for other forms of childhood maltreatment (Widom, 1995).

Given the significance of the problem of sexual victimization, finding methods for preventing sexual abuse is an urgent need. This chapter takes the approach that the management of the offender is one method of preventing sexual abuse. It focuses on mental health approaches to the management and treatment of sexual offenders.

CHARACTERISTICS

For the reader less familiar with the literature on sexual offenders, a brief review of relevant characteristics is provided. More detailed information regarding offender characteristics can be found in Weinrott (1996) and Barbaree, Hudson, and Seto (1993) for adolescent offenders, and Murphy and Smith (1996), Marshall (1997), and Hudson and Ward (1997) for adult offenders. The public in general and, unfortunately, many professionals have stereotyped views of what offenders are like. In reality, offenders vary significantly across most characteristics, such as IQ, socioeconomic status, personality, and psychopathology. Offenders range from those with superior IQs to the developmentally disabled and from physicians and lawyers to the chronically unemployed. They are very heterogeneous in terms of psychiatric disorders, with some showing major psychiatric disorders while others have little concomitant psychopathology. There seems to be no one personality type, and offenders can appear quite normal, can be shy and inhibited, or can be generally antisocial and aggressive. Attempts to find a specific general psychological profile have been unsuccessful (Erickson, Luxenburg, Walbeck, & Seely, 1987; Murphy & Peters, 1992). It also appears that, as a group, sexual offenders do not differ in terms of general personality patterns from other forensic populations (Quinsey, Arnold, & Pruesse, 1980). Some sexual offenders have significant histories of nonsexual criminal behavior, while others have little nonsexual criminal behavior (Greenfeld, 1997; Weinrott & Saylor, 1991).

Because of this heterogeneity, there have been attempts to look at subtypes of offenders to create more homogeneous groups. This has included complex typology systems (Knight & Prentky, 1990) and systems that more simply divide offenders based on characteristics of the offense.

The latter includes separating rapists from child molesters and further subdividing child molesters into incest and nonincest cases and those with male and female victims. Much of this chapter focuses on this subdivision. In general, rapists are more similar to general criminal populations than child molesters. They are more aggressive than passive and show more psychopathy or antisocial traits (Firestone, Bradford, Greenberg, & Serran, 2000; Hudson & Ward, 1997). There is some evidence that child molesters show more deficits in interpersonal skills and have less confidence in themselves interpersonally than rapists (Geer, Estupinan, & Manguno-Mire, 2000; Segal & Marshall, 1986). It is also commonly found that extrafamilial offenders against male children have the highest sexual recidivism rate and incest cases have the lowest recidivism rate. The pattern of recidivism also differs between rapists and child molesters. Rapists show a steady decline in recidivism with age, similar to general criminal populations. Extrafamilial child molesters show little decrease in recidivism until after the age of 50 (Hanson, 2002).

It has often been postulated that histories of sexual abuse have etiological significance in the development of sexual offenders. Again, however, the frequency of abuse in sexual offender populations is very much dependent on the subgroup studied. Hanson and Slater (1988) reviewed a number of studies and found that approximately 30% of adult sexual offenders reported being victims of sexual abuse, although this may be closer to 50% for those who offend against young males. Reviewing studies related to incest offenders, Williams and Finkelhor (1990) reported rates from 0 to 35% for sexual abuse and from 36 to 59% for physical abuse. In a national survey of individuals in state correctional facilities (Greenfeld, 1997), it was found that 11.8% of the general criminal population had histories of some type of abuse in childhood, while 19% of the rapists and 34% of other sexual offenders (which included many child offenders) reported some form of childhood abuse. One study did find high rates (62%) of sexual abuse in rapists (Dhawan & Marshall, 1996), although the sample size of rapists was relatively small ($n = 29$). Although nonincestuous offenders against children appear to have higher rates of abuse than the general population, it is not clear that this is true of rapists or incest offenders; the major finding appears to be for offenders against male children. It is also clear that most young males victimized do not become offenders, and almost no females who are abused become offenders.

One clear difference between sexual offenders and the general population is that the majority are male. Finkelhor (1984) reports that 5% of the molestation of females and 20% of the molestation of males were by females, although higher rates are at times reported (see Hunter & Mathews, 1997, for a review). Although not the focus of the current chapter, such data indicate that the primary prevention of sexual abuse may need to focus on those aspects of male psychosexual/psychosocial development that contribute to male sexually aggressive behavior.

Research suggests that certain categories of offenders report an early onset of deviant sexual arousal interests. The mean age of onset for nonincest offenders against male children was 18.2; for nonincest offenders against female children, 21.6; and for rapists, 21.8 (Abel, Osborn, & Twigg, 1993). Abel and Rouleau (1990) report that 50% of the nonincestuous offenders against male children had their onset before the age of 16, 40% of the nonincestuous offenders against female children had an onset before age 18, and 30% of rapists had an onset before the age of 18.

It has also been found that offenders have many more victims than officially known and that they tend to have multiple paraphilias[1] (Abel et al., 1987; Abel & Rouleau, 1990; Weinrott & Saylor, 1991). These studies used either a confidential interview or a confidential computerized interview to collect data. Abel et al. (1987) report that 225 offenders against female children, 155 offenders against male children, and 126 rapists reported 4,435 victims, 22,981 victims, and 882 victims, respectively. Studies using polygraphs have also shown increased reporting of victims after the polygraph examination for adult offenders (Hindman, 1988) and adolescent offenders (Emerick & Dutton, 1993; Harrison & Elliott, 1999). Another common finding among nonincestuous offenders against children is that they have a set deviant sexual arousal pattern when arousal is measured via penile plethysmography[2] in the laboratory (Freund & Watson, 1991; Harris, Rice, Quinsey, Chaplin, & Earls, 1992; Murphy & Barbaree, 1994). Data further suggest that incest cases do not typically show such deviant arousal patterns (Murphy & Barbaree, 1994). Data for rapists are mixed (Murphy & Barbaree, 1994), although there are clearly some rapists who are sexually attracted to violent sexual behavior (Harris et al., 1992).

The preceding does not cover all that is known about offenders, but has attempted to focus on issues that may be related to the management and the prevention of sexual abuse. First, our knowledge that sexual offending has an early onset suggests a strong need to target the adolescent sexual offender. There is some suggestion that young males who are abused may be at increased risk for sexual offending. Therefore adequate treatment services should be available for this population as a possible preventive strategy. Other data suggest that, at least among adolescent offenders, those who have been sexually abused tend to have more victims and an earlier onset, and may show more deviant sexual arousal patterns (Cooper, Murphy, & Haynes, 1996; Murphy, DiLillo, Haynes, & Steere, 2001).

Data related to the fact that offenders have multiple paraphilias and many more victims than is usually known have significant implications for management. First, in terms of investigation and prosecution, there should be no assumption that the offender has not abused other people, and this should be part of the investigative process. The existence of multiple paraphilias implies that the offense pattern of many offenders is not limited to victims of a specific gender or age. When offenders are monitored in the community, mistakes can be made if one assumes that a rapist would never molest a child, that a child molester would never rape, or that an incest father would not molest outside the home. One cannot assume that because the victim was a female child that the offender would be "safe" around male children.

CRIMINAL JUSTICE ROLE IN MANAGING
SEXUAL OFFENDERS AND RELATIONSHIP
TO OFFENDER TREATMENT

In the last 10–15 years there have been numerous approaches to improving the investigation of sexual abuse cases, including better law enforcement practices, special sex crimes units, improved child protective service investigations, and prosecutorial procedures that are more victim oriented (Bulkley, Feller, Stern, & Roe, 1996; Lanning, 1996; Myers, 1992; Nannetti & Greer, 1996; Portwood, Reppucci, & Mitchell, 1998; Righthand & Hodge, 1992).

There is no clear empirical data on the impact these procedures actually have on criminal justice outcome. However, the management of sexual offenders requires an effective child protective service and criminal justice system. Offenders cannot be "managed" if they are not identified, and few come forward voluntarily. Most offenders enter treatment after they have been identified by the criminal justice system or the child protective system. Unfortunately, only a small number of offenses are actually reported to authorities. Data from the National Crime Victim Survey indicate that for individuals 12 or older, only 32% of victims reported the offense to the police, with other sources suggesting even lower rates. Saunders, Kilpatrick, Hanson, Resnick, and Walker (1999), in a national probability sample, found that only 11.9% of child rape cases were reported to authorities. It is quite clear that a policy for reducing sexual victimization must address factors related to underreporting.

Once an offender is identified, a major component of the sexual offender management response is the parole and probation officer. Data from the Bureau of Justice Statistics for 1994 indicate that on any given day approximately 234,000 sexual offenders were under the auspices of correctional agencies. Sixty percent of these offenders were being supervised in the community by probation and parole (Greenfeld, 1997). Therefore, most sexual offenders are in the community, and most of those sent to prison will eventually return to the community.

English and colleagues (English, 1998; English, Pullen, & Jones, 1996, 1997) have described model policies and procedures for the management of sexual offenders in the community. This strategy is referred to as the containment model, which includes the parole/probation officer, the sexual offender treatment specialist, and the use of polygraphs. The polygraph examination is used both to encourage the offender to provide an honest history of his deviant sexual behavior and to monitor whether the offender is following his parole/probation and treatment requirements (Pullen, Olsen, Brown, & Amich, 1996). In addition, adequate knowledge of the range of any one offender's paraphilic behavior allows the development of a more individualized supervision plan. Knowledge that an individual, during treatment and supervision, is not following requirements and is placing himself in high-risk situations, such as contact with children, can trigger increased parole supervision and intensified treatment. As noted earlier, there is evidence that polygraph examinations do increase reporting of a range of deviant behaviors (Emerick & Dutton, 1993; Hindman, 1988). At this time, there is no empirical evidence that the addition of the polygraph examination to either treatment or supervision actually decreases recidivism, and no clear empirical evidence that the containment model actually reduces recidivism.

There are, however, uncontrolled studies from intensive supervision programs. A program in Maricopa County, Arizona, reports recidivism rates of 1.5% (cited in La Fond, 1998). They have lifetime probation, use of specialized treatment, specialized probation officers, and polygraphs. Berliner, Schram, Miller, and Milloy (1995) report that offenders sentenced to community placement under Washington state's special sexual offender sentence alternative had a relatively lower rearrest rate (6.1%) for sexual offenses. The majority of these individuals were in specialized sexual offender treatment; many providers in Washington frequently use polygraph examinations; and there tends to be a fairly well-integrated system between treatment providers and parole/probation. Although these studies were not controlled, the data at least support the notion that individuals under a coordinated management system have relatively low recidivism rates. Whether such rates would occur without such a coordinated system cannot be answered with current data.

REGISTRATION AND COMMUNITY
NOTIFICATION LAWS

The most recent developments in social policies to manage sexual offenders are sexual offender registries and community notification. At the current time, federal statutes, the Wetterling Act, and the federal Megan's Law (see Terry & Cling, Chapter 10, this volume) require all states to develop registration and notification procedures (Beckman, 1998; Sorkin, 1998) or lose federal law enforcement funds.

As is well known, these laws were prompted by horrible incidents, including the kidnapping of 11-year-old Jacob Wetterling, who is still missing, and the brutal killing of 7-year-old Megan Kanka. A third law, the Pam Lyncher Sexual Offender Tracking and Identification Act of 1996, established a national tracking and database system for sexual offenders and strengthened the previous Wetterling Act.

Washington state enacted the first community notification law in 1990, and by 1997, 47 states had community notification laws (Matson & Lieb, 1997). At the current time, all states have some type of community notification law, although they vary in how the data are accessed by the public. The U.S. Department of Justice has sponsored a national conference on sexual offender registers (1998) and has published a survey of sexual offender registry dissemination procedures (Adams, 2002). As of February 2001, 386,000 convicted sexual offenders were registered in 49 states and the District of Columbia (Adams, 2002). Data from Massachusetts were not included in the 2001 survey because at the time their registration procedure was stopped by a court injunction, which has since been resolved.

States vary on their approach to disseminating information. Washington, the first state to pass such a law, used a three-tier approach based on offender risk. Notification for those at the lower risk would be restricted to law enforcement officials, while those at highest risk would receive community-wide notification. For those in the moderate-risk category, notification is directed toward those at risk, such as schools or daycare, and may not be community wide (Matson & Lieb, 1997). However, since the inception of these laws more states are developing public accessible Web sites. In February, 2001, 29 states had public accessible Web sites of registered sexual offenders. According to the KlaasKids Foundation (*www.klaaskids.org*), 38 states currently have full public access Web sites.

There have been, and continue to be, legal challenges to these laws (Berliner, 1997; Finn, 1997; Sacco, 1998). Constitutional challenges have included cruel and unusual punishment, the ex post facto nature of these laws, double jeopardy, privacy issues, and due process. Although there have been mixed rulings, in the majority of cases it appears that courts are upholding these laws. The laws are not being seen as punishment but public protection, and the legal findings have indicated that the information provided in community notification is already public information.

In general, these laws have been viewed very positively by law enforcement (Matson & Lieb, 1996) and by the public (Phillips, 1998). However, some professionals have raised concerns (Freeman-Longo, 1996a, 1996b; Prentky, 1996). Issues have included the potential for violence against or harassment of the offenders, that the stress of notification could actually increase risk, and that these laws may lead to a sense of false security in the community and are unlikely to reduce recidivism for the offender motivated to reoffend. In terms of violence against offenders, although some incidents are reported, these are lower than expected. Matson and Lieb (1997) report a 3.5% incidence of harassment including one incident of an offender's house being burned. Finn (1997) reported that in Oregon less than 10% of offenders have experienced any type of harassment. Interviews with sexual offenders in Wisconsin who were registered indicated that 83% reported being excluded for housing, 57% reported loss of employment, and 57% reported threats or harassment (Zevitz & Farkas, 2000). The differences in these studies are mostly likely due to the sources of data, one being official reports (Oregon) and the other being reports from offenders (Wisconsin).

The question of whether the laws reduce recidivism is still to be determined. Washington compared reoffense rates (Schram & Milloy, 1995) in a group of offenders released prior to notification to a matched group of offenders after notification. There were no differences in sexual offense rearrest rates between groups at the end of a 54-month at-risk period. There were also no statistical differences between groups for rearrest for any offense. However, those on community notification were arrested more quickly, with a mean failure time of 25 months versus a mean failure time of approximately 62 months in the non-notification group.

The approach advocated in this chapter is the management of sexual offender risk, and in many ways registry and community notification can be seen as one aspect of the management of risk by making the public part of the offender surveillance system. However, as has been pointed out by those who have supported and developed these laws (Berliner, 1996; Lieb, 1996), they should only be seen as one part of the comprehensive approach to reducing sexual offending. The Association of the Treatment of Sexual Abusers (1996) has also developed a position statement that stresses the need for these laws to be part of an overall response. ATSA's position statement recommends that broad community notification be reserved for high-risk offenders and that validated risk assessment systems be employed in making decisions. ATSA's position paper raises concerns about the protection of sexual abuse victims due to confidentiality, and this is especially relevant for incest victims in states with broad community notification.

Community notification laws have provided an opportunity to educate the public about the realities of sexual offender risk and to make the public an ally in preventing sexual offending. However, for these laws to be effective it is likely that adequate resources will be needed to implement them. It also needs to be recognized that no one intervention is likely, by itself, to have a major impact on reducing recidivism. The public should not be lulled into a false sense of security because of the existence of such laws.

It should be recognized that approximately 1 of 7 sexual offenders in prison has a previous conviction for sexual offense; therefore, the majority of individuals in prison are there for their first offense (Greenfeld, 1997). Since offenders cannot be identified for community notification until they have been officially identified for an offense, it is clear that community notification will only be applicable to a small number of offenders.

TREATMENT APPROACHES TO THE MANAGEMENT OF SEXUAL OFFENDERS

Treatment is one component of an overall management approach to reducing recidivism in sexual offenders. This section initially outlines the context of and assumptions underlying sexual offender treatment and then describes components of comprehensive sexual offender treatment. For those seeking more details, there are multiple sources available that describe currently accepted treatment approaches to offenders (Laws & O'Donohue, 1997; Marshall, Laws, & Barbaree, 1990; Murphy & Smith, 1996).

Sexual offender treatment has developed into a subspecialty area within the mental health field, with its own ethical standards and principles of practice (Association for the Treatment of Sexual Abusers, 1997). Treatment of sexual offenders differs from the treatment of individuals with general mental health problems. First, the goal of treatment is to reduce recidivism, so, for most treatment programs, the "client" is the community rather than the individual being seen. Most programs work closely with protective services and parole/probation officers. Community safety is considered the priority of treatment, and external pressures through the courts are thought to enhance treatment (Association for the Treatment of Sexual Abusers, 2001). Individuals in sexual offender-specific programs are generally asked to waive confidentiality so that information can clearly be communicated to the various systems involved in their management. Offender treatment adopts a "no cure" philosophy, recognizing that the goal is lifelong control and management of the behavior (Association for the Treatment of Sexual Abusers, 2001).

Treatment is also sexual offender-specific rather than addressing more general psychological factors. That is, treatment tends to focus on specific sexual offender issues and generally follows a cognitive-behavioral model within a relapse prevention framework. Treatment focuses on the thoughts, feelings, and behaviors that tend to increase an individual's risk to reoffend.

Treatment begins with a comprehensive evaluation, usually referred to as a psychosexual evaluation. The evaluation involves interviews with the offender and, often, with significant others in the offender's life. A variety of psychological testing instruments are also generally administered. Many programs also try to assess deviant sexual interest through penile plethysmography (Murphy & Barbaree, 1994) or by the use of the Abel Assessment of sexual interest (Abel, Jordan, Hand, Holland, & Phipps, 2001). Penile plethysmography is the most widely researched method of assessing deviant arousal and involves using a gauge to measure change in penile size while the offender is presented with sexual stimuli through slides or audiotapes that describe sexual scenarios. These stimuli vary on the age and sex of the person depicted and can vary on amount of aggression depicted. The Abel Assessment is a newer, less well-researched method that assesses deviant interest by measuring the time the offender looks at slides of clothed males and females of various ages.

From the evaluation the clinician attempts to determine three general factors that are loosely drawn from the general correctional rehabilitation literature (Andrews & Bonta, 1998). The first factor is the determination of the risk of reoffense, which is generally based on what is termed static risk factors. These include previous sexual and nonsexual crimes, certain victim characteristics such as sex of victim and relationship of the victim to the offender, and offender characteristics such as age of the offender and history of previous adult relationships (see "Risk Assessment" section). This information is used to make decisions regarding whether treatment can be safely delivered in the community, intensity of treatment needed, and the degree of external monitoring or intensity of parole/probation supervision required.

The second factor is an assessment of the dynamic risk factors or treatment needs. These are characteristics of the offender that are related to both sexual and nonsexual reoffending that are changeable through therapeutic interventions. Commonly accepted treatment goals are included in Table 9.1. At the current time not all of these factors have empirical support, but they are accepted in the field as at least potentially or theoretically linked to recidivism. Not all offenders will have all of these factors, and treatment should be tailored to the specific treatment needs of the offender.

The final factor is responsivity. This is defined as delivering treatment that is consistent with the learning style of the offender (Andrews & Bonta, 1998). In sexual offender treatment, this means being cognizant of intellectual levels and potential learning disabilities, comorbid psychiatric disorders or personality disorders, and ethnic/cultural factors that will impact offender learning and change. It also means that therapist style should be conducive to change. Some perceive sexual offender treatment as being highly confrontational. Although offenders must be held accountable for their behavior, change is unlikely to occur if the therapist is perceived as being hostile to the offender. More recent data suggest that a therapist style that combines structure with empathic delivery may be most effective (Marshall & Serran, 2000).

One of the first components of treatment is specific targeting of the offender's denial and the attitudes or cognitions that support offending. One can view denial as a continuum, with denial on one end and complete honesty on the other end. In between these two poles offenders try to minimize what they have done and/or justify what they have done. Attitudes supportive of offending can be more general attitudes such as acceptance of rape myths (women secretly desire to be raped) to more specific justifications such as minimizations (I only did it once) or distortions (She was asking for it; It was sex education). These justifications are generally addressed within a group therapy format, many times using victim statements and police reports to challenge the offender's denial, minimizations, and distortions. In many programs, polygraph ex-

TABLE 9.1. Common Treatment Goals

- Decrease denial and attitudes supportive of offending.
- Increase understanding or risk factors and development of relapse prevention plans.
- Improve relationship and intimacy skills.
- Improve social competence.
- Increase victim empathy.
- Decrease sexual preoccupation.
- Decrease deviant sexual arousal.

aminations are used to further elicit details of offenses. In actual practice, most offenders will generally admit some aspects of the offense once they are in the group situation with other offenders who are admitting other offenses as well; the real focus is on the justifications for the offense.

There are a variety of group approaches to address the cognitions that support offending (Murphy & Carich, 2001). These techniques basically involve educating offenders regarding the role justifications play in maintaining their offending. This generally involves letting offenders know that the therapist knows they know right from wrong, but that they have developed methods to avoid negative feelings about their offending. These methods are the things they "say to themselves" to convince themselves that what they are doing is not wrong, not "too bad," or not their fault (Murphy & Carich, 2001). The next step is to help offenders identify the justifications they use, which usually begins in the group when they present their written history of their respective offenses. The therapist and group members identify when justifications are used. The therapist and group members then challenge the distortions, trying to assist each offender in seeing how the justifications he uses are irrational and in replacing the justifications with a more rational/realistic appraisal of his responsibility for offending.

Another goal of sexual offender treatment is for offenders to recognize factors that place them at risk to offend and to develop adequate relapse prevention plans to cope with risk factors. Risk factors can be environmentally based, such as babysitting, for a pedophile, or cruising late at night, for rapists, or can be more internal, such as anger, rejection, or interpersonal conflict. Recent theorizing and research (Hudson, Ward, & McCormick, 1999) suggests that there are two broad pathways to offending. The first is referred to as an avoidance pathway. Individuals who are following this pathway are actually trying to avoid offending. However, they may lack certain coping skills or use inappropriate skills to cope with negative emotional states or interpersonal conflict. For example, a rapist may have an argument with his wife and become angry, but he never discusses this with her. He may attempt to cope with the anger by going to a bar and drinking, which moves him closer to offending. Treatment for this group of offenders involves identifying high-risk situations and triggers to their offending. Once identified, the offender learns to avoid certain situations. However, more importantly, treatment focuses on strengthening or developing more healthy coping and general relationship skills.

The second pathway is referred to as an approach pathway and occurs in offenders who are not attempting to avoid offending. This pathway usually is seen in the more classic pedophile, where there is strong sexual attraction to children. For offenders who follow the approach pathway, there may be less focus on developing coping skills and more focus on developing environmental control, ensuring that there is adequate monitoring in the community and attempting to develop within the offender motivations not to offend. An important aspect of treatment is the development of behaviors and skills to replace the offending behavior. Therefore, with a pedophile one might focus on developing skills for establishing relationships with adults.

In actual practice, offender programs tend to look at two sets of risk factors. The first set comprises what are generally termed grooming behaviors, which refer to how the offender identifies victims, gets access to victims, manipulates and/or forces victims to engage in the sexual behavior. For example, the offender may get access to child victims by establishing relationships with women with children, or a rapist may identify potential victims by going to bars or by cruising certain neighborhoods late at night. The focus of treatment would then be avoiding these types of situations and ensuring that the parole officer was monitoring such situations. The second step would be attempting to identify whether there are any more "psychological" triggers to the offending. This usually is accomplished by having the patient "walk through" his life at the time the offending behavior was going on. The therapist and group members then try to identify any ongoing themes that seem to be associated with the offending. It may be noted that the offenses tend to occur when the offender is angry, depressed, feels rejected, or is experiencing interpersonal/relationship distress.

Once the offender's grooming process and other risk factors are identified, treatment moves to a focus on improving the offender's social competence and improving relationship and intimacy skills as outlined in Table 9.1. Treatment techniques for these areas are similar to those for other individuals who may have social skills or anger management deficits or who have difficulties developing relationships. These techniques tend to be psychoeducational, such as providing anger management training, assertiveness training, or relationship skills training. Generally these techniques involve offenders role playing various situations within the group setting, with therapist and group members giving them feedback on their skills.

As noted in Table 9.1, another potential area of focus is sexual preoccupation and/or deviant sexual arousal. Research has shown that sexual attraction to children, as measured by penile plethysmography, is the best predictor of recidivism (Hanson & Bussière, 1998). Not all sexual offenders experience deviant sexual arousal and, for example, most incest cases do not show deviant arousal in the laboratory. When deviant sexual arousal is identified through the use of penile plethysmography, specific behavioral treatments can be employed to reduce such arousal. Typical techniques include the use of odor aversion, covert sensitization, or satiation.

Odor aversion involves the pairing of deviant sexual stimuli with a noxious odor, which is usually ammonia. One approach in a laboratory situation would be for the offender to be presented with some type of deviant stimuli (a slide of a child or an audio description of sexual involvement with a child) and asked to self-administer the odor whenever arousal occurs. The offender would then be asked to use this technique outside of the therapy situation whenever he experienced a deviant sexual urge. Covert sensitization is a somewhat similar technique, although the deviant sexual fantasy is paired with some type of aversive imagery, rather than a noxious odor. For example, if the offender began thinking about sexual abuse, he would be trained to shift the imagery to thoughts of being in jail, thoughts of the impact on his family if he were arrested again, and, at times, thoughts of the impact of the abuse on victims. The third most commonly used technique is some form of what is referred to as satiation. Basically, in this technique, the offender is asked to masturbate to a nondeviant fantasy, which is usually recorded on a tape recorder to ensure that the fantasy is nondeviant. Following orgasm, the offender switches to his deviant fantasy and verbally repeats it for an extended period of time, usually 30–60 minutes. The theory is that the repetition of the deviant fantasy during a time when the offender is not aroused leads to boredom and extinction of the arousing properties of the fantasy. Generally, programs that use such techniques evaluate their effectiveness by measurement of deviant sexual arousal in the laboratory through penile plethysmography, as described earlier. However, it should be recognized that behavior in the laboratory may not reflect behavior in the natural environment. Although these behavioral techniques tend to reduce deviant arousal in the laboratory there is no guarantee these changes are permanent, and deviant arousal may return. It is important for offenders to recognize that these are self-control techniques that they may need to practice and reinforce throughout their lives.

For individuals whose sexual behavior is highly compulsive or whose deviant sexual arousal is difficult to control, certain pharmacological approaches can be used. Major classes of drugs include antiandrogens, which reduce male testosterone, and selective serotonin reuptake inhibitors, which are thought to work by reducing obsessive sexual thoughts (Bradford, 1997).

As a method of motivating offenders to "give up" their offending behavior, most programs involve components directed toward recognizing victim impact and developing victim empathy. This is approached in a number of ways, such as providing education regarding the impact of victimization, supplying readings from a victim standpoint, and using various victim-oriented videos. Although most programs address this issue, the data do not support a generalized empathy deficit in offenders (Marshall, Jones, Hudson, & McDonald, 1993). It may be that rather than having an empathy deficit, the offenders use various minimizations and distortions to avoid recognizing the impact their abuse has on their specific victim. Therefore, the goal of treatment is less focused on developing empathy than challenging the cognitions the offenders use to avoid facing the impact of their behavior.

The preceding material outlines general sexual offender-specific treatment issues. In addition, most programs try to involve significant others in the treatment process. One major treatment goal of managing offenders is to develop a support system around each offender that is aware of the offender's specific risk factors and offense process to assist the therapist in monitoring the offender outside of the group.

TREATMENT OUTCOME

There is a lack of consensus within the sexual offender field regarding whether there is adequate scientific evidence that treatment is effective (Marshall, 1993; Quinsey, Harris, Rice, & Lalumière, 1993), and the difficulties inherent in treatment outcome research with this population have been well described (Barbaree, 1997; Hanson, 1997). One of the major problems is the definition of recidivism, which usually is rearrest or reconviction for a new sexual offense. Because many sexual offenses are never reported, official recidivism records will underestimate true recidivism by some unknown factor. Official sexual offender recidivism data actually indicate rather low recidivism, making it difficult to show differences between treatment and nontreatment groups unless one has large samples and/or long follow-up periods, which is difficult.

Two early qualitative reviews (Furby, Weinrott, & Blackshaw, 1989; Marshall, Jones, Ward, Johnson, & Barbaree, 1991) reached somewhat different conclusions. The Furby et al. review found no evidence of treatment effectiveness and outlined many of the design problems in studies to date. Marshall et al. (1991), focusing on more recent cognitive-behavioral approaches, found support for treatment effectiveness in studies using cognitive-behavioral approaches or those using antiandrogens along with psychological treatments.

More recently, Alexander (1999) reviewed 79 sexual offender treatment outcome studies covering close to 11,000 subjects. Again, this was a qualitative review, but studies were subcategorized along a number of factors in order to look at those possibly related to treatment outcome.

One finding was that studies using a relapse prevention program produced reoffense rates of 7.2%; other types of treatment had recidivism rates of 13.9%; for no treatment groups, the rate was 17.6%. The relapse prevention treatments appeared especially effective for rapists and child molesters, where subjects receiving relapse prevention treatments had reoffense rates of around 8% versus 23–25% for untreated offenders.

A large meta-analysis of all offender treatment studies that had some type of control group (Hanson et al., 2002) supports this more qualitative review. When all 34 studies were included, there was a small effect for treatment, but significant variability among studies. When only the 17 studies with credible designs were included, there was also a significant treatment effect, with a recidivism rate of 9.9% for the treatment groups and 17.4% for the control group. There is also evidence that treatment is more effective with high-risk offenders (Gordon & Nicholaichuk, 1996), which would be consistent with the general correctional intervention literature.

In summary, at this time there is no definitive answer to the question of whether treatment effectiveness has been determined. However, the picture is not as grim as is sometimes assumed, and recent advances in treatment approaches seem to be showing promise in having at least a small impact on recidivism.

CIVIL COMMITMENT

Recently the use of civil commitment procedures to manage sexual offenders has reemerged. States are rapidly passing what are termed sexual predator statutes and, at the current time, 16 states have such statutes but only 15 are active (See Table 9.2). Virginia passed a statute but it has not been implemented (Doren, 2002). Washington State was the first to pass these new laws, and they have been held constitutional by the U.S. Supreme Court, *Kansas v. Hendricks*, 521 U.S. 346, 117 S. Ct. 2072, 138 L. Ed. 2d 501 (1997). In general, most states define "sexually violent predator" as an individual who has been convicted of a sexual offense who suffers from a mental abnormality or personality disorder (undefined) that makes a person more likely to engage in future sex-offending behavior. In a recent Supreme Court ruling, *Kansas v. Crane*, 534 U.S. 407, 122 S. Ct. 867, 151 L. Ed. 2d 856 (2002), the court has added that there must also be proof of "serious difficulty in controlling behavior." This finding reversed a Kansas State Supreme Court ruling that there must be a demonstration of total lack of control, which the

U.S. Supreme Court found unworkable and therefore appeared to reach a compromise with the "difficulty" standard.

These laws are applied at the end of sentence and require a court hearing. Table 9.2 provides some basic information about these laws in the 15 states where they are active. New Jersey actually has two laws, both which are listed. As can be seen, all states but three allow for a jury trial to determine if the individual is a sexual predator. The burden of proof is beyond a reasonable doubt in 12 of the states, while 3 require only clear and convincing evidence.

The determination of whether a person is a sexual predator usually requires that a person has been convicted of a sexual offense and has a mental abnormality or personality disorder that affects his likelihood of engaging in a future sex offense. As seen in Table 9.2, states vary on this likelihood standard, and it is rather vaguely defined. In practice, evidence is usually presented by mental health professionals in terms of psychiatric diagnoses and likelihood of reoffending. Likelihood of reoffending is usually guided by actuarial risk assessment instruments (see "Risk Assessment" section). As one can imagine, these trials are many times the "battle of experts."

If the individual is found to be a sexual predator, he is placed in a facility for rehabilitation. Although most states require periodic court review or allow the offender to request it, in practice the sentences are indeterminate. These laws are sometimes seen as "new," but they are in some ways a repeat of the old sexual psychopath laws that became popular in the 1930s but lost popularity in the 1960s (Group for the Advancement of Psychiatry, 1977; Lieb, Quinsey, & Berliner, 1998). These laws do appear on the surface somewhat different from the old psychopath laws in that they tend to be more narrowly crafted to apply to only the most dangerous offenders. The older psychopath laws were applied to a wider range of offenders, some who would not be considered predatory (Group for the Advancement of Psychiatry, 1977).

Mental health law scholars have been critical of these laws (La Fond, 1998; Winick, 1998). It is not the purpose of this chapter to cover all the legal arguments surrounding them. However, La Fond and Winick have questioned the civil nature of these laws and whether legislative intent was truly to develop a civil commitment process or to develop a preventive detention process. For this chapter, the concern with these laws is what role they play in the management of sexual aggressors, and what their limitations are. First, if the laws are applied in the fashion they appear to have been crafted, they will impact a very small number of offenders, although clearly a potentially highly recidivistic group. In addition, given the high-risk nature of this group, even the

TABLE 9.2. Selected Characteristics of Civil Commitment Statutes

State	Offenses likelihood standards	Standard of proof	Jury trial
Arizona	Likely to engage in sexual violence	Beyond a reasonable doubt	Yes
California	The person is a danger to the heath and safety of others in that he or she will engage in sexually violent criminal behavior	Beyond a reasonable doubt	Yes; unanimous
Florida	Likely to engage in acts of sexual violence	Clear and convincing evidence	Yes; unanimous
Illinois	Substantially probable that the person will engage in acts of sexual violence	Beyond a reasonable doubt	Yes
Iowa	Likely to engage in predatory acts constituting sexually violent offenses	Beyond a reasonable doubt	Yes; unanimous
Kansas	Likely to engage in predatory acts of sexual violence	Beyond a reasonable doubt	Yes; unanimous
Massachusetts	Likely to engage in a sex offense	Beyond a reasonable doubt	Yes; unanimous
Minnesota	Likely to engage in acts of harmful sexual conduct	Clear and convincing evidence	No
Missouri	More likely than not to engage in predatory acts of sexual violence	Beyond a reasonable doubt	Yes; unanimous
New Jersey (1994)	Likely to engage in acts of sexual violence	Clear and convincing evidence	No
New Jersey (1998)	Has a mental disorder that makes the person likely to engage in sexual violence	Clear and convincing evidence	No
North Dakota	Likely to engage in further acts of sexually predatory conduct	Clear and convincing evidence	No
South Carolina	Likely to engage in acts of sexual violence	Beyond a reasonable doubt	Yes; unanimous
Texas	Likely to engage in predatory acts of sexual violence	Beyond a reasonable doubt	Yes; unanimous
Washington	Likely to engage in predatory acts of sexual violence	Beyond a reasonable doubt	Yes; unanimous
Wisconsin	Substantially probable that the person will engage in acts of sexual violence	Beyond a reasonable doubt	Yes

Note. Adapted from Lieb & Matson (1998). Copyright ©1998 by the Washington State Institute for Public Policy. Adapted by permission.

most successful programs will likely have numerous failures, which could lead to a loss of political and public support for such laws. Failures in these programs may also impact the public's perception of the effectiveness of all treatment for sexual offenders.

These laws require that the offender be treated under "mental health" rules rather than "correctional" rules. Washington's sexual predator program was put under a federal special master for its failure to adhere to adequate mental health standards of care (La Fond, 1998) and was just recently released from the federal oversight. In addition, offenders will at some point be released, and issues of treatment in a least restrictive environment will clearly be future challenges to these laws. One can easily envision lawsuits, similar to those seen with the chronically mentally ill, requiring the development of alternative levels of care, such as group homes and transitional living situations. It is likely that the general public will be resistant to having these individuals placed in the community.

These laws are also extremely costly. The state of Washington spent over $6 million for 66 residents in 1997, while California will spend over $18 million instituting its program (La Fond, 1998). It is further estimated that an average predator trial can cost up to $100,000, a cost borne by the state. It also appears that for most programs it will cost around $100,000 per person per year to house and treat this population (La Fond, 1998; Lieb & Matson, 1998). This raises some concerns about whether these programs will distract from broader-based prison programs that target a larger number of offenders, and even whether they will remove resources from victim services. It is of interest that when California developed its program for sexual predators, it had no prison-based programs. In a 2000 survey of state correctional-based sexual offender programs, West, Hromas, and Wenger (2000) found that 39 states had some prison-based treatment programs. However, the capacities of these programs are limited, given the number of sexual offenders incarcerated. For example, Texas had over 25,000 incarcerated sexual offenders with a program capacity of only 307 offenders. This lack of capacity was repeated in most states. Becker and Murphy (1998) have pointed out that it seems quite countertherapeutic to allow offenders to spend a lengthy time in prison, probably reinforcing their deviant fantasies, before offering treatment.

A final implication of sexual predator laws, and in fact an implication of most approaches to managing an offender, is to develop adequate measures of risk to reoffend and developing measures of change that would indicate an individual is "safe" to return to the community. This will be addressed in the final section.

RISK ASSESSMENT

An issue underlying much of the management of sexual offenders, be it parole/probation supervision, community notification, mental health treatment, or sexual predator laws is the ability to accurately assess risk. It has been clearly established in the correctional field, as well as in the prediction of violence, that actuarial approaches consistently outperform clinical judgment (Andrews & Bonta, 1998; Borum, 1996; Mossman, 1994). In addition, as in the general criminology field (Andrews & Bonta, 1998), general psychological tests are very poor at predicting recidivism as compared to actuarial scales that focus on specific criminogenic factors (Hanson & Bussière, 1998).

Recently, the sexual offender field has had an explosion of empirically validated actuarial scales (Epperson, Kaul, & Huot, 1995; Hanson, 1998; Hanson & Thorton, 1999; Quinsey, Harris, Rice, & Cormier, 1998). In general, although these actuarial scales differ somewhat, they focus on two sets of factors, sexual deviancy and general criminal or antisocial tendencies/lifestyles. Sexual deviancy includes deviant sexual arousal, male victims, unrelated victims, and previous sexual offenses. More general criminological factors include age, previous noncriminal histories, early childhood behavioral problems, antisocial attitudes, and psychopathy. Many of these scales have improved predictive accuracy by 20–25% over chance.

These new instruments provide the sexual offender specialist with methods to make empirically informed decisions regarding risk. However, there are still some inherent problems. Although they can clearly identify groups of offenders at different risk levels, the decision of how to define "high-risk" is problematic. For example, if an offender's score on a risk assessment instrument places him in a group with a 50% risk of recidivism and a decision is made to civilly commit him, then this decision will theoretically be right 50% of the time and theoretically wrong 50% of the time. The decision to civilly commit is a public policy decision weighing individual rights versus societal protection and cannot be made on the basis of scientific evidence only (Becker & Murphy, 1998).

A second major problem is that current actuarial instruments are based almost solely on static factors, which are factors that are historical in nature and cannot change. Unfortunately, there are little data on dynamic factors that are amenable to change (Hanson, 1998; Hanson & Harris, 1998). Therefore, although evidence is accumulating to assist the sexual offender specialist in defining who may need the most intensive sexual offender management, there are few data to suggest when the level of management can be decreased. The ability to identify dynamic risk factors that are empirically related to decrease risk is a major challenge to the field at this time.

CONCLUSIONS

In this chapter, I have tried to outline a broad approach to the management of sexual offenders. Over the last 20 years the field has made significant advances in recognizing both its strengths and limitations. Although the data are far from perfect, there is at least a certain amount of hope that the combination of strong community supervision and monitoring along with more cognitive-behaviorally oriented treatments will reduce overall reoffense rates. The newer social control methods, such as registration, community notification, and to some extent sexual predator laws, are still untested. Given that if appropriately applied, these methods will probably only apply to a very small number of offenders, it is not clear that they will have a significant impact on overall victimization rates, although they do seem to provide a sense of well-being to the community. To the extent that methodologies are being developed to adequately manage sexual offenders in the community, a major challenge is the ability to identify larger numbers of offenders so that they can become part of the system and have treatment made available to them. As we have pointed out, prison programs that do exist do not have the capacity to treat the number of sexual offenders in prison. States may need to seriously consider whether putting more resources into programs in prisons and into parole/probation would reduce the future cost of reoffending.

A unique approach to reaching offenders and adults who are aware of offending is the STOP IT NOW! program in Vermont (Chasan-Taber & Tabachick, 1999). This program is a public media campaign that encourages abusers and adults to contact a confidential telephone number for information. Abusers can receive a confidential identification number that can be used to make an appointment with a sexual offender specialist for an evaluation without fear of being reported. In a 2-year period, 241 calls were received, and 23% of these were from abusers. Because of the confidential nature of the calls, it was difficult to track what offenders did. However, surveys of Vermont professionals working with adult sexual offenders indicated that 11 individuals self-reported, and surveys of child and adolescent specialists indicated that 39 adolescents and children with offending or sexual behavior problems entered treatment voluntarily. One wonders if such an approach were tried nationally, how many more offenders could be reached.

As a final comment, it is of interest to note the inherent tension between social control techniques such as community notification and approaches such as STOP IT NOW! Are offenders likely to come forward if they know that there is a risk of their community being informed of their behavior and their picture being placed on the Internet? The question is what methods will reduce the rate of victimization of women and children. Unfortunately, we do not currently have an answer to this question, but we may need to be open to options other than increased sanctions.

NOTES

1. Paraphilias are specific sexual disorders such as pedophilia, exhibitionism, voyeurism, fetishes, etc. Multiple paraphilias refer to individuals who have more than one paraphilia.
2. Penile plethysmography is a technique for direct measurement of an individual's erection response. The technique involves the subject placing a small band on his penis that measures changes in penile size while being exposed to specific sexual stimuli. Change in penile size is then recorded electronically.

REFERENCES

Abel, G. G., Becker, J. V., Mittelman, M. S., Cunningham-Rathner, J., Rouleau, J. L., & Murphy, W. D. (1987). Self-reported sex crimes of nonincarcerated paraphiliacs. *Journal of Interpersonal Violence, 2,* 3–25.

Abel, G. G., Jordan, A., Hand, C. G., Holland, L. A., & Phipps, A. (2001). Classification models of child molesters utilizing the Abel Assessment for child sexual abuse interest. *Child Abuse and Neglect, 25,* 703–718.

Abel, G. G., Osborn, C. A., & Twigg, D. A. (1993). Sexual assault through the life span: Adult offenders with juvenile histories. In H. E. Barbaree, W. L. Marshall, & S. M. Hudson (Eds.), *The juvenile sex offender* (pp. 104–117). New York: Guilford Press.

Abel, G. G., & Rouleau, J. L. (1990). The nature and extent of sexual assault. In W. L. Marshall, D. R. Laws, & H. E. Barbaree (Eds.), *Handbook of sexual assault: Issues, theories, and treatment of the offender* (pp. 9–21). New York: Plenum Press.

Adams, D. B. (2002). *Summary of state sex offender registries, 2001.* Washington, DC: U.S. Department of Justice, Bureau of Justice Statistics, NCJ 192265.

Alexander, M. A. (1999). Sex offender treatment efficacy revisited. *Sexual Abuse: A Journal of Research and Treatment, 11,* 101–116.

Andrews, D. A., & Bonta, J. (1998). *The psychology of criminal conduct* (2nd ed.). Cincinnati, OH: Anderson.

Association for the Treatment of Sexual Abusers. (1996). *Community notification position statement.* Beaverton, OR: Author.

Association for the Treatment of Sexual Abusers. (1997). *Association for the Treatment of Sexual Abusers professional code of ethics*. Beaverton, OR: Author.

Association for the Treatment of Sexual Abusers. (2001). *Practice standards for guidelines for members of the Association for the Treatment of Sexual Abusers*. Beaverton, OR: Author.

Barbaree, H. E. (1997). Evaluating treatment efficacy with sexual offenders: The insensitivity of recidivism studies to treatment effects. *Sexual Abuse: A Journal of Research and Treatment, 9*, 111–128.

Barbaree, H. E., Hudson, S. M., & Seto, M. C. (1993). Sexual assault in society: The role of the juvenile offender. In H. E. Barbaree, W. L. Marshall, & S. M. Hudson (Eds.), *The juvenile sex offender* (pp. 1–24). New York: Guilford Press.

Becker, J. V., & Murphy, W. D. (1998). What we know and do not know about assessing and treating sex offenders. *Psychology, Public Policy, and Law, 4*, 116–137.

Beckman, M. (1998). *Panel introduction*. Paper presented at the Proceedings of Bureau of Justice Statistics/SEARCH Conference on Sex Offender Registries. Sacramento, CA: SEARCH, The National Consortium for Justice Information and Statistics.

Berliner, L. (1996). Commentary: Community notification of sex offenders: A new tool or a false promise? *Journal of Interpersonal Violence, 11*, 294–295.

Berliner, L. (1997). Sex offenders: Policy and practice. *Northwestern University Law Review, 92*, 1203–1224.

Berliner, L., & Elliott, D. M. (1996). Sexual abuse of children. In J. Briere, L. Berliner, J. A. Bulkley, C. Jenny, & T. Reid (Eds.), *The APSAC handbook on child maltreatment* (pp. 51–71). Thousand Oaks, CA: Sage.

Berliner, L., Schram, D., Miller, L. L., & Milloy, C. D. (1995). A sentencing alternative for sex offenders: A study of decision making and recidivism. *Journal of Interpersonal Violence, 10*, 487–502.

Borum, R. (1996). Improving the clinical practice of violence risk assessment: Technology, guidelines, and training. *American Psychologist, 51*, 945–956.

Bradford, J. (1997). Medical interventions in sexual deviance. In D. R. Laws & W. O'Donohue (Eds.), *Sexual deviance: Theory, assessment, and treatment* (pp. 449–464). New York: Guilford Press.

Bulkley, J. A., Feller, J. N., Stern, P., & Roe, R. (1996). Child abuse and neglect laws and legal proceedings. In J. Briere, L. Berliner, J. A. Bulkley, C. Jenny, & T. Reid (Eds.), *The APSAC handbook on child maltreatment* (pp. 271–296). Thousand Oaks, CA: Sage.

Burman, M. A., Stein, J. A., Golding, J. M., Siegel, J. M., Sorenson, S. B., Forsythe, A. B., & Telles, C. A. (1988). Sexual assault and mental disorders in a community population. *Journal of Consulting and Clinical Psychology, 56*, 843–850.

Chasan-Taber, L., & Tabachnick, J. (1999). Evaluation of a child sexual abuse prevention program. *Sexual Abuse: A Journal of Research and Treatment, 11*, 279–292.

Cooper, C. L., Murphy, W. D., & Haynes, M. R. (1996). Characteristics of abused and nonabused adolescent sex offenders. *Sexual Abuse: A Journal of Research and Treatment, 8,* 105–119.

Dhawan, S., & Marshall, W. L. (1996). Sexual abuse histories of sexual offenders. *Sexual Abuse: A Journal of Research and Treatment, 8,* 7–15.

Doren, D. M. (2002). *Evaluating sex offenders: A manual for civil commitments and beyond.* Thousand Oaks, CA: Sage.

Emerick, R. L., & Dutton, W. A. (1993). The effect of polygraphy on the self report of adolescent sex offenders: Implications for risk assessment. *Annals of Sex Research, 6,* 83–103.

English, K. (1998). The containment approach: An aggressive strategy for the community management of adult sex offenders. *Psychology, Public Policy, and Law, 4,* 218–235.

English, K., Pullen, S., & Jones, L. (1996). *Managing sex offenders: A containment approach.* Lexington, KY: American Probation and Parole Association.

English, K., Pullen, S., & Jones, L. (1997). *Managing sex offenders in the community: A containment approach.* Washington, DC: U.S. Department of Justice.

Epperson, D. L., Kaul, J. D., & Huot, S. J. (1995, October). *Predicting risk for recidivism for incarcerated sex offenders: Updated development on the Sex Offender Screening Tool (SOST).* Poster session presented at the annual conference of the Association for the Treatment of Sexual Abusers, New Orleans, LA.

Erickson, W. D., Luxenburg, M. D., Walbek, N. H., & Seely, R. K. (1987). Frequency of MMPI two-point code types among sex offenders. *Journal of Consulting and Clinical Psychology, 55,* 566–570.

Finkelhor, D. (1984). *Child sexual abuse: New theory and research.* New York: Free Press.

Finkelhor, D., Hotaling, H., Lewis, I. A., & Smith, C. (1990). Sexual abuse in a national survey of adult men and women: Prevalence, characteristics and risk factors. *Child Abuse and Neglect, 14,* 19–28.

Finn, P. (1997, February). Sex offender community notification. *Research in Action* [newsletter]. Washington, DC: U.S. Department of Justice, National Institute of Justice.

Firestone, R., Bradford, J. M., Greenberg, D. M., & Serran, G. A. (2000). The relationship of deviant sexual arousal and psychopathy in incest offenders, extrafamilial child molesters and rapists. *Journal of the American Academy of Psychiatry and the Law, 28,* 303–308.

Freeman-Longo, R. E. (1996a). Invited Commentary: Feel good legislation. Prevention or calamity. *Child Abuse and Neglect, 20,* 95–101.

Freeman-Longo, R. E. (1996b). Prevention or problem. *Sexual Abuse: A Journal of Research and Treatment, 8,* 91–100.

Freund, K., & Watson, R. J. (1991). Assessment of the sensitivity and specificity of a phallometric test: An update of phallometric diagnosis of pedophilia. *Psychological Assessment: A Journal of Consulting and Clinical Psychology, 3,* 254–260.

Furby, L., Weinrott, M. R., & Blackshaw, L. (1989). Sex offender recidivism: A review. *Psychological Bulletin, 105,* 3–30.

Geer, J. H., Estupinan, L. A., & Manguno-Mire, G. M. (2000). Empathy, social skills, and other relevant cognitive processes in rapists and child molesters. *Aggression and Violent Behavior, 5,* 99–126.

Gordon, A., & Nicholaichuk, T. (1996). Applying the risk principle to sex offender treatment. *Forum on Corrections Research, 8,* 36–38.

Greenfeld, L. A. (1997). *Sex offenses and offenders: An analysis of data on rape and sexual assault.* Washington, DC: U.S. Department of Justice.

Group for the Advancement of Psychiatry. (1977). *Psychiatry and sex psychopath legislation: The 30s to the 80s.* New York: Mental Health Materials Center.

Hanson, R. K. (1997). How to know what works with sexual offenders. *Sexual Abuse: A Journal of Research and Treatment, 9,* 129–145.

Hanson, R. K. (1998). What do we know about sex offender risk assessment? *Psychology, Public Policy, and Law, 4,* 50–72.

Hanson, R. K. (2002). Recidivism and age: Follow-up data from 4,673 sexual offenders. *Journal of Interpersonal Violence, 17,* 1046–1062.

Hanson, R. K., & Bussière, M. T. (1998). Predicting relapse: A meta-analysis of sexual offender recidivism studies. *Journal of Consulting and Clinical Psychology, 66,* 348–362.

Hanson, R. K., Gordon, A., Harris, A. J. R., Marques, J. K., Murphy, W., Quinsey, V. L., & Seto, M. C. (2002). First report of the collaborative outcome data project on the effectiveness of psychological treatment for sex offenders. *Sexual Abuse: A Journal of Research and Treatment, 14,* 169–194.

Hanson, R. K., & Harris, A. (1998). *Dynamic predictors of sexual recidivism* (User Report 1998–01). Ottawa: Department of the Solicitor General Canada.

Hanson, R. K., & Slater, S. (1988). Sexual victimization in the history of sexual abusers: A review. *Annals of Sex Research, 1,* 485–499.

Hanson, R. K., & Thornton, D. (1999). *Static 99: Improving actuarial risk assessments for sex offenders.* (User Report 1999–02). Ottawa: Department of the Solicitor General Canada.

Harris, G. T., Rice, M. E., Quinsey, V. L., Chaplin, T. C., & Earls, C. (1992). Maximizing the discriminant validity of phallometric assessment data. *Psychological Assessment, 4,* 502–511.

Hindman, J. (1988). New insight into adult and juvenile sexual offenders. *Community Safety Quarterly, 1,* 3.

Hudson, S. M., & Ward, T. (1997). Rape: Psychopathology and theory. In D. R. Laws & W. O'Donohue (Eds.), *Sexual deviance: Theory, assessment, and treatment* (pp. 332–355). New York: Guilford Press.

Hudson, S. M., Ward, T., & McCormick, J. C. (1999). Offense pathways in sexual offenders. *Journal of Interpersonal Violence, 14,* 779–798.

Hunter, J. A., & Mathews, R. (1997). Sexual deviance in females. In D. R. Laws & W. O'Donohue (Eds.), *Sexual deviance: Theory, assessment, and treatment* (pp. 465–480). New York: Guilford Press.

Jones, L., & Finkelhor, D. (2001). *The decline in child sexual abuse cases.* Washington, DC: U.S. Department of Justice, Office of Juvenile Justice and Delinquency Prevention.

Knight, R. A., & Prentky, R. A. (1990). Classifying sexual offenders: The development and corroboration of taxonomic models. In W. L. Marshall, D. R. Laws,

& H. E. Barbaree (Eds.), *Handbook of sexual assault: Issues, theories, and treatment of the offender* (pp. 2 3–52). New York, NY: Plenum Press.

Koss, M. P., Woodruff, W. J., & Koss, P. G. (1990). Relation of criminal victimization to health perceptions among women medical patients. *Journal of Consulting and Clinical Psychology, 58*, 147–152.

La Fond, J. Q. (1998). The cost of enacting a sexual predator law. *Psychology, Public Policy, and Law, 4*, 468–504.

Lanning, K. V. (1996). Criminal investigation of suspected child abuse. In J. Briere, L. Berliner, J. A. Bulkley, C. Jenny, & T. Reid (Eds.), *The APSAC handbook on child maltreatment* (pp. 246–270). Thousand Oaks, CA: Sage.

Laws, D. R., & O'Donohue, W. (1997). Fundamental issues in sexual deviance. In D. R. Laws & W. O'Donohue (Eds.), *Sexual deviance: Theory, assessment, and treatment* (pp. 1–21). New York: Guilford Press.

Lieb, R. (1996). Commentary: Community notification laws. "A step toward more effective solutions." *Journal of Interpersonal Violence, 11*, 298–300.

Lieb, R., & Matson, S. (1998). *Sexual predator commitment laws in the United States: 1998 update*. Seattle: Washington State Institute for Public Policy.

Lieb, R., Quinsey, V., & Berliner, L. (1998). Sexual predators and social policy. *Crime and Justice: A Review of Research, 23*, 43–114.

Marshall, W. L. (1993). The treatment of sex offenders: What does the outcome data tell us? A reply to Quinsey, Harris, Rice, & Lalumière. *Journal of Interpersonal Violence, 8*, 524–530.

Marshall, W. L. (1997). Pedophilia: Psychopathology and theory. In D. R. Laws & W. O'Donohue (Eds.), *Sexual deviance: Theory, assessment, and treatment* (pp. 152–174). New York: Guilford Press.

Marshall, W. L., Jones, R., Hudson, S. M., & McDonald, E. (1993). Generalized empathy in child molesters. *Journal of Child Sexual Abuse, 2*, 61–68.

Marshall, W. L., Jones, R., Ward, T., Johnson, P., & Barbaree, H. E. (1991). Treatment outcome with sex offenders. *Psychology Review, 11*, 465–485.

Marshall, W. L., Laws, D. R., & Barbaree, H. E. (1990). *Handbook of sexual assault: Issues, theories, and treatment*. New York: Plenum Press.

Marshall, W. L., & Serran, G. A. (2000). Improving the effectiveness of sexual offender treatment. *Trauma, Violence and Abuse, 1*, 203–222.

Matson, S., & Lieb, R. (1996). *Community notification in Washington state: 1996 survey of law enforcement*. Olympia: Washington State Institute for Public Policy.

Matson, S., & Lieb, R. (1997). *Megan's law: A review of state and federal legislation*. Olympia: Washington State Institute for Public Policy.

Mossman, D. (1994). Assessing predictions of violence: Being accurate about accuracy. *Journal of Consulting and Clinical Psychology, 62*, 783–792.

Murphy, W. D., & Barbaree, H. E. (1994). *Assessments of sexual offenders by means of erectile response: Psychometric properties and decision making*. Brandon, VT: Safer Society Press.

Murphy, W. D., & Carich, M. S. (2001). Cognitive distortions and restructuring in sexual abuser treatment. In M. S. Carich & S. E. Mussack (Eds.), Handbook for sexual abuser assessment and treatment (pp. 65–76). Brandon, VT: Safer Society Press.

Murphy, W. D., DiLillo, D., Haynes, M. R., & Steere, E. (2001). An exploration of factors related to deviant sexual arousal among juvenile sex offenders. *Sexual Abuse: A Journal of Research and Treatment, 13*, 91–103.

Murphy, W. D., & Peters, J. M. (1992). Profiling child sexual abusers: Psychological considerations. *Criminal Justice and Behavior, 19*, 24–37.

Murphy, W. D., & Smith, T. A. (1996). Sex offenders against children: Empirical and clinical issues. In J. Briere, L. Berliner, J. A. Bulkley, C. Jenny, & T. Reid (Eds.), *The APSAC handbook on child maltreatment* (pp. 175–191). Thousand Oaks, CA: Sage.

Myers, J. E. B. (1992). *Legal issues in child abuse and neglect.* Newbury, CA: Sage.

Nannetti, C., & Greer, D. (1996). Investigating and prosecuting sex offenders. In K. English, S. Pullen, & L. Jones (Eds.), *Managing sex offenders: A containment approach* (pp. 8.1–8.8). Lexington, KY: American Probation and Parole Association.

Phillips, D. M. (1998). *Community notification as viewed by Washington's citizens.* Olympia: Washington State Institute for Public Policy.

Portwood, S. G., Reppucci, N. D., & Mitchell, M. S. (1998). Balancing rights and responsibilities: Legal perspectives on child maltreatment. In J. R. Lutzker (Ed.), *Handbook on child abuse research and treatment* (pp. 31–52). New York: Plenum Press.

Prentky, R. A. (1996). Commentary: Community notification and constructive risk reduction. *Journal of Interpersonal Violence, 11*, 295–298.

Pullen, S., Olsen, S., Brown, G., & Amich, D. (1996). Using the polygraph. In K. English, S. Pullen, & L. Jones (Eds.), *Managing sex offenders: A containment approach* (pp. 15.1–15.17). Lexington, KY: American Probation and Parole Association.

Quinsey, V. L., Arnold, L. S., & Pruesse, M. G. (1980). MMPI profiles of men referred for a pretrial psychiatric assessment as a function of offense type. *Journal of Clinical Psychology, 36*, 410–417.

Quinsey, V. L., Harris, G. T., Rice, M. E., & Cormier, C. A. (1998). *Violent offenders: Appraising and managing risk.* Washington, DC: American Psychological Association.

Quinsey, V. L., Harris, G. T., Rice, M. E., & Lalumière, M. L. (1993). Assessing treatment efficacy in outcome studies of sex offenders. *Journal of Interpersonal Violence, 8*, 512–523.

Read, J. P., Stern, A. L., Wolfe, J., & Ouimette, P. C. (1997). Use of a screening instrument in women's health care: Detecting relationships among victimization history, psychological distress, and medical complaints. *Women and Health, 25*, 1–17.

Rennison, C. (2002). *Criminal victimization 2001: Changes 2000–01 with trends 1993–2001.* Washington, DC: U.S. Department of Justice, Bureau of Justice Statistics, NCJ 194610.

Resnick, H. S., Kilpatrick, D. G., Dansky, B. S., Saunders, B. E., & Best, C. L. (1993). Prevalence of civilian trauma and posttraumatic stress disorder in a representative national sample of women. *Journal of Consulting and Clinical Psychology, 61*, 984–991.

Righthand, S., & Hodge, S. (1992). Agency and professional roles and responsibilities: The need for cooperation. In W. O'Donohue & J. H. Geer (Eds.), *The sexual abuse of children: Clinical issues* (Vol. 2, pp. 3–23). Hillsdale, NJ: Erlbaum.

Russell, D. E. H. (1984). *Sexual exploitation: Rape, child sexual abuse, and workplace harassment.* Beverly Hills, CA: Sage.

Sacco, D. T. (1998, April). *Arguments used to challenge notification laws—and the government's response.* Paper presented at the Proceedings of Bureau of Justice Statistics/SEARCH Conference on Sex Offender Registries. Sacramento, CA: SEARCH, The National Consortium for Justice Information and Statistics.

Saunders, B. E., Kilpatrick, D. G., Hanson, R. F., Resnick, H. S., & Walker, M. E. (1999). Prevalence, case characteristics, and long-term psychological correlates of child rape among women: A national survey. *Child Maltreatment, 4,* 187–200.

Schram, D. D., & Milloy, C. D. (1995). *Community notification: A study of offender characteristics and recidivism.* Olympia: Washington State Institute for Public Policy.

Segal, Z. V., & Marshall, W. L. (1986). Discrepancies between self-efficacy predications and actual performance in a population of rapists and child molesters. *Cognitive Therapy and Research, 10,* 363–375.

Sorkin, L. G. (1998, April). *The trilogy of federal statutes.* Paper presented at the Proceedings of Bureau of Justice Statistics/SEARCH Conference on Sex Offender Registries. Sacramento, CA. (SEARCH, The National Consortium for Justice Information and Statistics.)

Weinrott, M. R. (1996). *Juvenile sexual aggression: A critical review.* Boulder, CO: Center for the Study and Prevention of Violence.

Weinrott, M. R., & Saylor, M. (1991). Self-report of crimes committed by sex offenders. *Journal of Interpersonal Violence, 6,* 286–300.

West, M., Hromas, C. S., & Wenger, P. (2000). *State sex offender treatment programs: 50-state survey.* Colorado Springs: Colorado Department of Corrections.

Widom, C. S. (1995). *Victims of childhood sexual abuse: Later criminal consequences.* Washington, DC: U.S. Department of Justice.

Williams, L. M., & Finkelhor, D. (1990). The characteristics of incestuous fathers: A review of recent studies. In W. L. Marshall, D. R. Laws, & H. E. Barbaree (Eds.), *Handbook of sexual assault: Issues, theories, and treatment of the offender* (pp. 231–255). New York: Plenum Press.

Winick, B. J. (1998). Sex offender law in the 1990s: A therapeutic jurisprudence analysis. *Psychology, Public Policy, and Law, 4,* 505–570.

Wyatt, G. E. (1985). The sexual abuse of Afro-American and White-American women in childhood. *Child Abuse and Neglect, 9,* 507–519.

Zevitz, R. G., & Farkas, M. A. (2000). *Sex offender community notification: Assessing the impact in Wisconsin.* Washington, DC: U.S. Department of Justice, National Institute of Justice, NCJ 179992.

10 Megan's Law

New Protections against Sex Abuse

KAREN TERRY
B. J. CLING

Megan's Law, as well as new laws dealing with the further incarceration of sexually violent predators after they have served their jail terms (known as "sexual predator laws"), deal with the social issue of threat from convicted sexual offenders who are about to be released into the community. The public fears, with some justification, that pedophiles continue to want to molest children sexually, and that they are an invisible threat to their young neighbors. Children come to recognize and trust these offenders, who are often skilled at befriending children, and their parents do not realize that these neighbors are dangerous to the children, and are thus helpless to warn them. It is the context of this threat, and its actualization in a number of high profile cases, that has resulted in Megan's Law, which requires convicted and subsequently released sex offenders to register in their communities, thus notifying the police, other agencies, and at times the general public of their existence in their midst.

In 1989, residents of Tacoma, Washington, were shocked by one of the most disturbing crimes imaginable. A 7-year-old boy was raped, choked, stabbed, and sexually mutilated, left for dead with his penis severed. The culprit of this crime was Earl Shriner, a man with a 24-year history of criminal behavior, including sexual violence and murder. He

245

had just been released from prison, where he had spent most of his life since age 15. While serving his last sentence, he had bragged to others that he fantasized about sexual mutilation and murder. He went as far as to plan out his next offense, saying that when released he would kidnap and torture young boys in the woods.

There was nothing that the state could do to keep him incarcerated because he was serving a finite sentence. Once released, the state had no right to alert his neighbors to the nature of the risk he posed because there were no community notification statutes at that time. Two years after his release, he lured the young boy into the woods. Perhaps the most disturbing fact was that the boy lived in the same apartment building as Shriner. If the community had known about his extensive record of sexual abuse, it is possible that the attack could have been avoided.

Earl Shriner became a symbol of the need to reform the legal system in regard to sexual offenders. The state of Washington implemented the Community Protection Act in 1990, which consists of 14 different provisions allowing for better protection against sexual predators. However, this was a statewide system, and other, equally horrific crimes followed across the country. Some of the victims, such as Polly Klass,[1] became household names, though it was the murder of Megan Kanka that sparked a nationwide realization that protections against sexual offenders should exist on a federal level.

After the sexual assault and murder of Megan Kanka, New Jersey implemented "Megan's Law." This mandates registration and community notification of individuals who commit any type of sexual offense against an adult or a child. It does not encompass only offenders who torture, kidnap, or kill, but includes offenders with a wide range of offenses. Though enacted after a brutal crime against a child, Megan's Law aims to prevent recidivism from any type of sexual offender. Though we do not yet know if this legislation is effective, Megan's Law is one of several legislative steps toward protecting victims of sexual assault from potential recidivists.

VICTIMS OF SEXUAL OFFENSES

A sexual offense is a severe and intrusive violation against a person physically and emotionally. This is true regardless of the gender and age of the victim, or the relationship between the victim and offender. It is difficult to gauge the true rate of sexual victimization. Victim service agencies estimate that approximately one out of every three or four girls and one out of every seven boys is victimized in their lifetimes (see National Institute of Justice, 1992, p. 3, for a summary of victimization rates in the literature). Most sexual offense victims are young; one-third of known victims are under the age of 12 (National Report Series, 1999). Children who are sexually abused prior to age 12 are particularly likely to be abused by a family member or acquaintance (Langan & Harlow, 1994; National Report Series, 1999).

The rate of victimization appears to vary by age. Data from the National Incident-Based Reporting System (NIBRS) show that while male victims account for only 4% of adult sexual assault victims and 8% of victims ages 12–17 years, they account for one-quarter of sexual assault victims under age 12 (National Report Series, 1999). It is unclear whether males are victimized more at a young age than as adults or if this difference is the result of reporting variance, though it is likely a combination of both factors. Male victimization is likely to be under-reported even more than female victimization, making it difficult to estimate a true rate of sexual assault (Brochman, 1991; McMullen, 1992).

When sexual offenders choose their victims, most do not seem to single out a particular type because of static characteristics such as socioeconomic status or physical attributes. They may have preferences for age, though not all do. Some child molesters are situational, meaning that children are their victims because the molesters have easy access to them. Other child molesters are considered preferential, meaning that the primary object of their sexual attraction is a child (Groth, Longo, & McFadin, 1982). These offenders often have a preference for gender, particularly those who abuse adolescent boys. However, many child molesters and even some rapists may abuse any victim to whom they have access, regardless of gender (Groth & Burgess, 1980). In families with interfamilial child abuse, it is not unusual for the parent to abuse children of either or both sexes, depending on what is available.

Sexual offenders do target particular victims on dynamic terms. Most importantly, they tend to choose their victims based upon either proximity or vulnerability (in either a situational or emotional sense). Child molesters "groom" these vulnerable children in order to get them to comply with the abuse (Conte, 1991; Groth & Burgess, 1977; Pryor, 1996). Rapists also tend to target vulnerable victims, in particular, prostitutes, hitchhikers, individuals who are intoxicated, or those over whom they believe they can assert control. The methods by which they approach the potential victims depend upon their confidence in obtaining power over the individuals, and so they may employ tactics such as a con (the offender uses a ploy for accessibility, such as posing as a repairman), a blitz (direct physical assault), or a surprise approach (waits in hiding for the victim) (Hazelwood, Dietz, & Burgess, 1983, p. 3). It is primarily stranger rapists that use these tactics, though acquaintance rapists use similar tactics, such as encouraging or taking advantage of intoxication.

EFFECTS OF VICTIMIZATION

Sexual assault victims are likely to experience a range of physical and psychological reactions to sexual abuse. In terms of physical harm, less intrusive offenses such as touching through the clothing do not often result in physical injury. However, violent offenses that include intercourse may lead to injuries such as cuts, bruises and black eyes, or, at the extreme level, broken bones or injuries from weapons. Victims of rape and sexual assault are not likely to face an armed offender, however. They are less likely to do so than victims of any other violent offense, with approximately 6% of offenders threatening them with weapons (Rennison, 2001). The National Crime Victimization Survey (NCVS) shows that approximately one-quarter of all rape victims between 1992 and 1998 were physically injured during the sexual assault (Simon, Mercy, & Perkins, 2001, p. 2).

Some sexual assault survivors, particularly those abused over a period of time when they were children, may experience medically unexplained symptoms. This is referred to as "somatization," and some experts believe that somatisized injuries allow the victim to express emotional pain through physical symptoms (Nelson, 2001). Common physical symptoms for which there is no obvious cause include back pain, pelvic pain, and headaches; the victims also tend to have negative perceptions of their health (Calhoun & Atkeson, 1991; Walker et al., 1992). For example, Nelson (2001) shows a link between women who were forced to give an abuser oral sex as a child and physical symptoms as adults. The women in her sample complained of back pain, neck aches, and throat aches years after the abuse stopped, which she attributed to the fact that the abusers held the victims' heads back by pulling their hair so that the abusers could force their penis down the victims' throats.

Other physical problems resulting from sexual abuse include medical problems, including sexually transmitted diseases and pregnancy. Sexually transmitted diseases occur in up to 30% of rape cases, with human immunodeficiency virus (HIV) being transmitted in approximately 0.2% of the cases (Resnick, Acierno, & Kilpatrick, 1997). Pregnancy is also common, occuring in approximately 4.7% of rape cases (Resnick et al., 1997). Pregnancy resulting from rape causes psychological problems as well, since impregnated women must decide whether or not to carry the child through to term, and, if they do, whether to keep the child. These decisions can lead to psychological problems such as depression, anxiety, insomnia, or even mental illness (Frank et al., 1985).

The psychological effects of sexual abuse can be quite significant, whether the victim was an adult or child at the time of the offense. Many rape victims suffer a form of posttraumatic stress disorder, which Burgess and Holmstrom (1974) and later Burgess (1983) refer to as rape trauma syndrome (RTS). (For an in-depth discussion, see Cling, Chapter 2, this volume.) They describes this as a stress response pattern that follows unwanted sexual activity, including recurring recollection of the event, reduced involvement in the environment, and possibly hyper-alertness, disturbed sleep patterns, guilt about the incident, or avoidance of activities that arouse recollection. These symptoms occur in addition to other psychological problems, such as guilt, shame, fear, anxiety, stress, and fatigue (Burgess, 1995; Isley, 1991). Additionally, the victims may develop eating disorders, depression, dissociation, and suicidal feelings (Bass & Davis, 1988; Eby, Campbell, Sullivan, & Davidson, 1995; Resnick et al., 1997; Thompson, Wonderlich, Crosby, & Mitchell, 2001). These effects can be the same for men, women, and children (Burgess & Holstrom, 1974).

The most prevalent psychological reactions to sexual victimization are fear and anxiety, beginning with the fear created during the act itself, when victims may fear for their lives. This fear then leads to nervousness, specific anxiety about future sexual assaults, and ultimately a generalized anxiety (Calhoun & Atkeson, 1991, pp. 9–10). Many of those abused as children develop anxiety-related disorders, such as phobias, panic disorders, obsessive–compulsive disorder (OCD), and sleep disturbances (Lundberg-Love, 1999, p. 6). OCD is particularly prevalent as a washing ritual (Calhoun & Atkeson, 1991), symbolizing the cleansing of the victim from the abuse. Similarly, many women, particularly adolescents who were abused, resort to dangerous eating disorders and weight regulation practices. In particular, women practice bulimia, where they binge and purge repeatedly (Bass & Davis, 1988). Alcohol and substance abuse are also common, again with excessive bingeing.

Another frequent consequence of sexual abuse is depression, particularly if the abuse was ongoing and the perpetrator was someone close to the victim (Lundberg-Love, 1999). Calhoun and Atkeson (1991, p. 11) describe how victims are likely to experience a number of depressive symptoms immediately following the sexual assault, including crying spells, fatigue, feelings of guilt and worthlessness, a sense of hopelessness, and suicidal thoughts. They also tend to experience low self-esteem and self-blame, and they are likely to withdraw from social interaction, further perpetuating the cycle of depression.

Sexual abuse also affects how both child and adult victims develop and maintain relationships. Both male and female victims may experience sexual dysfunction as a result of the rape (Golding, 1996), particularly if they are experiencing long-term anxiety about the assault (Calhoun & Atkeson, 1991). Even if there is no physical dysfunction, victimization may result in altered sexual practices such as avoidance of sex, increased sexual activity, or loss of satisfaction with sex (Ellis, Atkeson, & Calhoun, 1981). Many victims go through a period of social adjustment immediately after the assault (Calhoun & Atkeson, 1991), and women in particular are likely to go through periods where they feel very angry with everyone close to them. While childhood sexual abuse may lead to sexual dysfunction for some women, it leads to sexual promiscuity for others (Thompson et al., 2001). For most victims, these effects are short-lived and will not continue to be long-term consequences of abuse (Calhoun & Atkeson, 1991), though healing once again depends upon the support systems for the individual.

Children who are victims of sexual abuse also experience many psychological problems and atypical behavior. The National Institute of Justice (1992, pp. 18–19) shows that children may experience the same problems as adults, including guilt, shame, anxiety, and fear, and physical consequences such as sexually transmitted diseases and somatic injuries. They also show poor self-esteem, self-blame, and a need to please others, which could result in long-term depression, destructive behavior, and suicidal thoughts. Like adults, children can experience serious psychological disorders such as multiple personalities, neuroses, and character disorders. Children also experience age-related problems, such as poor concentration in school, which often leads to failing grades. Additionally, they act out both physically and sexually, with antisocial or delinquent behavior and overt sexual behavior such as masturbation, for example. Though researchers have recognized similar characteristics in abused children as a group, a single diagnosis of "sexually abused child syndrome" has been all but discarded due to variance in victim and in type and length of abuse (National Institute of Justice, 1992, p. 20). (For an in-depth discussion of the effect of sexual abuse on children, see Olafson, Chapter 7, this volume.)

It is not just the person abused who suffers as a result of sexual assault. Secondary victims—parents, siblings, partners, peers, colleagues, and employers of those abused—are also significantly affected by the sexual abuse (Ward & Inserto, 1990). These individuals must help the primary victim to cope with the abuse and work through any psychological reactions that emerge.

In the case of child sexual abuse, the parents, particularly the mother, play an important role in the recovery of the child. For instance, if a woman discovers that her husband is abusing her daughter, she must help her daughter to recover. However, she must also cope with the fact that her daughter was being abused in the home, and that she knew the perpetrator of the crime. Also, she has to deal with the deterioration of the family unit as a result of the offense. Parents of abused children have varying levels of knowledge of the abuse and, as a result, have varying feelings of guilt, negligence, and responsibility once the abuse is known.

Parents and siblings of the victim both are likely to experience emotional reactions to the abuse, including denial, disbelief, remorse, regret, and even trauma. When the abuse is interfamilial, the family is likely to go through significant changes because in most cases either the victim or perpetrator will be removed from the home (Ward & Inserto, 1990). This uprooting will cause disruption for the entire family, and disruption may create emotional trauma for all involved—particularly the victim, who may feel responsible for the upheaval. The reaction toward the offender also varies; while some see the perpetrator as hateful and repugnant, others see him or her as sick and in need of help (Johnson, 1992).

The spouse or partner of a rape victim also plays a significant role in the recovery process. While some partners are fully supportive, sympathetic, and helpful to the victim, others become withdrawn or partially blame the victim for the offense (Baker, Skolnik, Davis, & Brickman, 1991; Ward & Inserto, 1990). Rape elicits a stronger negative reaction from partners than other violent crimes (Baker et al., 1991), which in some cases leads to feelings of vengefulness or a lack of support for the victim. Though many of the partners are supportive, problems may emerge in the relationship due to feelings of uncleanliness or unfaithfulness (Ward & Inserto, 1990, p. 82). The study by Baker et al. (1991) showed that female peers of sexual assault victims show the most positive and supportive attitudes toward the victims, and therefore this relationship is important for the victim who is recovering from the trauma.

BACKGROUND OF MEGAN'S LAW

In 1994, a 7-year-old girl named Megan Kanka was raped and killed by a recidivist pedophile living across the street from her. The perpetrator of this crime was Jesse Timmendequas, a twice-convicted pedophile with two previous convictions of sexual offenses against children. He lured Megan into his home with an invitation to see his new puppy, and she went into his home having no idea about his history. Jesse Timmendequas lived with two other convicted sexual offenders, all of whom had recently been released from prison. One of these men had even been arrested in that house for a sexual offense. Despite this history, the Kankas did not know that convicted child molesters lived on their street. Mrs. Kanka became an advocate for legislation mandating the notification of the community regarding the entry of sex offenders. She said that had she known about the history of Timmendequas, she could have warned Megan, and Megan would still be alive today.

Prior to Megan's death, only five states had laws mandating a system of registration and notification. Since that time, the federal government and all states have enacted their own versions of "Megan's Law," a system of registration and community notification. The federal law requires that each state enact a registry whereby convicted sexual offenders register their personal information with the police. If the states do not comply with this requirement, they can lose 10% of federal funding for state and local law enforcement. This federal law, called the Jacob Wetterling Crimes against Children and Sexually Violent Registration Program, is part of the Violent Crime Control and Enforcement Law of 1994. It is named after Jacob Wetterling, who was kidnapped while riding a bike with his friends near their home, and has not been seen since. But the Kankas felt that registration alone was an insufficient form of prevention, and they advocated active notification of the community about serious sexual offenders who are living in the neighborhood. On May 17, 1996, then-President Bill Clinton enacted the federal Megan's Law statute, which set notification guidelines for the individual states to follow.

REQUIREMENTS AND GUIDELINES OF MEGAN'S LAW

Though based upon a federal statute, every state has enacted its own version of Megan's Law, and the registration guidelines vary.[2] In every state, offenders are responsible for registering with the police if they commit an offense that is sexual in nature. An individual who commits such an offense must register for 10 years to life, depending upon the jurisdiction and risk level of the offender, and must report into the police or other designated state agency every year (or every 90 days, for those classified as high-risk offenders).

Though the statutes vary, the registration process is similar in most states. Upon conviction or release from a correctional institution, the sexual offender must go to the police or state agency and provide them with his or her residential address, a photograph, fingerprints, name and aliases, place of employment, and in some cases a DNA sample.[3] The agency then stores this information in a central registry for informational purposes for law enforcement and/or the community. To verify the address the offender submits, a letter is mailed to the residence given, and the offender is required to return the letter within a specified time period. If the letter is not returned or the offender does not register within the given amount of time, the offender has not complied with the statute and is subject to arrest. If the offender moves to a different address, he or she is required to reregister with the local agency in the new community.

The registration and notification system is based upon the concept of risk: The higher the risk of the offender recidivating, the higher his or her risk category is in the initial assessment process. All states vary in their risk assessment process, though most use specific registration guidelines to classify offenders into three tiers of risk level. This classification is based upon a number of factors, including type of offense, age and number of victims, level of force used, victim–offender relationship, and degree of contact with victim.

Level 1 offenders are the least serious and are considered a low risk to the community. Level 1 offenders may have abused someone without using physical force, have only touched someone on the outside of the clothing, have only one victim, have no serious psychological disorders (e.g., antisocial personality disorder), are not recidivist offenders, have no history of substance abuse or domestic violence, abused someone within the family (e.g., a sibling), or have strong community ties that render him unlikely to reoffend. Notification for Level 1 offenders is usually limited to law enforcement agencies, and information is not distributed to the community. Level 1 offenders generally register for 10–15 years, or may apply for expungement in states with lifetime registration after 10 years. They must check in with the registry agency annually to verify their address, or a letter is sent to their residence annually that must be returned for verification (Terry & Furlong, 2003).

Level 2 offenders pose a moderate risk to the community. They are not considered violent predators, but vulnerable members of the community should be notified of their presence. Examples of Level 2 offenders are those who have verbally but not physically threatened the victim, have had a previous relationship with the victim, have more than one victim, touched the victim under the clothing but have not penetrated the victim, have a history of substance abuse, or have no steady employment or strong community ties. For offenders classified in this category, notification is limited to law enforcement and any entity that may be at risk from this offender. For instance, if a child molester moves into the neighborhood, the registration agency would likely notify the schools, youth groups, community groups, church groups, day care facilities, and organizations such as the Boy Scouts/Girl Scouts. Also, some states look at Level 2 offenders on a case-by-case basis to determine whether the general community should be notified about the offender. This is the most common classification for sexual offenders (Terry & Furlong, 2003).

Level 3 offenders pose a high risk to the community. In some states they are labeled sexual predators or sexually violent persons. Level 3 offenders might have multiple victims, have assaulted a stranger, have abused a prepubescent child, penetrated the victim, have a history of psychological or mental disorders, have a substance abuse problem, have few community ties or no employment, or might not be participating in any treatment program. While Level 1 and 2 offenders usually only have to check in with the registration agency annually, Level 3 offenders check in every 90 days. Level 3 offenders are generally prohibited from living within a certain distance of schools, parks, or other recreational services, and the types of jobs they are allowed to maintain is limited. Additionally, it is these offenders about whom the community is notified (Terry & Furlong, 2003).

Notification can take place in several ways. The community can be notified by police officers going around to the various residences in the community, through flyers, through community meetings, through an 800 or 900 number, through a Web site, or by a CD-ROM. Information given to the community is the offender's photograph, address, type of offense, and class of offense (e.g., class B felony).

IS MEGAN'S LAW FAIR AND EFFECTIVE?

The purpose of registration and notification is twofold; it alerts the police to where the offender is living and also lets the community know if serious, repeat sexual offenders are living in the neighborhood. Registration aids the police in managing sexual offenders who are living in the community, as well as in their investigations when a sexual crime occurs. Because all sexual offenders are required to register, the names of all those living in the community appear on a central list, and the police can match the modus operandi of a current offense to those of offenders on the list. While registration aims to help the police, notification aims to assist the community by protecting society from known sexual offenders. The purpose of registration and notification is community protection, not retribution, though there have been many legal challenges as to whether the scope of registration goes past the realm of civil legislation and is therefore unconstitutional.

Megan's Law has faced many challenges in relation to privacy, double jeopardy, cruel and unusual punishment, retroactive application of a statute, and many other issues. In addition to these constitutional challenges, some argue that registration creates problems such as vigilantism, ostracism from the community, lower real estate values, and a false sense of security for the public. Because the community is only notified about Level 3 offenders, the list of offenders specified to the public is not representative of all sexual offenders. A spate of abductions in the summer of 2002 displayed another flaw in the premise of notification. Megan's Law is imposed locally, and it therefore does not allow for the fact that many child killers (and nonviolent child molesters) are mobile and can abduct or abuse children out of the registration catchment area.

The primary question the courts have addressed in terms of Megan's Law is whether registration and community notification constitute punishment. If so, Megan's Law could be considered unconstitutional on four bases: double jeopardy, ex post facto application of the law, bill of attainder, and cruel and unusual punishment. Double jeopardy, which is prohibited by the Fifth Amendment, protects an individual from being tried twice for the same crime. Protection against ex post facto application of a law means that an individual is not subject to punishment for a law that was enacted after the crime was committed. The Bill of Attainder clause prohibits infliction of punishment upon members of a group without judicial process. Finally, if registration and notification are punishment, then they must be proportionate to the offense committed, otherwise they are unconstitutional under the Eighth Amendment's prohibition against cruel and unusual punishment.

Because all four of these issues are related to punishment, the courts have regarded them together in several cases. No court has yet determined registration to be unconstitutional on the basis that it is punishment, though the courts have varied in their analysis of notification requirements. Most states have not prohibited notification, but the courts have put stringent requirements on the processes of notification and risk assessment. Hundreds of cases have gone through the courts; however, in March 2003, the Supreme Court decided two cases regarding registration and notification: *Connecticut Department of Public Safety v. Doe*, 123 S. Ct. 1160, and *Smith v. Doe*, 123 S. Ct. 1140. In these cases, the Court said that Megan's Law is not, in fact, punishment, thereby making moot the constitutional concerns about it. Additionally, the Court concluded that community notification through the posting of sex offenders' identifying information on the Internet is constitutional, despite the wide audience to whom this information is accessible.

There are also nonconstitutional concerns related to Megan's Law, such as vigilantism. The court does not recognize this as a serious obstacle to the law, however, as evidenced by the decision in *Doe v. Poritz*, 283 N.J. Super. 372, 661 A.2d 1335 (N.J. Super. 1995). The Court said it should not assume that the public will be punitive, and it should assume that the media will act responsibly with information that is disseminated about sexual offenders. The Court also stated that all community leaders and the media should emphasize the repercussions if the information released about offenders is used to punish rather than protect, as intended. Despite the warnings issued by most states about resulting repercussions, acts of vigilantism have occurred and have had some serious consequences because some individuals in the community lash out violently when they find out there are sexual offenders living in their midst. Worse yet, some sexual offenders give false addresses or do not update their addresses with the registering agency when they move, and innocent citizens are attacked. Though not too common, this is what happened to Thinh Pham, a 27-year-old Vietnamese refugee who had his front teeth knocked out by four men who thought he was a sexual offender. His address was listed on the Internet, even though the sexual offender who lived there previously moved months before.

Another problem with Megan's Law is the lack of compliance with it. Once released into the community, some sexual offenders abscond, or do not register, while others register with a fake address. If an offender fails to register, it is a punishable offense; however, with limited resources, few states can follow up on all offenders who do not comply with the law. It is difficult for local police departments, particularly in large cities, to monitor offenders after the initial registration period. If an offender absconds, a warrant is issued for his or her arrest, but this allows only for a reactive approach if the offender comes to the attention of officials for some other purpose.

The most significant problem with Megan's Law is that it gives parents a false sense of security. Sexual offenses are significantly underreported, and there are likely to be far more sexual offenders living in the community than are listed in the registry. The second problem is that sexual offenders on the register are often strangers to their victims, though the empirical studies and victimization surveys consistently show that sexual offenders tend to know their victims. Offenders who are strangers to their victims are almost always considered to be a higher risk to reoffend than those who were family members or acquaintances of their victims. Therefore, the strangers are most often assessed as Level 3 offenders and the community is notified of them. However, it leads to a misconception from the public that there are more stranger assaults than offenses by offenders known to the victim. As heinous as the death of Megan Kanka was, offenders such as Jesse Timmendequas are the most unusual type of sexual offender. Most child molesters are not violent, and children are far more likely to be abused by a family member than a stranger. Yet as a result of the registration and notification process, parents learn about the stranger offenders in the area and often only warn their children about particular strangers. They would be better served to educate their children about the general dangers of sexual offending rather than about specific individuals.

THE FUTURE OF MEGAN'S LAW:
IMPROVEMENTS AND OTHER LEGISLATION

Despite the challenges associated with Megan's Law, it is important to remember the general premise of the legislation: protection of the community and future victims. Crimes against children, particularly of a sexual nature, are tragic and distressing to the community at large. Even though studies have yet to show that Megan's Law is effective at preventing recidivism, it aims to give parents one tool to help in the fight against child sexual abuse. The question is, what can be done to make Megan's Law more effective?

One suggestion for improvement is the increase or redistribution of resources in order to better monitor compliance with Megan's Law. This would allow for the police to follow up on the information that offenders give them, and it would also allow them to track down offenders who are noncompliant. Another suggestion for improvement is community education. The community is rarely educated about sexual offenders and is often unaware that the majority of offenders know their victims. The media promulgates the image of "stranger-danger," publishing articles about "predators," "fiends," and "monsters." One possibility is to include general information about sexual offenses along with the notification about specific offenders.

Unfortunately, there are some sexual recidivists who, like Jesse Timmendequas, prey on children or vulnerable adults and yet are sentenced to finite terms of incarceration. There are now other protections against the most serious "sexual predators" who, under Sexually Violent Predator laws, can be civilly committed to a secure facility after they have completed their criminal sentence. These laws go well beyond Megan's Law in holding that violent sexual offenders should not be released at all into the community, and instead should be held civilly in mental hospitals for "treatment." These laws define a "sexually violent predator" as one who has been convicted of a sexual offense, and who has a "mental abnormality or personality disorder" that makes him likely to reoffend. These laws have a lower standard of psychological disorder than previously required for a finding of dangerousness under civil commitment laws (without the conviction of a sexual offense). In spite of a number of constitutional challenges, these laws have been upheld by the U.S. Supreme Court.[4] At this time, 16 states have such sexual predator statutes on their books. (See Murphy, Chapter 9, this volume, for more details.) Thus, it seems that society, at present, is trying to ensure the safety of its children through attempts to legally control convicted sexual offenders once they have been released. In the case of

Megan's Law, there is an intention to limit the free movement of potential sexual offenders, and in the case of sexual predator laws, an intention to effectively civilly incarcerate violent sexual predators. This has the positive effect of addressing problems caused by a certain group of known sexual offenders, some of whom are violent. However, it is unclear how well these laws control the offenders targeted by these laws, particularly Megan's Law. And because offenses are often perpetrated by offenders not included in these groups (i.e., not yet convicted), there is still the question as to how effective these laws are in significantly protecting children from future sexual assault.

NOTES

1. In 1993, Richard Allan Davis, a violent recidivist offender, kidnapped 12-year-old Polly Klaas from her own bedroom during a slumber party. This crime occurred in Petaluma, California, in a middle-class neighborhood. In the aftermath of the kidnapping, Polly was dubbed "America's child"; families throughout the United States recognized that this could happen anywhere.
2. For a detailed, state-by-state list of all statutes, guidelines, and case law related to Megan's Law, see Terry and Furlong (2003).
3. When offenders are released from prison, they often do not have a place to live. There are few establishments that house sexual offenders; even correctional programs such as halfway houses are often reluctant to take in sexual offenders, which leaves them with few choices of where to live once released. In some cities, public housing estates do not allow felons to live there, so no affordable housing is available for the sexual offenders. As a result of the lack of housing, many offenders are homeless or live in shelters. When this happens, there is no address for the offender.
4. *Kansas v. Hendricks*, 521 U.S. 346 (1997); *Seling v. Young*, 531 U.S. 250 (2001).

REFERENCES

Baker, T., Skolnik, L., Davis, R., & Brickman, E. (1991). The social support of survivors of rape: The difference between rape survivors and survivors of other violent crimes and between husbands, boyfriends, and women friends. In A. W. Burgess (Ed.), *Rape and sexual assault III: A research handbook*. New York: Garland.

Bass, E., & Davis, L. (1988). *Courage to heal*. New York: Harper & Row.

Brochman, S. (1991). Silent victims: Bringing male rape out of the closet. *The Advocate, 582*, 38–43.

Burgess, A. W. (1983). Rape trauma syndrome. *Behavioral Science and Law, 1*(3), 97–113.

Burgess, A. W. (1995) Rape trauma syndrome. In P. S. Searles & R. J. Berger (Eds.), *Rape and society*. Boulder, CO: Westview.

Burgess, A. W., & Holstrom, L. L. (1974). Rape trauma syndrome. *American Journal of Psychiatry, 131*, 981–986.

Calhoun, K. S., & Atkeson, B. M. (1991). *Treatment of rape victims: Facilitating psychosocial adjustment.* Elmsford, NY: Pergamon Press.

Conte, J. R. (1991). The nature of sexual offences against children. In C. R. Hollin & K. Howells (Eds.), *Clinical approaches to sex offenders and their victims.* West Sussex, UK: Wiley.

Eby, K. K., Campbell, J. C., Sullivan, C. M., & Davidson, W. S. (1995). Health effects of experiences of sexual violence for women with abusive partners. *Health Care for Women International, 16,* 563–576.

Ellis, E. M., Atkeson, B. M., & Calhoun, K. S. (1981). Sexual dysfunction in victims of rape. *Women and Health, 5,* 39–47.

Frank, P. I., Kay, C. R., Wingrave, S., Lewis, T., Osborne, J., & Newell, C. (1985). Induced abortion operations and their early sequelae. *Journal of the Royal College of General Practitioners, 35,* 175–180.

Golding, J. M. (1996). Sexual assault history and women's reproductive and sexual health. *Psychology of Women Quarterly, 20,* 101–121.

Groth, A. N., & Burgess, A. W. (1977). Motivational intent in the sexual assault on children. *Criminal Justice and Behavior, 4,* 253–264.

Groth, A. N., & Burgess, A. W. (1980). Male rape: Offenders and victims. *American Journal of Psychiatry, 137,* 806–810.

Groth, A. N., Longo, R. E., & McFadin, J. D. (1982). Undetected recidivism among rapists and child molesters. *Crime and Delinquency, 28,* 102–106.

Hazelwood, R. R., Dietz, P. E., & Burgess, A. W. (1983). *Autoerotic fatalities.* Lexington, MA: Lexington Books.

Isley, P. J. (1991). Adult male sexual assault in the community: A literature review and group treatment model. In A. W. Burgess (Ed.), *Rape and sexual assault III: A research handbook.* New York: Garland.

Johnson, J. T. (1992). *Mothers of incest survivors: Another side of the story.* Bloomington: Indiana University Press.

Langan, P. A., & Harlow, C. W. (1994). Child rape victims, 1992. In *Crime data brief.* Washington, DC: U.S. Department of Justice.

Lundberg-Love, P. K. (1999). The resilience of the human psyche: Recognition and treatment of the adult survivor of incest. In M. A. Paludi (Ed.), *The psychology of sexual victimization: A handbook.* Westport, CT: Greenwood Press.

McMullen, R. J. (1992). *Male rape: Breaking the silence on the last taboo.* London: GMP.

National Institute of Justice. (1992). *When the victim is a child* (2nd ed.). Washington, DC: U.S. Department of Justice, Office of Justice Programs.

National Report Series. (1999). *Juvenile justice bulletin: Children as victims.* Washington, DC: U.S. Department of Justice.

Nelson, S. (2001). Physical symptoms in sexually abused women: Somatization or undetected injury? *Child Abuse Review, 11,* 51–64.

Pryor, D. (1996). *Unspeakable acts: Why men sexually abuse children.* New York: New York University Press.

Rennison, C. M. (2001). Criminal victimization 2000: Changes 1999–2000 with trends 1993–2000. In *National crime victimization survey.* Washington, DC: Bureau of Justice Statistics.

Resnick, H. S., Acierno, R., & Kilpatrick, D. G. (1997). Health impact of interpersonal violence: Medicinal and mental health outcomes. *Behavioral Medicine, 23*, 65–78.

Simon, T., Mercy, J., & Perkins, C. (2001, June). *Injuries from violent crime, 1992–98*. Washington, DC: Bureau of Justice Statistics.

Terry, K. J., & Furlong, J. (2003). *Sex offender registration and community notification: A "Megan's Law" sourcebook* (2nd ed.). Kingston, NJ: Civic Research Institute.

Thompson, K. M., Wonderlich, S. A., Crosby, R. D., & Mitchell, J. E. (2001). Sexual victimization and adolescent weight regulation practices: A test across three community based samples. *Child Abuse and Neglect, 25*, 291–305.

Walker, E. A., Katon, W. J., Hansom, J., Harrop-Griffiths, J., Holm, L., Jones, M. L., Hickok, L., & Jemelka, R. P. (1992). Medical and psychiatric symptoms in women with childhood sexual abuse. *Psychosomatic Medicine, 54*, 658–664.

Ward, C., & Inserto, F. (1990). *Victims of sexual violence: A handbook for helpers*. Kent Ridge: Singapore University Press.

11 Maternal Violence

The Social Psychology
of Mothers Who Kill

JULIE BLACKMAN

When a woman is arrested, the stereotype of "woman as good" is already askew. When a woman is arrested because her child is dead, she is immediately subject to the harshest of prejudices—the disdain and condemnation reserved for bad mothers. Prejudice is, above all, a blinder. I hope, in this chapter, to enable the reader to see beyond the blinders and to acquire insight into why some girls and women cannot protect their offspring or are moved to do them harm.[1]

The ultimate goal of this chapter is to illuminate a path from insight to responsive action. What should happen to these women who have acted to end the lives of their children or who have failed to act to save them? What are the best courses of action in courtrooms for these mothers?

There is a special tension for me, as a feminist social psychologist, to pursue answers to these questions. The law accuses individuals. Little attention is paid to the contributions of that individual's social context. While practitioners in the justice system have a working awareness of the roles of race, class, and gender—and may consider these factors when they prepare oral arguments, prepare witnesses to testify, and select juries—the law is written as if individuals act and can be judged fairly without regard to these aspects of themselves. The separate and combined impacts of race, class, and gender on the individual and on those who will judge that individual exist outside what the law addresses. Other extraindividual factors also matter, most significantly, the nature and management of conflict and/or violence experienced and observed in family life. Because justice is best served when understanding is greatest, the courtroom's focus on individuals, plucked from their social histories and dropped into the language of legal statutes, makes it hard to serve justice and still follow the rules of criminal jurisprudence.

There are, of course, a few exceptions to this removal of the individual from her context. Insanity, which, as typically defined under the law, prevents the individual from appreciating the nature and consequences of his or her actions, is an exception to the general tendency to apply the law to all people, without variation. The introduction of expert testimony on the normal psychology of those accused of crimes—testimony on battered women or abused children, for example—has also served to bring social context to the courtroom, although with less impact than that which attaches to the insanity defense. There is no separate standard of responsibility under the law for battered women the way there is for those found to be not responsible by reason of insanity.[2]

Even so, the involvement of expert witnesses can help to redress the limitation in the law that decontextualizes those who are not mentally ill and are charged with criminal acts. It is right to see people in context (Blackman, 1989, 1990, 1994). Surely people are influenced by the power and resources that attach to their positions in society and their access to a nonviolent and supportive upbringing. There is no better predictor of bad acts than the emotional unrest that regularly follows from being deprived of access to the valued resources that are central to emotional well-being. Most instances of maternal violence can be better understood if one attends to the role of resources, social power, and social contact in the lives of those who commit these acts. This attention to context may or may not be exculpatory, but it is always explanatory and, therefore, important.

Further, please note that this chapter on arrested mothers cannot help but be a part of the persistent illusion that women can be understood as solo actors and that mothers are powerful (and therefore are properly deserving of high levels of ascribed responsibility) because they are mothers. This pertains no matter what else might be seen to detract from that power. Protestations and caveats notwithstanding, this is a chapter about mothers, not about fathers; about mothers, not about couples; about mothers, not about families; about mothers, not about poverty; about mothers, not about a society that has kept women down and then blamed them for not seeing the sky.

DEFINING THE PROBLEM:
WHO ARE MOTHERS WHO KILL?

Much of the literature in the United States on infanticide, like the court-room, is organized around a focus on the individual (Brouget & Brad-ford, 1990; D'Orban, 1979; Lewis, Baranoski, Buchanan & Benedek, 1998; Resnick, 1969, 1970; Silva et al., 1998). Recent increased atten-tion to culture notwithstanding, much of the empirical research ema-nates from psychiatrists or clinical psychologists, who are the specialists most likely to testify as expert witnesses in courtrooms. They are the professionals who tend to focus on the individual's mental status, rather than on more relational, cultural, or political concerns.

The most frequently cited starting points in the pursuit of a typology for mothers who kill were published in 1969 and 1970 by Resnick in the *American Journal of Psychiatry*. Resnick, a psychiatrist, reviewed 168 case reports of infanticide which occurred between 1751 and 1968. He asserted the importance of a distinction between neonati-cide, defined as the killing of a newborn on the first day of life, and filicide, which led to the death of a child after the first day.

He identified 37 cases of neonaticide and concluded that there were four explanations or "motives" for these killings. Mothers were de-scribed as either psychotic, altruistic (believing that killing the child will end some real or imagined suffering), acting unintentionally, or acting because the infant was unwanted. Resnick reported that neonaticidal women were younger, had fewer psychotic symptoms, and were more likely to kill their baby because it was unwanted. Others, after Resnick, have done research to test his model and his conclusions, finding a rather high level of support for the importance of distinguishing between neonaticide and filicide (Brouget & Bradford, 1990; D'Orban, 1979; Lewis et al., 1998).

Only recently have some within the community of those who study infanticide critiqued Resnick's typology (and those of his followers) as being overly narrow in its singular focus on the motives of the lethal par-ent. Work by Wilczynski (1997), Silva et al. (1998), Meyer and Ober-man (2001), and Spinelli (2003) have broadened Resnick's original typology (Meyer & Oberman, 2001; Silva et al., 1998; Spinelli, 2003; Wilczynski, 1997). For example Silva et al. (1998) wrote:

> These taxonomies are not comprehensive, and therefore they undermine any effort designed to develop well-integrated and systematic evalua-tions of child-killing behavior. Often the main limitation is the emphasis on categorizing the motivational characteristics of the individual perpe-

trator at the cost of failing to evaluate the relevant environmental factors in which the homicidal behavior takes place and the role that these play in the conscious and unconscious life of the perpetrators. (p. 1112)

Silva et al. proposed a "multilevel approach" for the classification of child-killing behavior, including psychiatric diagnostic factors (e.g., substance abuse), developmental factors, behavioral nonpsychopathological factors (e.g., unwanted children), and psychosociocultural/ecological factors (e.g., stressors).

Wilczynski, in her book *Child Homicide* (1997), identified risk factors in terms of eight clusters: demographic characteristics, social, psychiatric, victim characteristics, situational, prior family conflict, family history, and prior contact with agencies. Wilczynski concluded that those at risk for child homicide are most likely to have three main characteristics: many psychological problems, a negative view of their situation, and inadequate social and personal resources (Wilczynski, 1997, p. 5). Meyer and Oberman also have broadened the range of factors to be considered in their book, *Mothers Who Kill Their Children: Understanding the Acts of Moms from Susan Smith to the "Prom Mom"* (2001). Their research, based on over 200 recent cases of infanticide in the United States, led them to conclude the existence of five types of infanticide: neonaticide, assisted–coerced killing, neglect-related, mental illness-related, and abuse-related. Across these five types, they identified common themes, most important among them, the roles of isolation, stress, and the absence of social resources.

It is important to attend to culture and to the power differences that follow from culture in a society that treats some people much better than others, while expecting much more from mothers than from others, regardless of their culture or their access to power. The approach taken in this chapter continues in this new, broadening tradition.

THE FOUR CIRCUMSTANCES:
SEARCHING FOR MEANING

The central portion of this chapter is organized into four sections that follow from four different circumstances in which women get arrested for killing their children or for failing to protect their children who were killed by their abusive husbands. At the heart of these "circumstances" are the meanings attached to the actions that resulted in their deaths. Meanings follow from social context. Meanings reflect the individual's experiences within her social environment, resulting from her own history and place in the power hierarchy (see Fine & Carney, 2001).

The four circumstances are the following:[3]

1. Teenagers who committed neonaticide.
2. Women who killed their babies during the first few days or months due to postpartum psychosis.
3. Battered women whose abusive male partners killed their children.
4. Women who were themselves abused as children, whose neglectful or violent acts resulted in the deaths of their children.

In this section, I draw heavily from my own cases and from my personal contact with women who were arrested for killing their children or for failing to protect them from the violence of their partners. I have consulted with criminal defense attorneys on cases that reflect each of the four circumstances considered herein. I have included, in each of the four sections, examples of women's experiences and the contribution that an expert can make to enhancing insight into what these women have done. In a final, separate section, I discuss what appropriate responses might be with regard to each of these four circumstances.

The four circumstances that provide the centerpiece of this chapter include bits of my creative writing intended to show how these women might have felt. Actual descriptions of their cases are also included, to the extent that their views were expressed in the courtroom or received media coverage. In all but three of these cases, I evaluated the women and consulted with their attorneys. In one case, I testified as an expert witness at trial. In all these cases, whether I was involved or not, information included here comes from public sources or I have changed the names of the women involved.

The first two circumstances involve either very young women and/ or their very young children. These two sections have little to do with an actual relationship between the mother and child. As such, from a psychological perspective, the woman is more easily considered apart from her status as mother. She is nearly childless. She ends her mothering almost as soon as it begins. For these reasons, aspects of the individual, in particular, the extreme youth of neonaticidal mothers and the role of postpartum psychosis, are key to understanding the actions of these women. To the extent that, as a culture, we assign reduced responsibility to the young and the mentally ill, these factors introduce culture into the analysis of these kinds of infanticide. Even so, in my opinion, the role of race and class are reduced as significant factors for women who kill their babies immediately or shortly after birth.[4]

It is important to point out that these women are different from each other in many ways. They are brought together by circumstances that result in the deaths of their children—hence the title for this section. Even so, more than the circumstances unite them, their differences distinguish them. They vary in age, social class, race, the severity of the mental disorders from which they suffered, and the role extended periods of abuse by an intimate played in their lives.

Teenagers Who Committed Neonaticide

What Teenagers Who Commit Neonaticide Might Think during Pregnancy and at Birth

"Imagine a sinking feeling in the pit of your stomach. Imagine fearing that you are pregnant. Imagine terrible consequences: your childhood ended abruptly; disappointed, outraged family members; picketers hurling threats and blood-colored liquid in front of abortion clinics."

"Imagine wishing that this were not happening to you. Imagine pretending and then believing that it is not you, that you are not pregnant. Imagine giving birth anyway. The baby never cries. (You do not think to suction its lungs.) You throw the baby away. The baby is dead. A passerby finds your baby. Then, they find you and charge you with murder. Charge me with murder."

Two Teenagers in Denial: Amy Grossberg and Melissa Drexler

Two recent cases of babies born to teenage mothers in denial received a great deal of media attention. Their names are Amy Grossberg and Melissa Drexler. Both were white, from New Jersey, and teenagers at the time they gave birth. Amy was a freshman in college; Melissa, a senior in high school.[5]

AMY GROSSBERG

In November 1996, Amy Grossberg gave birth to a baby boy in a motel room in Delaware. Her boyfriend, Brian Petersen, was with her. They believed that the baby was stillborn and placed his body in a dumpster outside the motel. They were, at first, both charged with first-degree murder, punishable in Delaware by death. Held in jail for about 2 months, they were both released on bail to house arrest pending the resolution of their case.

Almost 2 years later, in July 1998, both pled guilty to manslaughter. Amy was sentenced to 30 months in prison. (Brian was sentenced to 24 months.) Amy was also sentenced to 5 years probation and ordered to serve 300 hours of community service working at clinics for pregnant teenagers. (It is hard to imagine a worse place for her to be, not only for her own emotional well-being and need to recover from her life's tragedy, but also because her experience can only add to the emotional burdens that are already great for pregnant teens.)

Judge Henry duPont Ridgely spoke to Amy: "If there's a disturbing aspect to your character, an unsettling trait as the time of childbirth neared, it was an egocentricity that blinded you to the need to seek help and to the intrinsic value of the life of the child" (in Hanley, 1998a). Here, Judge Ridgely rebuked Amy directly for her failure to do what good mothers are expected to do. Good mothers are the opposite of egocentric. Good mothers are selfless and will sacrifice their own needs for the needs of their children. Good mothers see the intrinsic worth of their children.

Amy, however, was not in a ready-to-mother state of mind during her pregnancy. Judge Ridgely quoted from letters Amy had written to Brian during her pregnancy. In these letters, Amy's fervent wish that she were not pregnant dominated her thinking: "All I want is for it to go away," and "I would do anything in the entire world if it just went away." She even wrote to God: "Don't let it go on any further" (Hanley, 1998a).

Like a child hoping against hope, praying for the impossible, Amy denied the reality of her pregnancy. Her defense lawyer, John Malik, offered this insight into Amy's thinking, "She put a premium on being the perfect daughter and she thought this would be a disappointment to her family" (in Hanley, 1998a).

MELISSA DREXLER

Melissa Drexler was already in labor when she left for her senior prom. Her water broke in the car on the way to the catering hall. She went directly into the bathroom, locked herself in one of the stalls and delivered a baby boy into the toilet. At her sentencing, she admitted that he had been born alive. This distinguished her admission from what Amy or Brian had confessed to. She pled guilty to aggravated manslaughter. Like Amy, Melissa admitted recklessness. Melissa's plea added the component of "extreme indifference to human life."

Judge John A. Ricciardi sentenced Melissa to 15 years in prison. Under New Jersey law still in effect at that time, this made her eligible for her first parole hearing after 2 years and 11 months.

Melissa's allocution followed the legal guidelines as she accepted responsibility for the death of her newborn son. Her defense attorney, Steven Secare, provided insight into her thinking. He described her as "immature, disoriented and frightened—in denial throughout her pregnancy and during the trip to the prom. Even though she had labor cramps before reaching the catering hall, 'there was no inevitability of birth' on her mind when she arrived." Mr. Secare said that Melissa made a "terrible, horrible, tragic mistake" (in Hanley, 1998b).

The assistant prosecutor, Elaine Leschot, rejected the idea that Melissa was in denial. Ms. Leschot went right to the heart of the bad mother rhetoric and described Melissa as "a selfish person who hid the pregnancy from her family and friends and refused to take responsibility to deal with it because of concerns that it would interfere with the fun of her senior year" (in Hanley, 1998b).

The Monmouth County Prosecutor, John Kaye, saw the problem differently: "There is no question from a psychological point of view that she was suffering from emotional stress and one of the keys in showing her mental condition was how she isolated herself from her family and from her boyfriend. She just denied it and continued to deny it" (in Smothers, 1998). Kaye added that, in his 15 years as county prosecutor, there had been 12 other cases of killings of newborns. All but one resulted in similar plea agreements. One woman, Patricia Giles, went to trial in 1987. She was convicted and sentenced to the maximum of 30 years in prison. Kaye's description of the legal prognoses for these women is consistent with my experience in this area. Most women know better than to go to trial in cases like these. Most plead guilty to avoid the wrath of jurors who are easily united in their fury against a bad mother—even when that mother is little more than a child herself.

QUESTIONS FOR AN EXPERT TO ADDRESS TO HELP THE FINDERS OF FACT

What would cause a teenager to be unaware of, to deny, or to fear her pregnancy? What would cause her to conceal the birth of her baby? What would cause her to throw her baby away?

ANSWERS: DENIAL AND FEAR OF PREGNANCY—PRIMITIVE BUT POWERFUL DEFENSE MECHANISMS

For teenagers, who are recent émigrés from childhood and may be immature under ordinary circumstances, pregnancy can lead to a disintegration of self. Teenagers are known risk-takers. Risk taking is facilitated by denying the possibility that harm can occur. Teenage girls who risk becoming pregnant may have no real, felt awareness that they actually could become pregnant. Confronting the truth of pregnancy and its normally inevitable consequence may be more than these girls can do.

It may seem, in retrospect, that these young women do things far more extraordinary than confronting the reality of their pregnancies. After all, Amy Grossberg went to a motel room to deliver her baby. Melissa Drexler endured the humiliation of having her water break on her way to the prom and the trauma of delivering her baby into the toilet of a public bathroom. These extraordinary choices and actions, however, were in service of a more pressing need—the need to believe that they were not really pregnant and would not really have babies.

Both of these very young women feared the judgment of others and sought psychological protection in denial. The fact that denial did not and could not serve them in the end made them no less eager to embrace it. Denial is not a rational defense mechanism. Denial is irrational. The answers denial provides are objectively incorrect, but knowing what is true can be intolerable.

It is surely pathological for these young women to deny what is true. At an unconscious level, there must be more. For some fleeting moments, these women may even know that they are pregnant and appreciate the meaning of this reality. However, fleeting knowledge is by definition, only momentary, and may leave little or no awareness in its wake when the defense mechanism of denial has done its work again.

We understand denial when someone is sick or dying. Then, we understand the fevered wish to believe that what is so is not so. It is only because we see motherhood as something to be valued that we reject the idea of denial as understandable. We fail to see that denial, while pathological, is also a frequently occurring self-protective strategy. The continua for denial (e.g., limited vs. far reaching, of great vs. small importance) are long. Sometimes denial is adaptive (e.g., people who must ride buses to get to work in Israel must engage in some measure of denial: "It won't happen here"). Sometimes denial is extreme and creates more problems than it solves.

Because denial is a primitive defense mechanism, more appropriate to children than to adults, many find these young mother-deniers to be not credible. In the United States, we find these deniers to be culpable. This is not so in England and other European countries where pathological behaviors that appear in tandem with childbirth are judged to be signs of mental illness, not of criminality. Amy Grossberg and Melissa Drexler would not have been prosecuted, convicted, or incarcerated under the laws of many other countries.

In the United States, these women are charged with murder and are often convicted and incarcerated. Consider, then, in the context of the laws of the United States, that for young women who dispose of their babies and are arrested, their denial takes on unusual properties in the courtroom. It is not unusual for defendants to deny criminal activity or for them to deny the events leading up to criminal activity. It is unusual for the very essence of the denial to be *self-defeating* instead of self-serving. It is one thing to deny something that may or may not be proved beyond a reasonable doubt, to deny something that may be subject to a range of alternative explanations. It is another thing to deny an extended pregnancy and the birth that is all but certain to follow from it. Self-defeating denial should not be confused with self-serving denial. The self-defeating denial that attends these pregnancies is all important for understanding the reactions of these young women in the aftermath of being discovered.

Denial eliminates or blunts emotion. Once discovered, the facts are revealed and the work of denial is brought to an abrupt end. The feelings that would have been present if denial were absent, however, do not spring to life. Therefore, these women maintain a child-like, flattened-affect self-presentation even after the babies' deaths are discovered. This is not a sign of their disregard for the intrinsic value of children, as Judge Ridgely insisted when he sentenced Amy Grossberg, but a sign that they never knew or felt for their children in utero. It was as if they never existed.

All the fears that were blanketed by denial came true. Their secrets were unmasked and, in these cases, widely publicized. As noted earlier, in this country we punish them, although, as Melissa Drexler's defense attorney Steven Secare pointed out, there are several countries in Europe that do not prosecute women whose babies die very soon after birth. They acknowledge pregnancy and birth-related emotional stresses and allow them to exculpate mothers in these circumstances (Atkins, Grimes, Joseph, & Liebman, 1999).

Infant Homicides: A Statistical Overview

Epidemiologist Mary Overpeck and her colleagues at the National Institute of Child Health and Human Development reported in the October 1998 issue of the *New England Journal of Medicine* that infant homicides were on the rise (Gilbert, 1998). They examined the death certificates of nearly 35 million babies born between 1983 and 1991 who died before their first birthday. In the population, there were 2,776 homicide victims. In 1996, homicide was the leading cause of death due to injury—accounting for almost one-third of such deaths. Of 100,000 births between 1988 and 1991, 8.9 died violent deaths. This same statistic had been 7.2 for the period from 1983 to 1987 (Overpeck, Brenner, Trumble, Trifiletti, & Berendes, 1998).

Five percent of babies killed were killed the day they were born. Half were killed within the first 4 months. The mother is most likely to be the one to kill the baby if the baby is 1 week old or younger. After that, male caregivers become the more likely perpetrators. After the age of 3, the majority of children killed are killed by someone unrelated to them.

The two biggest risk factors identified by these researchers were teenage mothers and being a latter-born child of a teenage mother. Babies fitting this description were 10 times as likely to be killed as the lowest risk group—firstborn children of mothers who were 25 years or older. Even so, only 17% of the victims had both of these leading risk factors, which indicates that other important factors are also at work. (Other infant risk factors included low birth weight, low gestational age, male sex, and low Apgar scores.)

Overpeck et al. (1998) advocated for such responsive actions as home visits by trained nurses during pregnancy and the first 2 years of life, as well as programs designed for pregnant adolescents with a specific focus on the prevention of severe and fatal abuse (p. 1215). Postpartum depression and domestic violence were both proposed by these researchers as important explanations to consider.

Insights from History

Mendlowicz, Rapaport, Mecler, Golshan, and Morales (1998) opened their article on neonaticidal mothers with a review of the history of infanticide. They noted that the public attitude toward the murder of newborns has changed over time and is different in different cultures.

> During the latter half of the first millennium B.C., the killing of newborns was not an uncommon practice in Greco-Latin civilization. In Athens . . . there was no law forbidding a free man to kill his . . . children. In Imperial Rome . . . a sentence of death could be imposed on the mother or the grandparents but not on the father.
>
> In contrast, ancient people . . . such as Egyptians, Hebrews and Germans, abhorred this crime: one Egyptian father who had killed his son was condemned to stay 3 days and 3 nights embracing the body of his deceased son, under the scrutiny of armed guards. (pp. 209–210)

In 1623, in England, the "Act to Prevent the Destroying and Murdering of Bastard Children" was established. The death penalty attached to the killing of newborns, and these laws required the mother to prove that the child was stillborn and not a victim of murder (Mendlowicz et al., 1998, p. 210). Two hundred years later, in 1823, the English reinstated the presumption of innocence for these mothers but retained the death penalty if convicted.

During those 200 years, other changes occurred in the legal view of single women who killed their babies. The founder of the Classical School of Penal Law, Count Beccaria, opined in 1764 that desperation and the fear of ostracism led women to kill their newborns. Beccaria believed that the act should be seen as culpable but understandable and should receive a lighter punishment than other killings he judged as heinous.

The Positivist School of Penal Law appeared in the late 1800s and relied on the work of two French psychiatrists, Esquirol and Marce, who saw a causal relationship among pregnancy, birth, and emotional upset. Thus, the murder of a newborn was attributed to the mother's abnormal state of mind.

According to Mendlowicz et al. (1998):

> This historical evolution has resulted in the current criminal legislation of most Western countries, which grants mothers who kill their newborns lighter punishments than those for murderers in general. Some of these codes justify this by attributing the crime to the shame felt by the single mother, while others presume that childbirth has deranged the parent. (p. 211)

Women Who Killed Their Babies during the First Few Days or Months Due to Postpartum Psychosis[6]

What Women Might Think When Postpartum Psychosis Hits

"The pregnancy is over. The baby is here. I know I should be happy, but I am not. I am overwhelmed by sadness. I will have to take care of this baby forever. I will have to listen to him cry day after day. I should be able to stop his crying, but what if I can't? He is crying now. Why won't he stop? I have to make him stop."

"The next thing I remember, I saw my hands holding a pillow over his face. Then, I realized something was happening to me again. It couldn't be, but it was. I felt that I was half there and half not there. I don't know why it happened. I never wanted to hurt my baby. I wanted a baby so much."

Two Women Who Smothered Their Babies: Marie Noe and Ann Green

Their marriages endured even though their babies kept dying. These women are not the kinds of women their husbands thought of as bad. They kept getting pregnant again and again as if this time the terrible problem, the urgency that led them to smother their children, would not recur.

MARIE NOE

In August 1998, a 70-year-old woman, Marie Noe, was arrested in Philadelphia and charged with smothering 8 of her 10 children. She used a pillow or soft object. The children, born between 1949 and 1967, were as young as 13 days and as old as 14 months when they died. One other pregnancy resulted in a stillbirth. A tenth child died of complications at birth.

After being freed on $500,000 bond, in June 1999, Marie Noe was sentenced to 20 years of probation, the first five of which were to be served under home confinement. She wore an electronic monitoring bracelet around her waist. Her husband's poor health was a factor in the plea agreement. Marie was also obliged to undergo treatment with a psychiatrist to determine the cause of her repeated infanticide (Associated Press, 1999).

ANN GREEN

Ann Green was a pediatrics nurse. She loved working with children. She smothered her first child, a girl, who died almost immediately. She smothered her second child, a boy, seemed to realize what she had done, and ran with him to the nearest hospital. He lingered there for several weeks before he died. She smothered her third child, a son, again realized what she was doing, and ran with him to the hospital. He survived.

Ann Green stood trial in New York County in 1988 for the deaths of her first two children and the attempted murder of her third. No longer acutely psychotic in the wake of pregnancy, she had herself voluntarily sterilized before the trial began. A relative adopted her surviving son and Ann's parental rights were terminated.

Ann testified about the reasons why she had smothered her children. They cried, they threw up, they had bowel movements, and she was made terribly anxious by this. Dr. Stuart Asch, a psychiatrist and an expert on postpartum psychosis and depression, testified and educated the jury about the reality of this mental illness. He described Ann as someone who was unable to appreciate fully the difference between what was real and what was not. He opined that she could not fully appreciate the meaning of her infanticidal acts. He believed that for her, smothering her babies meant undoing the birth process and stopping the bad things that were happening.

Asch testified that for women with postpartum psychosis, once the baby is unborn (killed), the mother is driven to repeat the process, to have a "good" baby and to prove her self-worth in this way. This leads to further pregnancies.

Asch saw a deeper underlying psychosis in women who killed their newborns this way. These mothers suffer from terrible self-images. They feel that they are bad, but that pregnancy and childbirth will make them good. Once the baby is born, however, it can never be the baby of their fantasy. Instead, the real baby is different and does bad things—like crying or throwing up. For these women, their defective, bad images of themselves reappear in their babies. This is intolerable and so they end their babies' lives.

The prosecutor argued that Ann was a murderer and had not been insane. Nor did she seem insane at the time of the trial. Why she would have smothered her own babies and then sought medical care for them was incomprehensible. The jury agreed that it was incomprehensible unless she had been insane. They found her not guilty by reason of insanity—postpartum psychosis.

QUESTIONS FOR AN EXPERT TO ADDRESS TO HELP THE FINDERS OF FACT

What would cause women to suffocate their babies? What preexisting factors give rise to postpartum psychosis?

AN ANSWER: POSTPARTUM PSYCHOSIS

Postpartum depression is a component of postpartum psychosis, though psychosis includes a more thoroughgoing break with reality. The essence of psychosis is that psychotic thinking trumps reality. People who are psychotic do not know what is real. They do not appreciate the nature and consequences of their actions. Legally and psychologically, postpartum psychosis is a form of insanity. Unlike other severe mental illnesses that strike adults, however, this one is sporadic and may abate without medication. It is primed by pregnancy, emerges at birth, and seems to disappear after the baby is dead. These women may lead remarkably "normal" lives, except for the fact that they smother their babies.

For example, when Marie Noe first admitted that she had caused the deaths of her children, her husband defended her. He said, "I've lived with this woman for 50 years. She was my life. That woman was not capable of doing such a thing. She wouldn't harm a fly" (Associated Press, 1999).

Even so, they are not entirely normal and are likely to show signs of psychotic thinking in other aspects of their lives. These signs, however, tend to be less dramatic and may never draw the sort of attention that follows from infanticide.

A study by Holden, Burland, and Lemmen (1996) included comparisons between women found to be criminally responsible for the murders of their children ($n = 8$) and those found not guilty by reason of insanity ($n = 20$). All of those found not guilty by reason of insanity described "psychotic motivations" for their actions. Common themes included the delusional conviction that the child was defective or monstrous in some way. Some reported that they heard voices which commanded them to kill the child. Some believed they were saving their child from an imagined disaster (e.g., undergoing torture).

Demographically, those mothers found to be not guilty by reason of insanity tended to be different from those found to be criminally responsible. Those found to be insane tended not to be young mothers. The majority were married and the children tended not to be newborns at the time of their deaths.[7] A majority attempted suicide after they acted against their child (Holden et al., 1996).

Battered Women Whose Abusive Male Partners Killed or Injured Their Children

Insights from the Old Testament

The story of the binding of Isaac is the first story told every Jewish New Year. It is the story of Abraham's belief in one God, a belief so strong that he heeds God's demand that he sacrifice his son, Isaac. Isaac was not Abraham's only son. He was Sarah's only son. Abraham had fathered a son with Hagar. When he and Sarah finally conceived Isaac, though, he forced Hagar and her son, Ishmael, to leave. Ishmael is the father of Islam. Sarah and Abraham did not have this son easily. Sarah was 90 years old when she finally gave birth to Isaac. In Hebrew, *yitzhak* ("Isaac" in English) means "laughed." Sarah laughed when Isaac was born, with the joy of having a son after so many years of wanting a child.

Abraham did not tell Sarah what God had commanded him to do. He took Isaac up on Mount Moriah to sacrifice him to his God. Only after Isaac had been restrained and Abraham was about to kill his son did God relent. God sent an angel to Abraham. Although God had spoken to Abraham in the past, he sent an angel to stay Abraham's hand. The angel called twice to Abraham, and Isaac's life was saved. God never spoke to Abraham again (Kulwin, 1998). Abraham and Isaac returned to Sarah.

In the very next part of the Old Testament, Sarah dies. While there is no specific link between Abraham's near-killing of her son and Sarah's death, it may be that the juxtaposition of Isaac's near death and Sarah's real death has meaning. Perhaps we are to believe that the news of what Abraham was prepared to do to her only son brought an end to her life.

For women whose male partners kill their children, the harm to these women is enduring. Often, they are also the victims of this man's violence, as well as the victims of violence when they were children. They frequently are arrested, prosecuted, and convicted for being complicit or worse in the harm done to their children. Fine and Carney (2001) provide an insightful analysis of the ways in which women are made responsible not only for serving their families but also for policing them:

> Young, scared and isolated . . . women . . . who fail to protect their children from violence are held accountable for the actions of husbands or boyfriends who are often much stronger and much more powerful than themselves. Their failure, then, is not only to protect their children. Rather, it is to effectively manage their homes and their co-inhabitants. When the men in their lives become violent, the women, who either voluntarily or through force, renounce the cultural obligation to manage, become punishable as well. (p. 7)

What Women Might Think When Men Batter Them and Their Children

> "What now? What now? If I look away, will he stop beating my son? If I get in the way, he will beat us both. What now? What now? He says my son acts bad. He's got to teach him a lesson. Don't feed him, he says. So, I don't. Don't go to him, he says. So, I don't. I don't. I can't stop him anyway. He's stronger than I am. I yell at my son, too. Why can't he behave? If he just kept quiet."

Jennifer Hall

Jennifer Hall's (a pseudonym) boyfriend had beaten her and had beaten her son many times. Jennifer did seek medical care for herself, going for prenatal visits during her pregnancy with her daughter. She did not seek medical care for her son. She was aware of his injuries but feared that if doctors saw him they would take him away from her. Jennifer had spent time in the foster care system herself. As a young child, she watched as her mother's boyfriend shot and killed her mother.

Andrew was 3 when he died. Her boyfriend put her child's body in the refrigerator. Jennifer stayed in the apartment, then, as she had in the past. She wept quietly. She pleaded with her boyfriend not to take the boy from her, especially not now. For days, this mother kept vigil over her dead son.

One night, though, she slept, and in the morning he was gone.

Then, only then, she became frantic. She went to the police and said that her boy was missing. They never found his body but they arrested her anyway. They did not arrest her boyfriend, who she said had killed her boy. He denied it, and there was no proof because there was no body. Also, Jennifer's story was filled with inconsistencies and things that could not have been true. For example, she reported that her 3-year-old son had scalded himself in the shower and that she had had to hit him to keep him from burning himself.

Urbelima Emiliano

One of 11 children, Urbelima left her family and came into the United States from Mexico hidden underneath a blanket in the back seat of a car. She traveled to a suburb of New York City and began to work as a housekeeper and a factory worker. Two of her brothers had come before her and they worked as gardeners in her new town.

A man from her hometown came to visit her one day and, before he left, he raped her. Urbelima had been a virgin and felt that she had to continue her relationship with this man who had taken her virginity. Soon, she was pregnant. Urbelima returned to her hometown, where she became reacquainted with an old boyfriend. He wanted to marry her. She told him of her pregnancy but he said it did not matter.

They returned to the United States and married. Only a few months later, Urbelima gave birth to a baby girl at a local hospital. She and her daughter and husband took a taxi home from the hospital. When they arrived at her house, her husband took the baby from her as he helped her out of the car. He carried the baby behind the house and he placed her in a hole he and his brother had dug in the backyard. While Urbelima cried, he covered the baby with dirt and placed a heavy stone on top of her. He dragged Urbelima into the house and threatened to kill her if she told anyone.

Urbelima hardly left the house after that. Her husband went to work but Urbelima did nothing. She did not tell her brothers about what had happened. Soon, she was pregnant again. At about 3 months, she went back to the same hospital for her first prenatal visit. The nurse noticed from her records that she had given birth recently and asked Urbelima about the baby. Urbelima began to cry and told the nurse that her husband had buried her baby in the backyard.

Urbelima was arrested, as was her husband. They were tried separately. Both of them were convicted of murder. Urbelima was sentenced to 25 years to life in prison. Before her trial, she had already given birth to another girl—this one with Down syndrome. When this infant was brought to see her during her incarceration, she held this child with so much tenderness that the psychologist who evaluated her mothering skills was persuaded that Urbelima had not been a part of her husband's plan to kill her firstborn child. The jury did not believe this expert. They did not believe me when I testified that Urbelima lived in fear of her husband, and they did not believe Urbelima.

Urbelima's inability to protect her child at the moment of its burial was made evil by her failure to speak out afterwards. For Urbelima, however, it was all over when the heavy stone was laid upon her baby. What she did next would not bring her baby back, so next she did nothing.

Sherry Andrews

Sherry Andrews (a pseudonym) was raised in the foster care system. Finally, when she was about 12 years old, the system sent her home. Her mother was an alcoholic who got into a fight with another woman and was pushed to her death from a rooftop. Sherry's father abused her sexually. Sherry's boyfriend also abused her. Sherry had three children when they entered a shelter for battered women. They stayed there for 18 months, until the program closed. Sherry and her children were sent home—back to the boyfriend who had beaten her. They had two more children together. He beat Sherry and he beat the children. David, their middle child, was beaten to death. Sherry and her boyfriend both went to prison. Sherry pled guilty to assault charges. Her boyfriend pled guilty to manslaughter. She is out of prison now. Her surviving children remained in foster care. She fought to regain custody of her daughter, who was the youngest of her children. She lost that fight and her parental rights were terminated. She was afraid of her sons, who were young teenagers by the time she got out of prison. She did not seek custody of them. She gave birth to another daughter after her release from prison. This daughter was taken from her and placed in a foster home.

THE QUESTION FOR AN EXPERT TO ADDRESS TO HELP THE FINDERS OF FACT

What would cause a battered woman to fail to protect her children—to see them become the victims of abuse and neglect—even to see them killed?

AN ANSWER: THE AFTEREFFECTS OF HISTORICAL VIOLENCE AND FEAR OF CONTEMPORARY VIOLENCE

Part of the answer is in the name: battered women. Women are diminished by battering, and made less than they would be were they not fearful and in pain. In addition, many battered women were abused as children, too, so that the reference point for good treatment that might have come from a nonviolent upbringing is missing. The missing reference point for good treatment applies not only to themselves but extends to their children. Not having been treated kindly when they were children, these women may have little feeling for the importance of treating their children kindly.

I remember a conversation I had with a woman who was incarcerated as a result of the death of one of her children. Three of her surviving children were brought to visit her once a month. I asked her if she hugged her children when they came to visit. She said that she did not. No one had ever hugged her as a child so she did not feel comfortable hugging her children. It was as if she did not know how to hug them, and could not see this behavior as appropriate for her.

Each of us carries within ourselves a sense of what feels right, of what is familiar. There is no guarantee that what feels right is also right in a moral sense. What feels right is little more than what a person has repeatedly experienced, especially what she experienced as a child.

There is so little real protection afforded children. Families are whatever they happen to be—kind or cruel, nurturing and empathic or not (Blackman, 1990, 1994, 1996). Children get born and raised by chance, and in that lottery much is determined. Children not rescued soon enough or not rescued at all from abject neglect or abuse will not recover fully. They will not get a second chance to craft what is familiar to them. Their brains will not get ready a second time for the imprinting that is the work of the very young brain.

Whatever abused children learn later about kindness in intimate relationships will come to them like a second language learned after the brain's plasticity for the acquisition of language has hardened. Just as people who acquire new languages after the age of 12 or so will speak with an accent, so abused children, treated well later, will understand this kindness as a second-order experience. For abused children/adults, kindness must piggyback precariously on the more familiar and ingrained cruelty—in this analogy, their native language. First-order experiences, those that happen first in life and make their indelible mark, are never erased, although they may be overwritten.

In this sense, then, women who were abused as children are especially vulnerable as adults to abuse by their partners. The violence that is made familiar to them during their childhoods serves to make them less likely to notice and to reject the early warning signs of danger in their adult relationships. If violence is rendered ordinary, or at least is seen as inescapable, then it is scarcely worth noticing or reacting to the signs of yet another violent relationship. Particularly for those women who see violence everywhere—in all the families they know—the thought of escape or the precautionary measures that might avoid violence altogether can only seem useless.

When violence does occur in their adult relationships, when these women have children who also become the victims of violence, they may be unable to see the alternatives that would free them and their children. The pursuit of a violence-free life may seem as likely to succeed as a climb to the top of Mt. Everest without a guide, oxygen, or equipment. Why would a woman undertake such a Herculean effort, especially when she has to take care of her children?

It may seem that there is an inherent contradiction here. Is a woman "taking care" of her children when they are being abused by her partner? The answer may be yes. She is taking care of them to the best of her ability—given the absence of those interpersonal essentials that would enable her to see and to aspire to the summit of a safe family life. Without a guide, oxygen, or equipment, however, it may be better to hunker down and wait for the violence to end than to go forth into the unknown. Going anywhere else would have to feel like going nowhere— going to an unattainable place.

In these cases, though, the woman cannot be the final arbiter of what constitutes taking care. The reality that eludes her is there even if she does not see it. Before it is too late, her children need what the Mt. Everest climber needs: a guide—a mentor who models nonviolence; oxygen—the right to breathe freely and without fear at home; and equipment—the resulting behaviors that will equip her to be a better parent than her parents were.

When battered women take care of children who are being battered and the violence is discovered, the importance of the woman's history is likely to pale beside her status as an adult. Adult expectations will attach to her regardless of the nature of her childhood. Then it will be important to understand her fear of the abuser and the extent to which contemporary, everyday fear diminishes a mother's ability and opportunity to act to keep her children safe from harm (Blackman, 1989).

Much has been written about battered women as mothers. Some of the early work described these women as traditionalists in their marriages, which by extension rendered them "good mothers" (Walker, 1979). Recent research by Sullivan, Nguyen, Allen, Bybee, and Juras (2000) offered support for this view. Their research with 80 battered mothers and their 7–11-year-old children showed that these mothers and children both described the mothers as emotionally available and more likely to use noncorporal punishment than corporal punishment. However, the batterers' abuse of mothers had a direct impact on the children's "behavioral adjustment."

While these findings are encouraging with regard to mothering by battered women, the fact that the batterers' violence against mothers harms the children complicates these families. Battered mothers must try harder to repair the damage done to the children, when they are themselves suffering. Often, the violence is simply too severe and the mothers are overwhelmed.

Mary Ann Dutton (1987), a clinical psychologist, described the impairment that follows from abuse and the attendant risks of putting an unfair amount of weight on the psychological state of the individual removed from her right context. She wrote:

> The BWS (Battered Woman Syndrome) is a collection of specific characteristics and effects of abuse on the battered woman. Not all women who are battered suffer from the BWS, but those who do typically are less able to respond effectively to the violence against them. Consequently, they become psychologically entrapped in a violent relationship. (p. 40)

As to the criticism that BWS points an isolating finger of blame at the individual and makes women responsible for stopping the violence against them, instead of assigning responsibility to societal factors, Dutton (1987) argued that BWS enables researchers to recognize the devastating impact of battering on women. This, she argued, is a contribution that serves not only the community of helping professionals but also instructs juries and judges when battered women are tried for acts that can be best understood in the context of the violence they have endured (p. 45).

From the perspective of feminism, with attention to the overwhelming contribution of social factors, attributions of responsibility become complex when, in restrictive courtroom settings, we must talk about the mothers whose partners killed their children. Things get even more complicated when we turn our attention to those women who killed their children through their own acts of commission or omission.

Women Who Were Themselves Abused as Children, Whose Neglectful or Violent Acts Resulted in the Deaths of Their Children

What Women Who Kill Their Children Might Think

"Leave me alone. Always crying, always wanting something. Waking me up early. Acting hungry. Leave me alone. I can hardly take care of myself. Nobody's around to help me. Listening to you bellyache all night. Shut up! Just shut up! Stealing food, stealing my sleep, making a mess. You are nothing but trouble and more trouble. If you won't shut your mouth, I'll shut it for you."

Two Women Whose Neglectful or Violent Acts Resulted in the Deaths of Their Children: Tabitha Walrond and Kelly Boyd

TABITHA WALROND

On May 19, 1999, in the Bronx, Tabitha Walrond was convicted of criminally negligent homicide in the death of her 2-month old son. He had starved to death. The jury was out less than 3 hours after a trial that had lasted for more than 3 weeks. She was acquitted of the more serious charge of second-degree manslaughter. Ms. Walrond's defense focused on the idea that she had been "a devoted mother unaware that her surgically reduced breasts were producing insufficient milk for her first-born child . . . misguided by her own mother and rebuffed by the health-care system when she sought medical care for her son, because he lacked a Medicaid card" (Bernstein, 1999).

Autopsy photographs showed a skeletal baby. One juror commented, "No matter what, she was the mother. She was failed, but she should have been strong enough to do more." Another said that the emaciated condition of the baby made its need for care too severe to miss. He said, "It was definitely negligence" (Bernstein, 1999, p. B1).

Robert Johnson, the Bronx County District Attorney, knew what this mother should have done: "How can you imagine any mother seeing her child like that and not absolutely jumping up and down in the emergency room saying, 'Look at my child?' " (p. B8).

In the end, the jury concluded that Tabitha Walrond should have known better than to believe her mother, who advised her that the baby was just thin and that he would fill out. The prosecutor summed it up this way: "It comes down to responsibility and accountability" (p. B8).

KELLY BOYD

Kelly Boyd (a pseudonym) and her two younger siblings were abandoned by their mother as young children. Discovered alone in an apartment, their mother's mother became their guardian. They were poor and the children often went without necessities.

Kelly gave birth to two sons, Michael and Thomas, who were both fathered by Clarence Tyler. Michael was born while Kelly was in 12th grade. She received a certificate from the high school for young mothers.

Kelly denied any abuse in her family of origin, although she admitted to at least one episode of abuse by Clarence to her aunt.

In October 1989, when Thomas died, Kelly had been working two jobs, 5 days a week. That day, Kelly was home alone with her children. Thomas got up early, at about 6:00 A.M., and went into the kitchen. He pulled a chair up to a counter, climbed up and took a pepper box. He shook pepper onto the floor. He fell and Kelly heard this. She went into the kitchen, wiped off his face, and sent him back to bed. She returned to bed herself. Thomas went to play with the pepper again. As punishment, Kelly shook the contents of the pepper box into his mouth. He began to choke, so she gave him water. The water caused the pepper to swell, and about an hour later, Thomas died.

In October 1989, Kelly was arrested and indicted for murder in the second degree. Kelly was convicted of criminally negligent homicide.

QUESTIONS FOR AN EXPERT TO ADDRESS TO HELP THE FINDERS OF FACT

What would cause a mother to put her child's life at risk—to allow him or her to become malnourished, to waste away? What would cause a mother to punish her child with such vigor that he died?

AN ANSWER: THE AFTEREFFECTS OF CHILD ABUSE AND NEGLECT

As suggested earlier, the very best predictor of maternal behavior that has lethal consequences is the mother's history of abuse when she was a child. I have yet to meet a woman whose actions resulted in her child's death who was not herself a victim of serious and persistent abuse as a child.

Leonard Shengold's (1989) *Soul Murder: The Effects of Childhood Abuse and Deprivation* is a powerfully written book about the enduring damage caused by child abuse, written by a psychiatrist. He pointed out two of the most profound contributors to the continuation of lethal and near-lethal abuse of children. First, violent mothers are not only their children's tormentors. They are also their rescuers. Second, to acknowledge one's mother as a torturer is so painful that many abused children distort what they remember and are, in effect, brainwashed.

Shengold (1989) wrote:

> If the victim is in the tormentor's absolute power, the child can turn for rescue and relief only to the tormentor, making for an intense need to see the torturer as good and right and to identify with the torturer; where this need is reinforced by a parental claim to godlike, benevolent parental rightness . . . the child *must* lose all knowledge of what has happened and responsibility for how he or she has been made to feel; this means

that any sense of a separate identity is compromised. The child submits
to and becomes like the righteous parent. (p. 22)

In this confounding of righteousness and cruelty in childhood, the
basis for later cruelty is created. Without independent, objective knowledge of what is right and fair treatment for children, adult victims of
child abuse are all but destined to repeat what was done to them.[8]
Abusive mothers may experience anger that feels righteous. So deep is
the harm they have suffered, that the violence they enact may feel justified.

Nor is it so strange for them to think that violence can do good. Violence, being used for supposedly valued ends, is epidemic everywhere.
Might makes right. This lesson is taught around the world. Perhaps, for
mothers with little or no real social power, with no access to the riches
that others enjoy, the abuse of their children is their only chance to feel
mighty and right. Furthermore, until the beating that results in the
child's death, what these mothers do to their children may be no different from what their mothers did to them.

CONCLUSIONS: WHAT TO DO AND
UNDER WHAT CIRCUMSTANCES TO DO IT

For women who come to the attention of the courts because of their
roles in their children's deaths, the question of what to do exists within a
context of punishment. The criminal courts offer no aid. An acquittal
means these women go back to the lives they came from with the added
stigma of having been a part of their own children's deaths.[9] A conviction most often means prison time.

Families are notably dangerous environments, especially for the
weak. Children and women are the most frequent victims. In intimacy
and in privacy, there exists the potential for a great range of human emotions. While some of these emotions come from the very best within us,
some of them are lethal.

When women appear in courtrooms because their children have
died, it is most important to consider their social-psychological context.
Poverty, youth, mental illness, race discrimination, and the inequities inherent in societal ascriptions to gender all deserve a place in our efforts
to secure justice.

Meyer and Oberman (2001) wrote:

Infanticide is not a random, unpredictable crime. Instead, it is deeply
imbedded in and is a reflection of the societies in which it occurs. The
crime of infanticide is committed by mothers who cannot parent their

child under the circumstances dictated by their unique position in place and time. These circumstances vary, but the extent to which infanticide is a reflection of the norms governing motherhood is a constant that links seemingly disparate crimes. (p. 2)

For teenagers who are arrested for neonaticide, their context is often best illuminated in light of the impact of society's expectations of them. Not wanting to be judged harshly by others, they deny their pregnancies or the reality of birth at the pregnancy's inevitable end. While we might wish more maturity for these girls, it is worthwhile to account for their real maturational stage of development. For girls who are immature, their only hope may seem to come from making the baby disappear. The loss of these babies must be seen in the light of the child-mothers' stalled emotional development. While we might wish an easy adolescence on all girls, reality is not so easy. Girls trapped by their fears and undermined by their denial deserve a measure of leniency that follows from their youth. Surely the death of these infants, discovered in spite of their denial, will haunt them. Sometimes, publicity is punishment enough.

For older women who kill newborns, postpartum psychosis has provided an explanation that has lessened punishment for these women throughout much of history. Even in contemporary times, in other countries, women are not brought to trial for these acts of insanity. Here, women are brought to trial and, unless they can convince a jury or a judge that they were moved by forces that were not rational, they may be convicted and sent to prison. Again, punishment does little to protect society. Treatment and attentive, supportive care for mother and child during the first year might prevent these tragedies.

Women whose children are killed by their batterers are most clearly the victims of prejudice. Unable to stop the violence against them or their children, these women may be doubly condemned—first, for their failure to have a good family and, second, for their failure to police their violent men (see Fine & Carney, 2001). The real powerlessness of battered women is ignored in favor of the urge to assign blame to mothers when their children die. Maternal instinct is supposed to override all else. Of course, this cannot be so. Beaten women are rarely phoenixes. They cannot rise from their own misery to be resourceful, agentic, and protective. It is unrealistic for society to expect the physically abused to raise themselves up. Especially for women who are poor and of color, the routes to a safer life may be truly foreclosed. For those of us who reside on the other side of the roadblocks to safety, it is important to know how high the barriers are and how likely it is that escape will be impossible.

When women kill their children after the first day of life, context is most likely to illuminate, but not exculpate. Even so, the childhood experiences of these women deserve attention. As we struggle to bring peace to families and to transform these high risk zones into safe places, the circumstance of mothers whose actions result directly in their children's deaths underlines how desperately we need to redress social injustice and how linked children's fates are to the happenstances of their births. Children born to poor young women of color, children born to women who were beaten as children, children born to women who saw their mothers get beaten by their fathers, and children born to women who use drugs or alcohol to quiet their pain have little chance to see safety in their own lives. These children are at risk even before their mothers first lay a hand on them and, in this sense, it is important for the courts to see the role of larger forces in the lives of individual women.

As we acknowledge the risks to children that follow from the social histories and the places of their mothers in society, we start on a path that is more humane, more inclusive, and more likely to save the lives of children. As the courts give more attention to the influences of context on the individual, we are more likely to see the context of punishment tempered by insight and leniency. The courts can play a more therapeutic role in the lives of these defendants, can remove batterers from the home, can require treatment for victims of family violence and for those who are drug and alcohol dependent, and can act more affirmatively to remove children from violent families and to place them in safer homes.

Little attention has been paid to the role of low social power in increasing the likelihood of infanticide, particularly when domestic violence is implicated. Important exceptions to this focus on the individual appear in work by feminist historians, anthropologists, sociologists, and social psychologists. (See, for example, Fine & Weis, 1998a, 1998b; Gordon, 1990; Scheper-Hughes, 1992). To my knowledge, however, this work has not made its way into courtroom settings. The words that would account explicitly for the influences of race, class, gender, and the lower power that attaches to being nonwhite, poor, and female are typically absent from what has been judged to be acceptable expert testimony when mothers are on trial. In part, this chapter is intended to help broaden the scope of relevant factors so that when these mothers are arrested and judged for their actions against their children, they are seen in the context that best accounts for the reality of their desperation, depression, fear, and anger.

The dearth of helping resources that accompany poverty, the disadvantages that follow from being nonwhite in a society that practices prejudice and discrimination, the disintegration of person and family that results from drugs, alcohol, and disease, and the high level of privacy afforded families all work together to make women raised with violence more dangerous as mothers. When children born to these mothers die, we should not be surprised (Blackman, 1994).

Nor should we blame them for our failure to intervene on their behalf when they were children. Knowing where to draw the line of responsibility that will separate the guilty from the not guilty is no easy matter when we must confront the fact that so many children raised in violent homes are never rescued. How can we expect these mothers to be anything but deeply troubled? How do we fairly hold them accountable for what they were born into? At least at first, it was not their fault.

When these women act in ways that result in the deaths of their children (or in their near deaths), it is incumbent upon us—even at this worst of times—to see these women over time. They must not be judicially dismembered, separated from their childhoods, lest we punish them for having been punished. Figuring out how to punish them for the harm they have done, when they have endured so much harm themselves, is a particularly thorny problem.

We cannot expect people to know more than they are taught, to see rescue when they are lost. It is tragic that, as a society, we make our most enduring commitment to the provision of resources (e.g., food, shelter) after the worst has happened. For some women, prison is the best and safest place they have ever lived. The community support, the presence of a system in which each person's place is noted (no one can be invisible in prison), the opportunity to be rewarded within that structure, and courses that teach alternatives to violence and better parenting skills, can create an oasis of calm for women whose lives were chaotic.

Good programs must be in place so that the courts can send people in need to these programs. We need to act affirmatively to create supportive communities for women and their children outside prison walls, before tragedies occur. We need to foster productive interdependence among women with few resources and between women with little and those who have much. Particularly as governmental resources shrink, it will be important for individuals and private agencies to make real commitments of time and money to the provision of resources to poor, violence-prone families. Then, in the context of their lives, and in the context of our caring, mothers whose acts caused or contributed to their children's deaths, and their surviving children may finally have the chance they need to live in safety.

NOTES

1. The lesser attention paid to men in this chapter occurs because this is a chapter about mothers. Even so, it is worth noting that the nurturing aspects of the "good father" stereotype are still underdeveloped in contemporary American culture. Men who violate this stereotype violate a more amorphous and less firmly rooted value. As Nancy Chodorow (1978) wrote:

> Women mother. In our society, as in most societies, women not only bear children. They also take primary responsibility for infant care, spend more time with infants and children than do men, and sustain primary emotional ties with infants. . . . Though fathers and other men spend varying amounts of time with infants and children, the father is rarely a child's primary parent. (pp. 1–2)

Although Chodorow wrote these words more than 25 years ago, they are no less true today.

2. The fact that some states' laws now allow for a verdict of insane but still responsible complicated this distinction and has enabled states to criminalize and to incarcerate those who are found to be insane. Even so, people found to be insane and responsible (whatever that means) have been judged in terms of different criteria than those found to be guilty or not guilty in a context of combined responsibility and sanity.

3. As described in the preceding section, early typologies emphasized mental illness; later typologies emphasized social factors. The typology of circumstances proposed here belongs with the latter group. Even so, attention to both sides of the dichotomy between social factors and psychosis is important. The actions of mothers whose children die as a result of abuse and neglect have always been and will always be overdetermined. Sometimes, psychosis and society both help to explain a mother's acts.

4. I do not mean that poverty does not contribute to decreased access to medical care (and therefore to abortions and counseling), or that different race/ethnicity groups do not view young motherhood differently. Nor do I mean to suggest that women who kill infants are treated the same in the courtroom regardless of their place in the culture. There, race and class play significant roles in verdicts and sentences. Before they reach the courtroom, however, their youth and mental illness are, in my view, the more significant factors in helping us to understand their lethal acts.

5. While race and class may not shed much light on what causes teenagers to dispose of newborns, race and class certainly play a role in what happens next. When it comes to mothers implicated in their children's deaths, white women attract high levels of media attention. Amy Grossberg, for example, was interviewed by Barbara Walters. Hedda Nussbaum, the mother of an older child who died at home after being assaulted by her adoptive father, Joel Steinberg, received more media attention than any mother of a dead child ever has. This intense interest in white women who fail as mothers can only be attributable to racism and perhaps to a stereotyping of Jewish mothers that makes the deaths of their children more newsworthy. It is news when white women—especially white, Jewish women—do it. Such women are supposed to know better, to see their access to power and to opportunities to avoid devastation. Women of color never get the same sort of media attention.

6. From *http://womensissues.about.com/library/blwyntkppp.htm*:

> The defining factor of post partum psychosis is that the patient suffers a break with reality and becomes delusional. She may show signs of post partum depression, but she will also have feelings of suspicion and distrust of the people around her. She may also begin to believe that there is something wrong with her child, including a belief that the child is divine or demonic. Common symptoms include: fear of being alone, hostility, overactivity, anger or aggression, severe depression, unexplained crying, hallucinations, delusions, and paranoia. Post partum psychosis symptoms generally present themselves within the first 4 weeks after giving birth, but can appear up to 90 days after delivery. Preliminary studies also indicate that if a mother has suffered from PP during one pregnancy there is a 20-25% chance that she may suffer from it in subsequent pregnancies. The cause is unclear. Some possible factors being discussed among physicians include the change in hormones, psychological and social insecurity, and/or the release of substances in the breast-milk which can influence the mental functions and somatic conditions.

See also the fourth edition of the *Diagnostic and Statistical Manual of Mental Disorders* (1994), where "postpartum onset specifier" is a subcategory of mood disorders:

> In general, the symptomatology of the postpartum Major Depressive, Manic, or Mixed

Episode does not differ from the symptomatology in nonpostpartum mood episodes and may include psychotic features. A fluctuating course and mood lability may be more common in postpartum episodes. When delusions are present, they often concern the newborn infant (e.g., the newborn is possessed by the devil, has special powers, or is destined for a terrible fate). In both the psychotic and non-psychotic presentations, there may be suicidal ideation, obsessional thoughts regarding violence to the child, lack of concentration and psychomotor agitation. (American Psychiatric Association, p. 386)

7. The most recent case to receive national attention involved Andrea Yates, a Texas mother who drowned her five young children as a result of postpartum psychosis. Yates claimed to have heard Satan's message that her children had to be killed if they were to be saved. See *http://writ.news.findlaw.com/colb/20020327.html* for "The Andrea Yates Verdict: A Nation in Denial about Mental Illness," by Sherry Colb. Andrea Yates was convicted of murder; her insanity defense was rejected. She was sentenced to 40 years in prison.

8. It is, of course, the case that some abused children do not grow up to be abusers themselves. Two key factors in preventing child victims from becoming adult abusers of children appear to be intelligence and the significant presence of a mentor during the individual's childhood. In *Soul Murder*, Shengold (1989) wrote about a number of men who rose above violent beginnings and achieved great fame (e.g., Anton Chekhov). The fact that they achieved fame, however, does not necessarily mean that they were nonviolent with their children. By virtue of their intellect and talent, they were able to transform their miserable childhood experiences into memorable literary works.

9. The exception is the not guilty by reason of insanity verdict, which would lead to placement in a psychiatric facility.

REFERENCES

American Psychiatric Association. (1994). *Diagnostic and statistical manual of mental disorders* (4th ed.). Washington DC: Author.

Associated Press. (1999, June 29). Mother sentenced to probation for killing eight of her children. *New York Times*, p. A12.

Atkins, E. L., Grimes, J. P., Joseph, G. W., & Liebman, J. (1999). Denial of pregnancy and neonaticide during adolescence: Forensic and clinical issues. *American Journal of Forensic Psychology, 17*(1), 5–33.

Bernstein, N. (1999, May 20). Bronx woman convicted in starving of her breastfed son. *New York Times*, pp. B1, B8.

Blackman, J. (1989). *Intimate violence: A study of injustice*. New York: Columbia University Press.

Blackman, J. (1990). Emerging images of severely battered women and the criminal justice system. *Behavioral Sciences and the Law, 8*, 121–130.

Blackman, J. (1994). At the frontier: In pursuit of justice for women. In B. D. Sales & G. R. VandenBos (Eds.), *Psychology in litigation and legislation: Master lecturers* (pp. 141–173). Washington, DC: American Psychological Association.

Blackman, J. (1996). What would an ideal world look like for young children and their families? In E. J. Erwin (Ed.), *Putting children first: Visions for a brighter future for young children and their families*. Baltimore: Brookes.

Brouget, D., & Bradford, J. M. W. (1990). Homicidal parents. *Canadian Journal of Psychiatry, 35*, 233–237.

Chodorow, N. (1978). *The reproduction of mothering: Psychoanalysis and the sociology of gender*. Berkeley: University of California Press.

D'Orban, P. T. (1979). Women who kill their children. *British Journal of Psychiatry, 134,* 560–571.

Dutton, M. A. (1987). The battered woman syndrome. In D. J. Sonkin (Ed.), *Domestic violence on trial: Psychological and legal dimensions of family violence*. New York: Springer.

Fine, M., & Carney, S. (2001). Women, gender and the law: Toward a feminist rethinking of responsibility. In R. Unger (Ed.), *Handbook of the psychology of women and gender* (pp. 338–409). New York: Wiley.

Fine, M., & Weis, L. (1998a). Crime stories: A critical look through race, ethnicity, and gender. *Qualitative Studies in Education, 11*(3), 435–459.

Fine, M., & Weis, L. (1998b). *The unknown city: The lives of poor and working-class young adults*. Boston: Beacon Press.

Gilbert, S. (1998, October 27). Infant homicides found to be rising in the U.S. *New York Times*, p. F10.

Gordon, L. (1990). Family violence, feminism and social control. In E. C. DuBois & V. L. Ruiz (Eds.), *Unequal sisters: A multi-cultural reader in U.S. women's history*. New York: Routledge.

Hanley, R. (1998a, July 10). Teen-agers get terms in prison in baby's death. *New York Times*, p. A1.

Hanley, R. (1998b, October 30). Woman gets 15 years in death of newborn at prom. *New York Times*, p. B1.

Holden, C. E., Burland, A. S., & Lemmen, C. A. (1996, Spring). Insanity and filicide: Women who murder their children. *New Directions for Mental Health Services, 69,* 25–34.

Kulwin, Rabbi C. M. (1998, September 12). [Sermon.] Temple B'nai Abraham, Livingston, NJ.

Lewis, C. F., Baranoski, M. V., Buchanan, J. A., & Benedek, E. P. (1998). Factors associated with weapon use in maternal filicide. *Journal of Forensic Science, 43*(3), 613–618.

Mendlowicz, M. V., Rapaport, M. H., Mecler, K., Golshan, S., & Morales, T. M. (1998). A case-control study on the socio-demographic characteristics of 53 neonaticidal mothers. *International Journal of Law and Psychiatry, 21*(2), 209–219.

Meyer, C. L., & Oberman, M. (2001). *Mothers who kill their children: Understanding the acts of moms from Susan Smith to the "Prom Mom."* New York: New York University Press.

Overpeck, M. D., Brenner, R. A., Trumble, A. C., Trifiletti, L. B., & Berendes, H. W. (1998). Risk factors for infant homicide in the United States. *New England Journal of Medicine, 339*(17), 1211–1216.

Resnick, P. J. (1969). Child murder by parents: A psychiatric review of filicide. *American Journal of Psychiatry, 126,* 325–334.

Resnick, P. J. (1970). Murder of the newborn: A psychiatric review of neonaticide. *American Journal of Psychiatry, 126,* 1414–1420.

Scheper-Hughes, N. (1992). *Death without weeping: The violence of everyday life in Brazil*. Berkeley: University of California Press.

Shengold, L. (1989). *Soul murder: The effects of childhood abuse and deprivation.* New Haven, CT: Yale University Press.

Silva, J. A., Leong, G. B., Dassori, A., Ferrari, M. M., Weinstock, R., & Yamamoto, J. (1998). A comprehensive typology for the biopsychosociocultural evaluation of child-killing behavior. *Journal of Forensic Science, 43*(6), 1112–1118.

Smothers, R. (1998, August 21). Guilty plea by mother, 20, in prom death. *New York Times,* p. B1.

Spinelli, M. G. (2003). *Infanticide: Psychosocial and legal perspectives on mothers who kill.* Washington, DC: American Psychiatric Association.

Sullivan, C. M., Nguyen, H., Allen, N., Bybee, D., & Juras, J. (2000). Beyond searching for deficits: Evidence that physically and emotionally abused women are nurturing parents. *Journal of Emotional Abuse, 2*(1), 51–71.

Walker, L. (1979). *The battered woman.* New York: HarperCollins.

Wilczynski, A. (1997). *Child homicide.* New York: Oxford University Press.

Epilogue

This book attempts to deal with the tripartite topic of sex, violence, and women (and their children), looking at it from the three-way intersection of the fields of psychology, law, and women's studies. The book does not introduce new individual subject areas. Rather, it brings together all these topics under one heading for the first time and, I hope, provides an introduction to this area that has fascinated me since as a psychologist and a feminist I entered the field of law.

In looking back over the areas covered, rape, spousal abuse, and child sexual abuse seem to be the most pressing issues for investigation and exploration in terms of how these wrongs can be addressed and, most importantly, stopped. Next, I feel that areas such as stalking, particularly non-violent stalking, and sexual harassment are less life-threatening, although important, and deal more with the quality of life for women in our society. Lastly, I feel that treatment, problems with treatment, and corrections when treatment fails (such as Megan's law and sexual predator laws) help us as a society. However, in terms of urgency of study they perhaps come after the extreme harms perpetrated against women. Also, as a separate issue, the ways women have been warped and may harm their own children is, although not common, important in its own right.

I hope that this book serves as a model for investigation of other areas not included here. For example, child sexual abuse in the church is a topic that is, unfortunately, still being unearthed. Child abuse is another area, separate from spousal abuse (although often co-occurring), that could be addressed as a forensic psychology issue with a feminist aspect. In addition, battered women are often blamed for not stopping the child abuse perpetrated by their battering spouses. They may be held legally accountable for the abuse meted out even though they are unable to control their out-of-control spouses, who are terrorizing and beating them as well. Within the area of child abuse, the special area of child custody in the face of child and spousal abuse also deserves attention. It is frankly startling that battering husbands often apply for custody of their children and, amazingly, succeed in court as well. Other topics, perhaps just coming to light, which have an impact on women and children in violent and sexually violent ways, are potential items for future investigation as well.

In sum, this book focuses attention on this new area of interconnection, and invites psychologists, lawyers, and feminists to join in addressing and ultimately stamping out these harms.

Index